Gestational Diabetes: Causes, Diagnosis and Treatment

Gestational Diabetes: Causes, Diagnosis and Treatment

Edited by Eden Kerr

AMERICAN
MEDICAL PUBLISHERS
www.americanmedicalpublishers.com

American Medical Publishers,
41 Flatbush Avenue,
1st Floor, New York,
NY 11217, USA

Visit us on the World Wide Web at:
www.americanmedicalpublishers.com

ISBN: 978-1-63927-117-7

Cataloging-in-Publication Data

Gestational diabetes : causes, diagnosis and treatment / edited by Eden Kerr.
p. cm.
Includes bibliographical references and index.
ISBN 978-1-63927-117-7
1. Diabetes in pregnancy. 2. Diabetes in pregnancy--Etiology. 3. Diabetes in pregnancy--Diagnosis.
4. Diabetes in pregnancy--Treatment. I. Kerr, Eden.

RG580.D5 G47 2022

618.364 6--dc23

Table of Contents

Preface

The world is advancing at a fast pace like never before. Therefore, the need is to keep up with the latest developments. This book was an idea that came to fruition when the specialists in the area realized the need to coordinate together and document essential themes in the subject. That's when I was requested to be the editor. Editing this book has been an honour as it brings together diverse authors researching on different streams of the field. The book collates essential materials contributed by veterans in the area which can be utilized by students and researchers alike.

The condition when a woman develops high blood sugar levels during pregnancy without prior diabetes is known as gestational diabetes. It increases the risk of pre-eclampsia and depression. Mothers having gestational diabetes may give birth to babies having jaundice and low blood sugar after birth. It can also cause stillbirth. Babies born in this condition are often too large and are at a higher risk of being overweight. A lack of insulin in the insulin resistance setting causes gestational diabetes. Other most common risk factors include previously having gestational diabetes, a family background of type 2 diabetes and polycystic ovarian syndrome. The diagnosis of gestational diabetes is based on blood testing. It is treated with a diabetic diet, exercise and insulin injections. This book provides comprehensive insights into gestational diabetes. It presents researches and studies performed by experts across the globe. It will serve as a valuable source of reference for graduate and post graduate students.

Each chapter is a sole-standing publication that reflects each author's interpretation. Thus, the book displays a multi-facetted picture of our current understanding of application, resources and aspects of the field. I would like to thank the contributors of this book and my family for their endless support.

Editor

1

Intercellular Adhesion Molecule and Endogenous NOS Inhibitor: Asymmetric Dimethylarginine in Pregnant Women with Gestational Diabetes Mellitus

Elżbieta Poniedziałek-Czajkowska, Radzisław Mierzyński, Dariusz Szymula, Bożena Leszczyńska-Gorzelak, and Jan Oleszczuk

Chair and Department of Obstetrics and Perinatology, Medical University of Lublin, Jaczewskiego 8, 20-954 Lublin, Poland

Correspondence should be addressed to Radzisław Mierzyński; radek@bg.umlub.pl

Academic Editor: Ilaria Campesi

Objective. The aim of the study was to evaluate the concentrations of soluble intercellular adhesion molecule-1 (s-ICAM-1) and endogenous NOS inhibitor, asymmetric dimethylarginine (ADMA), as markers of endothelium dysfunction in patients with gestational diabetes mellitus (GDM). *Patients and Methods.* The levels of s-ICAM-1 and ADMA were analysed in the group of 56 patients with GDM and compared to 25 healthy pregnant women. The concentrations of s-ICAM-1 and ADMA were measured in serum using ELISA tests. *Results.* The groups did not differ by baseline descriptors: age (30.75 ± 6.32 versus 28.50 ± 4.95 years, NS) and gestational age (28.96 ± 2.85 versus 29.12 ± 2.96 hbd, NS). The patients with GDM were more obese (BMI 27.93 ± 7.02 versus 22.34 ± 4.21 kg/m^2, $p = 0.032$) and had higher concentration of C-reactive protein (6.46 ± 6.03 versus 3.18 ± 3.83 mg/L, $p = 0.029$). In the GDM group the level of ADMA was lower (0.38 ± 0.17 versus 0.60 ± 0.28 μmol/L, $p = 0.001$) and the level of s-ICAM-1 was significantly higher (289.95 ± 118.12 versus 232.56 ± 43.31 ng/mL, $p = 0.036$) compared to controls. *Conclusions.* The pregnant women with GDM are characterized by higher concentration of s-ICAM-1 that reflects the activation and dysfunction of the endothelial cells. The decreased ADMA level in GDM patients seems to be preventive in the limitation of NO synthesis caused by the impaired insulin action and the endothelial dysfunction.

1. Introduction

The physiological pregnancy induces insulin resistance (IR) which appears to result from a combination of increased maternal adiposity and the insulin-desensitizing effects of placental hormones [1]. It is suggested that there are some possible etiological mechanisms responsible for GDM development. Women with GDM are often obese so processes linking the obesity to insulin resistance and/or promoting obesity are likely to play an important role. There is a lot of evidence that endothelial dysfunction may be responsible for IR. It is defined as the partial or complete loss of balance between vasoconstrictors and vasodilators, growth promoting and inhibiting factors, proatherogenic and antiatherogenic factors, and procoagulant and anticoagulant factors [2]. Most frequently the term "endothelial dysfunction" has been used to refer to the impaired endothelium-dependent relaxation caused by loss of nitric oxide (NO) bioactivity in the vessel wall [3]. Nitric oxide not only produces vasodilation, but also participates in various processes that are beneficial to the vasculature, such as reduction of the vascular smooth muscle cell migration and growth, platelets aggregation and thrombosis, and monocytes and macrophages adhesion and inflammation. One of the methods of assessment of endothelial function is to measure the levels of endothelial activation markers, such as soluble vascular cell adhesion molecule (sVCAM), soluble intercellular adhesion molecule (sICAM), endothelin 1 (ET-1), E-selectin, and others, such as markers of the coagulation/fibrinolysis and low-grade inflammation. sICAM-1 is a member of the immunoglobulin superfamily that mediates its functional activity through binding to leukocyte 2-integrins. The sICAM-1 molecule is functionally involved in the regulation of adhesion of leukocytes to the endothelium as well as leukocytes migration [4]. Both the impairment of glucose tolerance and type 2 diabetes are characterized by higher plasma levels of sICAM [5]. The bioavailability of nitric oxide is a key factor for the development of endothelial dysfunction and, furthermore, it seems to play an important role in the development of insulin resistance. Insulin itself, in addition to its metabolic actions, has a direct influence on the endothelium and smooth muscle cells and increases the skeletal muscle blood flow in healthy, insulin-sensitive people. Endothelium-derived NO synthase (eNOS) regulates blood flow to insulin-sensitive tissues (i.e., skeletal muscle, liver, and adipose tissue), and its activity is impaired in insulin-resistant individuals. The inhibition of eNOS disturbs microvascular recruitment and blunts muscle glucose uptake in response to insulin [6]. There is growing evidence that the increased level of eNOS inhibitor, asymmetric dimethylarginine (ADMA), which is a posttranslationally modified form of arginine, contributes to the endothelial dysfunction and diminishes endothelium-related vasodilatation [7]. The raised ADMA plasma concentration may contribute to the vascular defect observed in the IR and is associated with abnormalities closely related to this syndrome such as hypertriglyceridemia, hyperglycaemia, and hypertension. The ADMA level is positively correlated with the impairment of insulin-mediated glucose disposal in nondiabetic, normotensive individuals [8]. During normal pregnancy ADMA diminishes, but it increases in women with preeclampsia [9]. A clear correlation with endothelial dysfunction has been reported in women with high levels of ADMA at the beginning of pregnancy [10].

Both ADMA and s-ICAM-1 are thought to be the markers of endothelial dysfunction. Extensive literature on their role in various pathologies in humans is available but so far there has been little evidence related to their significance in GDM. Thus, the aim of this study was to analyse the serum levels of ADMA and s-ICAM-1 as the markers of endothelium dysfunction in patients with gestational diabetes.

2. Patients and Methods

Fifty-six women with GDM and 25 healthy pregnant women were included in the study, which was performed in the Department of Obstetrics and Perinatology at Medical University of Lublin. All of them signed informed consent to participate in the study, which had previously been approved by the Bioethical Review Board of the Medical University in Lublin. The inclusion criteria were as follows: gestational age between 24th and 34th week as determined on ultrasound examination before 20th week of gestation, first prenatal visit before 8th week, singleton pregnancy, and gestational diabetes mellitus first diagnosed in the current pregnancy before completion of 28 weeks of gestation. The exclusion criteria were as follows: prepregnancy diabetes mellitus, any form of hypertension, prepregnancy and gestational hypertension, preeclampsia, chronic renal disease, intrauterine growth retardation, liver diseases, inflammation, and infectious diseases; patients with positive urine or vaginal culture were also excluded from the study as well as cigarette smokers. The oral glucose tolerance test (OGTT) with 75 g of glucose in compliance with WHO standards was performed in all women participating in the study and in the control group between 24th and 28th week of gestation. The gestational diabetes mellitus was diagnosed on the basis of the following WHO criteria: fasting ≥92 mg/dL (5.1 mmol/L), at 1st hour ≥180 mg/dL (10.0 mmol/L) and at 2nd hour ≥153 mg/dL (8.5 mmol/L) [11].

The glucose concentration was measured in venous blood plasma with the use of glucose oxidase method (Cormay, Poland). The ADMA, s-ICAM-1, C-reactive protein levels were assessed. The blood samples for research tests were taken from patients who were fasting together with the samples for routinely performed laboratory tests. The samples were allowed to clot for at least 30 minutes before centrifugation at 1000 G, which was continued for 20 minutes. Serum has been removed and then frozen at −70°C. The s-ICAM-1 concentration was measured by means of the sandwich enzyme immunoassay technique (Human sICAM-1 Immunoassay, R&D Systems Inc. Minneapolis, USA) as well as the ADMA level (ADMA direct ELISA Kit, Immundiagnostik AG, Bensheim, Germany). CRP concentration was measured with high-sensitivity CRP assay (CRP HS ELISA, DRG International, Inc., USA). Body mass index (BMI) calculation was based on the weight measurement at the first prenatal visit before 8th week of gestation.

The study group was compared to the control one with respect of maternal age, gestational age at the entry to the study, parity, BMI, CRP levels, and glucose levels at each hour of OGTT as well as s-ICAM-1 and ADMA concentrations. Correlations between ADMA and s-ICAM-1 and BMI, CRP, and glucose levels at each hour of OGTT were analysed.

The Statistica 5.5A for Windows (StatSoft, Poland) was used for data analysis. The elements of descriptive statistics were used. Data was presented as mean ± standard deviation. The Shapiro-Wilk test for normal distribution of data and one-tailed Student's t-test, or (in unequal variance) the Cochran-Cox test (absence of normal distribution and nonparametric data), and the Mann-Whitney U test were performed. The Spearman rank test was employed for searching correlations between variables. The statistical significance was defined as $p < 0.05$.

3. Results

The studied groups did not differ with regard to the baseline descriptors: age, gestational age when included to the study, and parity (Table 1). Patients with GDM were more obese than the controls (BMI 27.93±7.02 versus 22.34 ± 4.21 kg/m^2, $p = 0.032$) and had higher concentration of C-reactive protein (6.46 ± 6.03 versus 3.18 ± 3.83 mg/L, $p = 0.029$) (Table 1). The glucose levels during OGTT fasting, at 1st and 2nd hour of test, were significantly higher in GDM group (0′: 93.35 ± 18.28 versus 78.88 ± 6.62 mg/dL, $p = 0.001$; 1′: 181.50 ± 21.29 versus 107.29 ± 22.60 mg/dL, $p < 0.000001$; 2′: 165.39 ± 29.42 versus 83.89±28.13 mg/dL, $p < 0.000001$) (Table 2). The level of ADMA was lower in GDM group in comparison with the controls (0.38 ± 0.17 versus 0.60 ± 0.28 μmol/L, $p = 0.001$), but the level of s-ICAM-1 was significantly higher in patients

TABLE 1: Characteristics of group with GDM and control.

	GDM group $N = 56$	Control group $N = 25$	p
Age (years)	30.75 ± 6.32	28.50 ± 4.95	NS
Gestational age (hbd)	28.69 ± 2.85	29.13 ± 2.96	NS
Parity	2.14 ± 1.22	1.88 ± 1.09	NS
BMI (kg/m^2)	27.93 ± 7.02	22.34 ± 4.21	$p = 0.032$
CRP (mg/L)	6.46 ± 6.03	3.18 ± 3.83	$p = 0.029$

GDM: gestational diabetes mellitus.
BMI: body mass index.
CRP: C-reactive protein.
p: statistical significance.
NS: statistically not significant.

TABLE 2: ADMA, s-ICAM-1, and glucose levels in GDM and control group.

	GDM group $N = 56$	Control group $N = 25$	p
ADMA (μmol/L)	0.38 ± 0.17	0.60 ± 0.28	$p = 0.001$
s-ICAM-1 (ng/mL)	289.95 ± 118.12	232.56 ± 43.31	$p = 0.036$
Glucose (mg/dL)			
0′	93.35 ± 18.28	78.88 ± 6.62	$p = 0.001$
1′	181.50 ± 21.29	107.29 ± 22.60	$p < 0.000001$
2′	165.39 ± 29.42	83.89 ± 28.13	$p < 0.000001$

GDM: gestational diabetes mellitus.
ADMA: asymmetric dimethylarginine.
s-ICAM-1: soluble intercellular adhesion molecule-1.
p: statistical significance.

with GDM (289.95 ± 118.12 versus 232.56 ± 43.31 ng/mL, $p = 0.036$) (Table 2).

No correlations were found between ADMA and s-ICAM-1 levels and BMI, CRP, and glucose levels both fasting and at the 1st hour of OGTT in the GDM patients as well as in the control ones. A marked, but statistically insignificant, correlation of ADMA level and the glucose level at the 2nd hour of OGTT was observed in patient with GDM (Table 3).

4. Discussion

The insulin resistance increases during pregnancy and in the third trimester, and it is comparable to this observed in type 2 diabetes. It is partly related to the growth of adiposity, but its sudden drop right after delivery is suggestive of an important role of placental hormones acting as antagonists of insulin. Development of GDM only in some pregnant women indicates the role of other factors like prepregnancy insulin resistance observed in obesity and/or endothelium dysfunction. Being overweight before conception adds an already existing insulin resistance (both hepatic and peripheral) to the normal changes of the glucose tolerance present in late gestation. There is a 40% reduction in peripheral insulin sensitivity in obese pregnant women and insulin response to an intravenous glucose load is reduced in obese women in comparison with lean pregnant ones [12]. Obesity was found to be associated with the elevated s-ICAM-1 levels [13]. We

TABLE 3: Correlation between ADMA and s-ICAM-1 levels and BMI and CRP levels and glucose levels in OGTT in patients with GDM and control group.

	GDM				Control			
	ADMA		s-ICAM-1		ADMA		s-ICAM-1	
	R	p	R	p	R	p	R	p
BMI	−0.067	NS	0.309	NS	0.160	NS	−0.397	NS
CRP	0.058	NS	0.261	NS	−0.290	NS	0.094	NS
Glucose								
0′	−0.156	NS	−0.090	NS	−0.148	NS	−0.071	NS
1′	−0.167	NS	−0.050	NS	−0.205	NS	0.240	NS
2′	0.326	$p = 0.05$	0.285	NS	−0.368	NS	0.011	NS
ADMA			−0.044	NS			0.122	NS

GDM: gestational diabetes mellitus.
BMI: body mass index.
CRP: C-reactive protein.
ADMA: asymmetric dimethylarginine.
s-ICAM-1: soluble intercellular adhesion molecule-1.
R: Spearman correlation's coefficient.
p: statistical significance.
NS: statistically not significant.

observed that patients with GDM were overweight and had significantly higher concentration of s-ICAM-1 compared to healthy controls. They also had significantly higher levels of C-reactive protein. No correlation was noted between the s-ICAM-1 levels and BMI, CRP levels, or glucose levels in OGTT either in GDM or control group. These results suggest activation and dysfunction of endothelial cells as well as the inflammation in course of GDM. In vitro, insulin was shown to decrease ICAM-1 expression [14]. In type 2 diabetic patients, s-ICAM-1 levels were found to be increased [15]. In the large Nurses' Health Study that included 121,700 subjects, s-ICAM-1 level was predictive for the incidence of diabetes [16]. Therefore, it might be postulated that not only obesity, inflammation, or glucose metabolism impairment's degree could result in endothelium activation in GDM. There is little evidence about s-ICAM role in GDM; most studies reveal the significance of s-ICAM-1 as predictor of type 2 diabetes in women with previous GDM. It was shown that, despite resolving of previous metabolic anomalies, higher levels of ICAM and VICAM were observed after delivery in women with previous GDM compared to healthy ones. This appears to suggest persistent endothelium dysfunction which coexists with an increased future cardiovascular risk [17]. ICAM-1 and VICAM-1 have been reported to predict the development of type 2 diabetes in women irrespective of other known risk factors including abdominal obesity or CRP levels as a marker of inflammation [16]. There is a lot of evidence emphasizing the predictive role of ICAM i VICAM in early identification of patients in whom preeclampsia develops [4, 18].

In NO synthesis, insulin and ADMA have opposite roles. There is a growing evidence that increased level of ADMA contributes to the endothelial dysfunction and diminishes endothelium-related vasodilatation. ADMA inhibits eNOS and diminishes NO synthesis, whereas insulin is known to have a direct vasodilatory effect mediated through stimulation of NO production in the endothelial cells [19]. In the insulin-resistant state, the ability of insulin to stimulate NO production in the endothelium is diminished. It may be assumed that the excess of ADMA can suppress insulin-related vasodilatation and promotes insulin resistance development [20]. In this study it was shown that patients with GDM are characterized by significantly lower levels of ADMA when compared to healthy pregnant women. No correlations were found between ADMA level and BMI, CRP level, and glucose levels fasting at 1st hour of OGTT. A marked but statistically insignificant correlation of ADMA level and the glucose level at 2nd hour of OGTT was observed. There is a lot of evidence that raised ADMA concentrations may contribute to the vascular pathology observed in the insulin resistance [8, 21]. There is published data indicating that ADMA concentrations are significantly higher in GDM patients in comparison with the healthy controls [22, 23]. Therefore, in this context the results of this study, which showed lower ADMA levels in GDM group, appear to be surprising. However, it was also suggested that chronic hyperglycaemia might downregulate mechanisms implicated in ADMA production or stimulate its metabolism [24]. According to the study of Anderssohn et al. the relationship between ADMA and diabetes seems to be ambiguous and partly related to type and stage of DM [25].

In the course of physiological pregnancy ADMA levels decline even with an elevated concentration of total cholesterol, LDL and HDL cholesterol, and triglycerides. Pathological stimuli such as hyperglycaemia, inflammatory cytokines, hyperhomocysteinaemia, infectious agents, and oxidized low-density lipoprotein (LDL) may reduce activity of degrading ADMA enzyme, dimethylarginine dimethylaminohydrolase (DDAH), and allow ADMA to accumulate [8, 26]. Lower ADMA levels during normal pregnancy may be explained with increase in DDAH activity [27] or they may be reflective of the physiological adaptation to pregnancy, irrespective of the disturbances of glucose tolerance [23]. Our observations are similar to the results of study presented by Takaya et al. who found that the level of ADMA was significantly lower among children with diabetes and obesity compared to control subjects and that ADMA concentrations were inversely correlated with serum glucose level. It has been suggested that limited ADMA synthesis could be protective against the endothelial cell dysfunction caused by hyperglycaemia which is partly related to the limited NO synthesis [28].

It has been postulated that hyperglycaemia could decrease ADMA levels through the restricted ADMA synthesis or through enhancing its metabolism by the enzyme DDAH [29]. Additionally, it is widely known that the prolonged impact of high glucose levels on endothelial cells increases NO synthase expression and superoxide anion generation [30]. Thus, some other factors responsible for ADMA lowering in pregnancy should be taken into consideration. It has been proven that estrogens that have antioxidant properties may increase the activity of DDAH what is accompanied by a reduced release of ADMA. The estrogens synthesis increases as pregnancy progresses, but some other factors should be considered as causative since ADMA concentration in GDM is even lower than in healthy pregnancy [31]. It may be presumed that lowering ADMA levels in GDM patients might result from excellent glucose control after GDM diagnosis. Das et al. observed that the strict control of hyperglycaemia decreases the serum ADMA levels [32]. Consequently, a hypothesis could be formulated that decreased ADMA levels in GDM could be preventive in the limitation of NO synthesis due to impaired insulin action.

5. Conclusions

Pregnant women with GDM are characterized by higher concentration of s-ICAM-1 which reflects the activation and dysfunction of the endothelial cells. The decreased ADMA level in GDM patients seems to be preventive in the limitation of NO synthesis caused by the impaired insulin action and the endothelial dysfunction.

Conflict of Interests

The authors declare no conflict of interests.

Acknowledgment

This study was supported by Medical University of Lublin, Grant no. 332.

References

[1] T. A. Buchanan and A. H. Xiang, "Gestational diabetes mellitus," *The Journal of Clinical Investigation*, vol. 115, no. 3, pp. 485–491, 2005.

[2] A. A. Quyyumi, "Endothelial function in health and disease: new insights into the genesis of cardiovascular disease," *American Journal of Medicine*, vol. 105, no. 1, pp. 32S–39S, 1998.

[3] H. Cai and D. G. Harrison, "Endothelial dysfunction in cardiovascular diseases: the role of oxidant stress," *Circulation Research*, vol. 87, no. 10, pp. 840–844, 2000.

[4] S.-Y. Kim, H.-M. Ryu, J. H. Yang et al., "Maternal serum levels of VCAM-1, ICAM-1 and E-selectin in preeclampsia," *Journal of Korean Medical Science*, vol. 19, no. 5, pp. 688–692, 2004.

[5] K. Matsumoto, Y. Sera, H. Nakamura, Y. Ueki, and S. Miyake, "Serum concentrations of soluble adhesion molecules are related to degree of hyperglycemia and insulin resistance in patients with type 2 diabetes mellitus," *Diabetes Research and Clinical Practice*, vol. 55, no. 2, pp. 131–138, 2002.

[6] M. A. Vincent, E. J. Barrett, J. R. Lindner, M. G. Clark, and S. Rattigan, "Inhibiting NOS blocks microvascular recruitment and blunts muscle glucose uptake in response to insulin," *The American Journal of Physiology—Endocrinology and Metabolism*, vol. 285, no. 1, pp. E123–E129, 2003.

[7] J. T. Kielstein, B. Impraim, S. Simmel et al., "Cardiovascular effects of systemic nitric oxide synthase inhibition with asymmetrical dimethylarginine in humans," *Circulation*, vol. 109, no. 2, pp. 172–177, 2004.

[8] K. Y. Lin, A. Ito, T. Asagami et al., "Impaired nitric oxide synthase pathway in diabetes mellitus: role of asymmetric dimethylarginine and dimethylarginine dimethylaminohydrolase," *Circulation*, vol. 106, no. 8, pp. 987–992, 2002.

[9] M. López-Alarcón, I. Montalvo-Velarde, V. S. Vital-Reyes, J. C. Hinojosa-Cruz, A. Leaños-Miranda, and A. Martínez-Basila,

"Serial determinations of asymmetric dimethylarginine and homocysteine during pregnancy to predict pre-eclampsia: a longitudinal study," *BJOG: An International Journal of Obstetrics & Gynaecology*, vol. 122, no. 12, pp. 1586–1592, 2015.

[10] P. N. Alpoim, L. C. Godoi, L. G. Freitas, K. B. Gomes, and L. M. Dusse, "Assessment of L-arginine asymmetric 1 dimethyl (ADMA) in early-onset and late-onset (severe) preeclampsia," *Nitric Oxide*, vol. 33, pp. 81–82, 2013.

[11] WHO, "Diagnostic criteria and classification of hyperglycaemia first detected in pregnancy," WHO/NMH/MND 13.2, 2013.

[12] P. M. Catalano, L. Huston, S. B. Amini, and S. C. Kalhan, "Longitudinal changes in glucose metabolism during pregnancy in obese women with normal glucose tolerance and gestational diabetes mellitus," *American Journal of Obstetrics and Gynecology*, vol. 180, no. 4, pp. 903–916, 1999.

[13] H. Ito, A. Ohshima, M. Inoue et al., "Weight reduction decreases soluble cellular adhesion molecules in obese women," *Clinical and Experimental Pharmacology and Physiology*, vol. 29, no. 5-6, pp. 399–404, 2002.

[14] T. Hamaguchi and M. Namba, "Insulin therapy in diabetic patient with hypertension," *Nippon Rinsho*, vol. 61, no. 7, pp. 1238–1244, 2003.

[15] N. Takeuchi, T. Kawamura, A. Kanai et al., "The effect of cigarette smoking on soluble adhesion molecules in middle-aged patients with Type 2 diabetes mellitus," *Diabetic Medicine*, vol. 19, no. 1, pp. 57–64, 2002.

[16] J. B. Meigs, F. B. Hu, N. Rifai, and J. E. Manson, "Biomarkers of endothelial dysfunction and risk of type 2 diabetes mellitus," *The Journal of the American Medical Association*, vol. 291, no. 16, pp. 1978–1986, 2004.

[17] S. Bo, S. Valpreda, G. Menato et al., "Should we consider gestational diabetes a vascular risk factor?" *Atherosclerosis*, vol. 194, no. 2, pp. e72–e79, 2007.

[18] E. Abe, K. Matsubara, H. Ochi, M. Ito, K. Oka, and K. Kameda, "Elevated levels of adhesion molecules derived from leukocytes and endothelial cells in patients with pregnancy-induced hypertension," *Hypertension in Pregnancy*, vol. 22, no. 1, pp. 31–43, 2003.

[19] K. Kuboki, Z. Y. Jiang, N. Takahara et al., "Regulation of endothelial constitutive nitric oxide synthase gene expression in endothelial cells and in vivo: a specific vascular action of insulin," *Circulation*, vol. 101, no. 6, pp. 676–681, 2000.

[20] M. Montagnani and M. J. Quon, "Insulin action in vascular endothelium: potential mechanisms linking insulin resistance with hypertension," *Diabetes, Obesity and Metabolism*, vol. 2, no. 5, pp. 285–292, 2000.

[21] H. Matsuoka, S. Itoh, M. Kimoto et al., "Asymmetrical dimethylarginine, an endogenous nitric oxide synthase inhibitor, in experimental hypertension," *Hypertension*, vol. 29, no. 1, pp. 242–247, 1997.

[22] M. Akturk, A. Altinova, I. Mert et al., "Asymmetric dimethylarginine concentrations are elevated in women with gestational diabetes," *Endocrine*, vol. 38, no. 1, pp. 134–141, 2010.

[23] B. Telejko, A. Zonenberg, M. Kuzmicki et al., "Circulating asymmetric dimethylarginine, endothelin-1 and cell adhesion molecules in women with gestational diabetes," *Acta Diabetologica*, vol. 46, no. 4, pp. 303–308, 2009.

[24] M. L. Marcovecchio, B. Widmer, C. Turner, D. B. Dunger, and R. N. Dalton, "Asymmetric dimethylarginine in young people with Type 1 diabetes: a paradoxical association with HbA_{1c}," *Diabetic Medicine*, vol. 28, no. 6, pp. 685–691, 2011.

[25] M. Anderssohn, E. Schwedhelm, N. Lüneburg, R. S. Vasan, and R. H. Böger, "Asymmetric dimethylarginine as a mediator of vascular dysfunction and a marker of cardiovascular disease and mortality: an intriguing interaction with diabetes mellitus," *Diabetes and Vascular Disease Research*, vol. 7, no. 2, pp. 105–118, 2010.

[26] J. Leiper, J. Murray-Rust, N. McDonald, and P. Vallance, "S-nitrosylation of dimethylarginine dimethylaminohydrolase regulates enzyme activity: further interactions between nitric oxide synthase and dimethylarginine dimethylaminohydrolase," *Proceedings of the National Academy of Sciences of the United States of America*, vol. 99, no. 21, pp. 13527–13532, 2002.

[27] J. Murray-Rust, J. Leiper, M. McAlister et al., "Structural insights into the hydrolysis of cellular nitric oxide synthase inhibitors by dimethylarginine dimethylaminohydrolase," *Nature Structural Biology*, vol. 8, no. 8, pp. 679–683, 2001.

[28] J. Takaya, Y. Tanabe, Y. Kuroyanagi, and K. Kaneko, "Asymmetric dimethylarginine is negatively correlated with hyperglycemia in children," *Endocrine Journal*, vol. 62, no. 6, pp. 551–556, 2015.

[29] B. Ellger, M. C. Richir, P. A. M. Van Leeuwen et al., "Glycemic control modulates arginine and asymmetrical-dimethylarginine levels during critical illness by preserving dimethylarginine-dimethylaminohydrolase activity," *Endocrinology*, vol. 149, no. 6, pp. 3148–3157, 2008.

[30] F. Cosentino, K. Hishikawa, Z. S. Katusic, and T. F. Lüscher, "High glucose increases nitric oxide synthase expression and superoxide anion generation in human aortic endothelial cells," *Circulation*, vol. 96, no. 1, pp. 25–28, 1997.

[31] Z. Dai, H.-Q. Zhu, D.-J. Jiang, J.-L. Jiang, H.-W. Deng, and Y.-J. Li, "17β-Estradiol preserves endothelial function by reduction of the endogenous nitric oxide synthase inhibitor level," *International Journal of Cardiology*, vol. 96, no. 2, pp. 223–227, 2004.

[32] U. N. Das, G. Repossi, A. Dain, and A. R. Eynard, "L-arginine, NO and asymmetrical dimethylarginine in hypertension and type 2 diabetes," *Frontiers in Bioscience*, vol. 16, no. 1, pp. 13–20, 2011.

2

Maternal Dietary Patterns and Gestational Diabetes Risk

Fatemeh Sedaghat,[1] Mahdieh Akhoondan,[2] Mehdi Ehteshami,[2] Vahideh Aghamohammadi,[3] Nila Ghanei,[1] Parvin Mirmiran,[4] and Bahram Rashidkhani[2]

[1]Department of Basic Medical Sciences, Faculty of Nutrition Sciences and Food Technology, National Nutrition and Food Technology Research Institute, Shahid Beheshti University of Medical Sciences, Tehran, Iran
[2]Department of Community Nutrition, Faculty of Nutrition Sciences and Food Technology, National Nutrition and Food Technology Research Institute, Shahid Beheshti University of Medical Sciences, Tehran, Iran
[3]Department of Paramedical Sciences, Ahvaz Jundishapur University of Medical Sciences, Ahvaz, Iran
[4]Nutrition and Endocrine Research Center, Research Institute for Endocrine Sciences, Shahid Beheshti University of Medical Sciences, Tehran, Iran

Correspondence should be addressed to Bahram Rashidkhani; rashidkhani@yahoo.com

Academic Editor: Eusebio Chiefari

Background. Maternal dietary patterns play an important role in the progress of gestational diabetes mellitus (GDM). The aim of the present study was to explore this association. *Method.* A total of 388 pregnant women (122 case and 266 control) were included. Dietary intake were collected using a food frequency questionnaire (FFQ). GDM was diagnosed using a 100-gram, 3-hour oral glucose tolerance test. Dietary pattern was identified by factor analysis. To investigate the relation between each of the independent variables with gestational diabetes, the odds ratio (OR) was calculated. *Results.* Western dietary pattern was high in sweets, jams, mayonnaise, soft drinks, salty snacks, solid fat, high-fat dairy products, potatoes, organ meat, eggs, red meat, processed foods, tea, and coffee. The prudent dietary pattern was characterized by higher intake of liquid oils, legumes, nuts and seeds, fruits and dried fruits, fish and poultry whole, and refined grains. Western dietary pattern was associated with increased risk of gestational diabetes mellitus before and after adjustment for confounders (OR = 1.97, 95% CI: 1.27–3.04, OR = 1.68, 95% CI: 1.04–2.27). However, no significant association was found for a prudent pattern. *Conclusion.* These findings suggest that the Western dietary pattern was associated with an increased risk of GDM.

1. Introduction

Gestational diabetes mellitus (GDM), defined as any degree of glucose intolerance with onset during pregnancy, is a common complication, and its prevalence ranges between 7 and 14% worldwide [1].

Incidence of GDM among Iranian women living in urban areas has been reported similar to developing countries [2–5]. However, with the prevalence of type II diabetes increasing across the world and considering that the prevalence of GDM is thought to shadow that of type II diabetes, we expect to see a rise in GDM incidence during the coming years [3].

Thus, it is crucial to detect modifiable risk factors that may contribute to the prevention of GDM. Food and dietary factors have been reported to affect glucose homeostasis, and diet may be associated with GDM risk factors [6, 7]. Several studies found a positive association between GDM risk and intake of total fat [8, 9], saturated fat [10, 11], and an inverse relation between the risk of GDM and polyunsaturated fat [10, 12]. In contrast, no significant association was found between total dietary, saturated, and polyunsaturated fat intake and the risk of GDM in another study [13].

However, most previous studies have traditionally focused on the role of the single food items [14], nutrients [15, 16], or food groups [17, 18]. Considering the limitations of these kinds of studies, such as neglecting the interactions and synergistic effects of nutrients [19], detecting dietary patterns offers a comprehensive and complimentary method in investigating the relationship between diet and disease risk [20]. Dietary patterns are population specific and are influenced by sociocultural factors and food availability [20]. The results of recent systematic reviews showed that adherence to a healthier dietary pattern, like Mediterranean dietary pattern, and reducing the intake of sugar sweetened cola, potatoes, fatty foods, sweets, and food with high heme iron content can decrease the incidence of GDM, especially in women at higher risk and before getting pregnant [7, 21]. However, the majority of the studies to date have been conducted in western populations [17, 22, 23]. Conversely, studies investigating dietary patterns in relation to GDM in Asian women, who are at a much greater risk of developing GDM compared to others ethnics, are sparse [24, 25]. Due to the growing trend of gestational diabetes and a shortage of research on the effect of dietary patterns on the prevention of GDM in Asian women, this study aimed to investigate the association between prepregnancy dietary patterns and risk of GDM in Iranian women.

2. Materials and Methods

2.1. Participants. This hospital-based case-control study was conducted in Tehran, a province of Iran at high-risk of diabetes. Cases ($n = 123$) with pregnant women aged 18–40 years who visited major general hospitals in different regions of Tehran (11 million inhabitants) were included. Pregnant women were screened for gestational diabetes between the 24th and 28th weeks of gestation with a 50 g, 1 hr glucose challenge test (GCT). If the screening test was positive (blood glucose greater than 130 mg per ml), diagnostic testing was performed using a 100 g, 3-hour oral glucose tolerance test (OGTT). Women meeting the Carpenter and Coustan criteria [26], fasting 5.3 mmol/l, 1 h 10.0 mmol/l, 2 h 8.6 mmol/l, and 3 h, 7.8 mmol/l, were diagnosed with GDM (any two values at or above established thresholds).

Controls were pregnant women ($n = 268$) whose GCT tests at 24–28 weeks of pregnancy were in the normal range. The exclusion criteria were multiple pregnancies, history of gestational diabetes or diabetes (prepregnancy), and undergoing a weight-reduction diet one year before pregnancy. Furthermore, controls were followed up until the end of pregnancy. If they developed GDM, they were excluded from the study. In this study, two controls were recruited within the same medical center for each case. Controls were matched to cases on age (within 5 years). During analysis, three patients (1 case and 2 controls) with extreme energy intakes that probably reflected careless completion of the dietary questionnaire (below or above the mean ± 3 SD for log-transformed calories; cutpoints: 244 kcal and 5284 kcal) were excluded. The final sample for statistical analysis was 122 cases and 266 controls.

Informed consent was obtained from each participant prior to enrollment. The study protocol was approved by the ethics committee at the National Nutrition and Food Technology Research Institute of Shahid Beheshti University of Medical Science.

2.2. Dietary Intake. One year before pregnancy, dietary intake of all participants were collected through validated semi-quantitative food frequency questionnaires (FFQs) by trained interviewers. The FFQ consisted of 147 food items, including some of the most common Iranian meal recipes, and has been previously shown to be valid and reproducible for use in Iranian adults [27]. Subjects were asked to mention their consumption frequency of a given serving of each food item during the past year, on a daily, weekly, monthly, or yearly basis. Common household measures (measuring cups, spoons, and palm of hand) were used for better estimation of the real portion consumed by the subjects [28]. Portion sizes consumed from each food item were then converted to daily gram intake using the household scales [28]. In addition to the daily energy, macronutrient and micronutrient consumption for participants was calculated using the United States Department of Agriculture Food Composition Databases (USDA FCT). However, for some dairy products such as Kashk, wild plum, mint, sweet canned cherry, and sour cherry that are not listed in the USDA FCT, Iranian FCT was used alternatively [28].

2.3. Assessment of Nondietary Exposures. Information on age, prepregnancy weight, education level, socioeconomic status, cigarette smoking, family history of diabetes, and taking supplements were obtained from all cases and controls by trained professional interviewers using a questionnaire. The weight of each subject was measured with minimum clothing, and 100 g sensitivity and height was measured with using a nonstretch tape-meter fixed to a wall and was recorded to the nearest 0.5 cm. Body mass index (BMI) was computed subsequently by the formula (weight in kg)/(height in meter)^2.

Physical activity level before pregnancy and average time per day spent on different intensity activities was evaluated using a validated self report-based questionnaire [29] and was expressed as metabolic equivalents hours/day (METs-h/d) in which nine different MET levels were ranged on a scale from sleep/rest (0.9 METs) to high-intensity physical activities (>6 METs). By multiplying the time spent on each activity level by the MET value of each activity, the MET-time for an activity was computed. Based on questionnaire data, we estimated a total activity score by adding the specific activities together.

2.4. Statistical Analysis. All analyses were performed using the Statistical Package for Social Sciences software version 16 (SPSS Inc., Chicago, IL, USA), and a two-sided p value < 0.05 was considered significant. The Kaiser–Meyer–Olkin test (KMO = 0.7) indicated adequacy of sampling. Bartlett's test

Table 1: Food groupings used in the dietary pattern analysis.

Food groups	Food items
Refined grains	White breads (lavash, baguettes), rice, pasta, noodles, biscuits
Fast foods	Sausages, bologna (beef), pizza
Potatoes	Potatoes (cooked and fried potatoes, French fries)
Salty snacks	Crackers, potato chips, corn puffs, pickled vegetables
Mayonnaise	Mayonnaise
Sugar sweetened beverages	Soft drinks, synthetic fruit juices
Eggs	Eggs
Vegetables	Lettuce, spinach, green leafy vegetables, onions, cucumber, turnip, cabbage, cauliflower, kale, eggplant, squash, celery, green pepper, garlic, mushrooms, green peas, green beans, broad beans, carrots, pumpkin, tomatoes, tomato sauce
Whole grains	Iranian dark breads, barley, corn, bulgur
Fruits and dried fruits	Apple, orange, tangerine, date, melon, watermelon and Persian melon, cantaloupe, banana, lemon, lime, apricots, grapes, cherries, strawberries, pomegranates, kiwi, grapefruit, persimmons, pear, peach, plums, nectarine, mulberry, fig, dried fruits, and natural fruit juices
Poultry and fish	Chicken, canned tuna fish, and every kind of fish
High fat dairy	Whole fat milk, cocoa milk, whole fat yoghurt, concentrated and creamy yoghurt, cream cheese, kashk, ice cream
Low-fat dairy	Low-fat milk, plain yoghurt, cheese, and yoghurt drink
Jam and tinned fruits	Jam, honey, and tinned fruits
Liquid oils	Vegetable oils, olives, and olive oil
Solid fats	Butter, margarine, cream, hydrogenated vegetable oils, and animal fats
Sweet snacks	Cakes, cookies, Iranian confectioneries (gaz, sohan, noghl), confections, sugars, chocolates, candies
Red meats	Beef, lamb, hamburger, ground meat
Organ meats	Liver, heart, kidney, tongue, feet, head, tripe, and brain
Tea and coffee	Tea, coffee
Nuts and seeds	Walnuts, almonds, hazelnuts, pistachios, peanuts, and roasted seeds
Legumes	Lentils, beans, chickpea, split peas, and soya beans

of sphericity was significant ($p < 0.001$) indicating that factor analysis was suitable for the data.

For identifying the dietary patterns, food items obtained from the FFQ were categorized into 22 groups based on the similarity of nutrients (Table 1). Principal component analysis was used to identify major dietary patterns based on the 22 food groups. Two interpretable factors were retained based on the Scree test [19]; an orthogonal rotation procedure, the Varimax rotation, was then applied to simplify the factor structure facilitating interpretation. The labeling of derived factors was done on the basis of interpretation of the data and of the earlier literature. The factor score for each pattern was calculated by summing intakes of food groups weighted by factor loading, and individuals were assigned a factor score for each dietary pattern [19].

Two dietary pattern scores were divided into two categories based on the medians. To evaluate the differences in distribution of categorical variables, chi-square test was applied. To assess the differences in distribution of continuous variables across the dietary pattern score categories, independent sample t-test was used in case of normality, and Mann–Whitney test was used where the distribution of variables were not normal. Unconditional logistic regression was used in estimating odds ratio (OR) with 95% confidence interval (CI) after controlling for confounding variables (prepregnancy weight, gestational age, physical activity, family history of diabetes, housing ownership, and building area).

3. Results

Table 2 compares the characteristics of 122 cases and 266 controls. By design, age was similar in both groups (29.7 years versus 29.6 years in controls and cases, resp.). Cases had higher prepregnancy BMI and family history of diabetes compared to controls, while gestational age and physical activity were higher significantly in the control group ($p < 0.001$). Controls reported higher building area and housing ownership. No significant differences were observed for maternal age, energy intake, smoking status, and education status.

Factor-loading matrix for the 2 retained factors is shown in Table 3. Two dietary patterns were derived with eigenvalues above 2 from the scree plot, as well as factor loadings using factor analysis; these two patterns accounted for 19.4% of the total variation in food intakes. Dietary patterns

TABLE 2: Characteristics of patients in an Iranian GDM case-control study between 2009 and 2010, Tehran, Iran.

Characteristics	Controls $N = 266$	Cases $N = 122$	p value[a,b]
Age (years), mean ± SD	29.76 ± 4.26	29.64 ± 4.52	0.81
Gestational age (week), mean ± SD	31.19 ± 3.53	29.39 ± 4.74	<0.0001
Prepregnancy BMI (kg/m^2), mean ± SD	24.64 ± 3.32	27.25 ± 3.82	<0.0001
Energy intake (kcal), mean ± SD	2672 ± 706	2818 ± 755	0.06
Physical activity (METs-h/d), mean ± SD	21.75 ± 26.37	12.92 ± 16.43	0.001
Family history of diabetes, n (%)	89 (33.46)	66 (54.55)	<0.0001
Supplement use a year before pregnancy, n (%)	84 (31.58)	45 (37.19)	0.28
Smoking exposure, n (%)	24 (9.02)	8 (6.61)	0.42
Education (%)			0.35
Illiterate and primary	29.7	24.4	
High school	41.3	48.8	
Diploma and over	29.0	26.8	
Housing ownership (yes), (%) History of abortion, n (%)	79.2	20.8	0.002
Building area (m^2)	69	75	0.03

[a]Values are presented either as mean ± SD or n (%) for quantitative and qualitative variables, respectively; [b]chi-square test and independent sample t-test were applied for categorical variables and continuous variables, respectively; $n = 388$.

TABLE 3: Factor loadings matrix for the major dietary patterns identified by factor analysis in an Iranian GDM case-control study between 2009 and 2010, Tehran, Iran ($n = 388$).[a]

Food groups	Western dietary pattern	Prudent dietary pattern
Refined grains	—	0.24
Fast foods	0.22	—
Potatoes	0.32	—
Salty snacks	0.44	—
Mayonnaise	0.43	0.27
Sugar sweetened beverages	0.40	—
Eggs	0.29	
Vegetables	—	—
Whole grains	−0.24	0.35
Fruits and dried fruits	—	0.51
Poultry and fish	—	0.43
High-fat dairy	0.34	—
Low-fat dairy	−0.21	—
Jam and tinned fruits	0.50	—
Liquid oils	—	0.69
Solid fats	0.38	—
Sweet snacks	0.48	—
Red and processed meats	0.23	0.21
Organ meats	0.31	—
Tea and coffee	0.25	—
Nuts and seeds	0.28	0.58
Legumes	−0.38	0.59
Explained variance (%)	10.3	8.9

[a]Values < 0.20 were excluded for simplicity.

were denoted "Western" and "prudent" according to previous studies. The "Western" dietary pattern had high positive factor loadings for sweet snacks, jam and tinned fruits, mayonnaise, sugar-sweetened beverages, salty snacks, solid fats, high-fat dairy, potatoes, organ meats, eggs, red and processed meat, and tea and coffee, as well as negative factor loading for low fat dairy, legumes, and whole grains. The "prudent" dietary pattern had high positive factor loadings for liquid oils, legumes, nuts and seeds, fruits and dried fruits, fish and poultry whole, and refined grains.

Characteristics of the study participants across median categories of the dietary pattern scores are shown in Table 4. BMI, family history of diabetes, parity, and energy intake was higher in pregnant women with higher scores of "Western" dietary pattern compared to those with lower scores ($p < 0.05$). Women with higher scores of the "prudent" dietary pattern had higher energy intake and education level compared to those with lower scores ($p < 0.05$).

The ORs and their 95% CI for GDM by the median of dietary pattern scores are displayed in Table 5. Risk of developing GDM among women in the second median of "Western" dietary pattern scores was higher compared to the first median (OR = 1.97, 95% CI: 1.27–3.04). After adjusting for prepregnancy weight, gestational age, physical activity, family history of diabetes, housing ownership, and building area, the association was still significant (OR = 1.68, 95% CI: 1.04–2.27). However, no significant association was found between "prudent" dietary pattern scores and risk of GDM.

4. Discussion

In the present study, we identified two distinct dietary patterns among participants: Western dietary pattern (high in sweets, jams, mayonnaise, soft drinks, salty snacks, solid

TABLE 4: Participants' characteristics according to dietary pattern scores in an Iranian GDM case-control study between 2009 and 2010, Tehran, Iran.

Characteristics	Western dietary pattern[a]		Prudent dietary pattern[a]	
	Low	High	Low	High
Age (years)	29.6 ± 4.3	29.8 ± 4.4	29.6 ± 4.3	29.8 ± 4.4
p value[b]	0.5		0.8	
Prepregnancy BMI (kg/m^2)	25.1 ± 3.5	25.9 ± 3.8	25.6 ± 3.9	25.4 ± 3.5
p value	0.02		0.54	
Gestational age (week)	30.5 ± 3.9	30.8 ± 4.1	30.5 ± 3.9	30.8 ± 4.1
p value	0.56		0.50	
Energy intake (kcal)	2489 ± 673	2984 ± 787	2275 ± 549	3194 ± 684
p value	<0.001		<0.001	
Family history of diabetes (%)	34.4	46.6	40.3	40.5
p value	0.02		0.85	
Smokers (%)	1.5	0	0.5	1.1
p value	0.24		0.62	
Physical activity (%)				
Low	49.0	51.0	54.6	45.4
High	51.0	49.0	45.4	54.6
p value	0.65		0.56	
Education (%)				
Illiterate and primary	5.5	8.3	9.7	4.1
High school	18.7	23.7	26.5	15.8
Diploma and over	75.8	68.0	63.8	80.1
p value	0.49		0.005	

[a]Low category comprises below median values, and high category corresponds to above median values; [b]values are presented either as mean ± SD or (%) for quantitative and qualitative variables, respectively; $n = 388$.

TABLE 5: Unadjusted and adjusted odds ratios (OR) and 95% confidence intervals (CI) for gestational diabetes mellitus by median categories of dietary patterns in an Iranian GDM case-control study between 2009 and 2010, Tehran, Iran.

	Cases, *n* (%)	Controls, *n* (%)	Unadjusted OR (95% CI)	Adjusted OR[b] (95% CI)
Western dietary pattern[a]				
Low	48 (39.0)	150 (55.8)	1.00 (reference)	1.00 (reference)
High	75 (61.0)	119 (44.2)	1.97 (1.27–3.04)	1.68 (1.04–2.72)
Prudent dietary pattern[a]				
Low	63 (51.2)	133 (49.4)	1.00 (reference)	1.00 (reference)
High	60 (48.8)	136 (50.6)	0.93 (0.60–1.42)	0.97 (0.61–1.56)

[a]Low category comprises below median values, and high category corresponds to above median values; [b]adjusted for confounding variables (prepregnancy BMI, gestational age, physical activity, family history of diabetes, housing ownership, and building area); $n = 388$.

fat, high-fat dairy products, potatoes, organ meat, eggs, red meat, processed foods, tea and coffee and low-fat dairy product, and whole grains) and prudent dietary pattern (which includes high intake of liquid oils, legumes, nuts and seeds, fruits and dried fruits, fish and poultry whole, and refined grains). Western dietary pattern was positively associated with an increased risk of gestational diabetes, after adjustment for potential confounders. However, there was no significant association between healthy dietary pattern and risk of GDM.

Healthy dietary patterns have consistently been associated with a reduced risk of type 2 diabetes mellitus (T2DM); however, few studies have investigated the association between prepregnancy dietary patterns and risk of GDM [17, 22, 23], and to our knowledge, only few has been conducted in Asian females [24, 25].

In a large prospective cohort study in 3063 pregnant Chinese women, no significant association was found between prudent pattern and GDM risk, while the sweets and seafood pattern was associated with an increased risk of GDM [25].

Our findings are further supported by the findings from the Nurses' Health Study II [17]. Women in the highest quintile of Western dietary pattern were associated with increased likelihood of GDM compared to those women in the lowest quintile [17].

Pregnancy is characterized by progressive hyperlipidemia, insulin resistance, and a deterioration of glucose tolerance as the pregnancy advances to the third trimester [30]. Prior evidence suggests that women who develop GDM have altered functions of β-cells and insulin resistance, compromising their capacity to deal with the metabolic challenges of pregnancy [17, 22, 30]. The Western dietary pattern and a dietary pattern similar to that were associated with a significant increase in fasting insulin and C-peptide levels and higher plasma glucose concentrations in healthy individuals [31].

Red and processed meats as one of the main components of the Western dietary pattern are sources of saturated fat, heme iron, nitrosamines, and other constituents which have been associated with beta cell damage, oxidative stress, and insulin resistance as well as incident GDM [17, 22]. Toxicity effects of nitrosamines which are produced by the reaction of nitrite (commonly used as a preservative in processed meats) with amine compounds has been reported in deterioration of beta cell function, increased lipid peroxidation and proinflammatory cytokine activation [32]. In addition, early limited N-nitrosodiethylamine (NDEA) exposures play critical roles in the pathogenesis of major insulin resistance diseases including T2DM in animal models [33]. Furthermore, advanced glycation end products (AGEs) produced during the heating process in red meat and high-fat products are suggested as another possible mediator of association between red and processed meat and GDM [34]. Moreover, it has been observed that high intakes of saturated and trans fatty acids by reducing insulin binding ability to its receptors and impairing glucose transport could be one of the important risk factors triggering GDM [21, 35].

Another potential explanation is related to a high consumption of sugar-sweetened beverages contributing to a high glycemic load (GL) diet leading to inflammation, insulin resistance, and impaired β-cell function [14, 30]. In addition, soft drinks contain caramel colouring which are rich in AGEs promoting inflammatory mediators that might be important in the development of diabetes, such as C-reactive protein and TNF-α [34]. It is also plausible that low intakes of whole grains in Western dietary pattern can contribute to GDM risk. Whole grains are high in insoluble fiber which delay gastric emptying and slow absorption of glucose, resulting in a small increment in insulin levels [6, 30].

On the other hand, some studies have shown an inverse relationship between a healthy dietary pattern and GDM [17]. The effects of a healthy dietary pattern on reducing risk of GDM may be due to a lower dietary energy density and glycemic load and higher amount of fruits and vegetables rich in antioxidants and phytochemicals, dietary fiber, and micronutrients such as magnesium and vitamin C [22, 30]. In our study, in line with some other studies [25], no significant association was found between healthy dietary pattern and gestational diabetes. This probably could be due to the presence of rice and refined grains in our healthy dietary pattern since rice and refined grains are Iranian staple foods [36]. It seems that the adverse effects of refined grains (high glycemic index and low fiber content) on glucose metabolism outweigh other benefits of healthy dietary pattern identified in our study.

Discrepancies between results of studies could be referring to differences in study design, sample size, food questionnaire, definition, and number of the food groups. Since dietary patterns reflect the culture, food preferences, and environmental factors (such as food availability), it can be expected that different dietary patterns are identified in different populations and time periods [19]. Dietary patterns derived from factor analysis capture the effect of the combination of many interacting and synergic foods facilitating the application of nutritional findings for public health recommendations and providing dietary guidelines which might be useful in the prevention of diseases. To our knowledge, the present study is the first one in a Middle-Eastern country to report the association between major dietary patterns and GDM. Studies in developing countries can provide unique opportunities to assess the relation between dietary patterns and GDM risk. Generally, where economic resources are severely restricted, food intake is strongly linked to income, so that even small economic differences are directly reflected in dietary intakes [37]. Other strengths of this analysis are that we were able to control for several potential confounders such as physical activity, prepregnancy BMI, and gestational age. In addition, high participation rate in this study, as 100% of cases and 97% of controls who were initially invited to participate in the research were retained in the final analyses, decreased the risk of selection bias. Since cases were more likely to have changed their diets due to the disease symptoms, the incident cases of GDM were registered in the present study to reduce the possibility of recall bias. One other strength is that the study was conducted in a province with a very high point prevalence of GDM [4].

The study has several limitations. First, because of the observational nature of the current study, we cannot rule out the possibility of residual confounding by unmeasured factors such as abnormal metabolic factors. However, significant associations remained after carefully controlling for major well-documented risk factors for GDM. Second, the results of factor analysis approach might be affected by several arbitrary but important decisions including the number of factors to extract, the components labelling, the method of rotation, and even their interpretation [38]. Third, since dietary intake was assessed using FFQ, measurement errors were unavoidable which can cause underestimation of associations. However, the FFQ applied in this study has relative good reproducibility and validity among the Iranian population [27], and we also excluded subjects overreporting their energy intakes. Fourth, due to the case-control study design, we cannot provide evidence of a causal relationship between prepregnancy dietary patterns and the risk for GDM.

Finally, the sample size of this study was small and the study was only conducted on women living in Tehran city. These could limit the generalization of study results to the entire Iranian population.

5. Conclusion

Overall, we found strong associations between Western dietary pattern and higher GDM risk, while no association was found between prudent pattern and GDM. However, case-control studies may prove an association but these do not demonstrate causation. As a result, these findings need to be confirmed in future prospective studies for etiological purposes to identify whether improving maternal's dietary pattern adherence before pregnancy is associated with a decreased risk of GDM.

Conflicts of Interest

None of the authors had any personal or financial conflicts of interest.

Authors' Contributions

Fatemeh Sedaghat and Mahdieh Akhoondan contributed equally to this article.

Acknowledgments

The present study was financially supported by the National Nutrition and Food Technology Research Institute (NNFTRI) of Shahid Beheshti University of Medical Sciences, Tehran, Iran. The authors are thankful to all other investigators, staffs, and participants of this study.

References

[1] Association AD, "Diagnosis and classification of diabetes mellitus," *Diabetes Care*, vol. 37, Supplement 1, pp. S81–S90, 2014.

[2] F. Atashzadeh Shoorideh, "Frequency of gestational diabetes and its related factors in pregnant women in prenatal clinics of educational hospitals, in Tehran (Oct 2000-March 2002)," *Journal of Rafsanjan University of Medical Sciences*, vol. 5, no. 3, pp. 175–180, 2006.

[3] A. Hossein-Nezhad, Z. Maghbooli, A.-R. Vassigh, and B. Larijani, "Prevalence of gestational diabetes mellitus and pregnancy outcomes in Iranian women," *Taiwanese Journal of Obstetrics and Gynecology*, vol. 46, no. 3, pp. 236–241, 2007.

[4] M. Jafari-Shobeiri, M. Ghojazadeh, S. Azami-Aghdash et al., "Prevalence and risk factors of gestational diabetes in Iran: a systematic review and meta-analysis," *Iranian Journal of Public Health*, vol. 44, no. 8, pp. 1036–1044, 2015.

[5] B. Larijani, "A review on the prevalence of gestational diabetes mellitus (GDM) in different regions of Iran," *Journal of Diabetes and Metabolic Disorders*, vol. 8, p. 7, 2009.

[6] D. Shin, K. W. Lee, and W. O. Song, "Dietary patterns during pregnancy are associated with risk of gestational diabetes mellitus," *Nutrients*, vol. 7, no. 11, pp. 9369–9382, 2015.

[7] M. Donazar-Ezcurra, C. López-del Burgo, and M. Bes-Rastrollo, "Primary prevention of gestational diabetes mellitus through nutritional factors: a systematic review," *BMC Pregnancy and Childbirth*, vol. 17, no. 1, p. 30, 2017.

[8] R. G. Moses, J. L. Shand, and L. C. Tapsell, "The recurrence of gestational diabetes: could dietary differences in fat intake be an explanation?," *Diabetes Care*, vol. 20, no. 11, pp. 1647–1650, 1997.

[9] V. Wijendran, R. B. Bendel, S. C. Couch et al., "Maternal plasma phospholipid polyunsaturated fatty acids in pregnancy with and without gestational diabetes mellitus: relations with maternal factors," *The American Journal of Clinical Nutrition*, vol. 70, no. 1, pp. 53–61, 1999.

[10] S. Bo, G. Menato, A. Lezo et al., "Dietary fat and gestational hyperglycaemia," *Diabetologia*, vol. 44, no. 8, pp. 972–978, 2001.

[11] K. Bowers, D. K. Tobias, E. Yeung, F. B. Hu, and C. Zhang, "A prospective study of prepregnancy dietary fat intake and risk of gestational diabetes," *The American Journal of Clinical Nutrition*, vol. 92, no. 2, pp. 446–453, 2012.

[12] Y. Wang, L. H. Storlien, A. B. Jenkins et al., "Dietary variables and glucose tolerance in pregnancy," *Diabetes Care*, vol. 23, no. 4, pp. 460–464, 2000.

[13] J. S. Radesky, E. Oken, S. L. Rifas-Shiman, K. P. Kleinman, J. W. Rich-Edwards, and M. W. Gillman, "Diet during early pregnancy and development of gestational diabetes," *Paediatric and Perinatal Epidemiology*, vol. 22, no. 1, pp. 47–59, 2008.

[14] L. Chen, F. B. Hu, E. Yeung, W. Willett, and C. Zhang, "Prospective study of pre-gravid sugar-sweetened beverage consumption and the risk of gestational diabetes mellitus," *Diabetes Care*, vol. 32, no. 12, pp. 2236–2241, 2009.

[15] C. Zhang, C. Qiu, F. B. Hu et al., "Maternal plasma 25-hydroxyvitamin D concentrations and the risk for gestational diabetes mellitus," *PLoS One*, vol. 3, no. 11, article e3753, 2008.

[16] K. Bowers, E. Yeung, M. A. Williams et al., "A prospective study of prepregnancy dietary iron intake and risk for gestational diabetes mellitus," *Diabetes Care*, vol. 34, no. 7, pp. 1557–1563, 2011.

[17] C. Zhang, M. B. Schulze, C. G. Solomon, and F. B. Hu, "A prospective study of dietary patterns, meat intake and the risk of gestational diabetes mellitus," *Diabetologia*, vol. 49, no. 11, pp. 2604–2613, 2006.

[18] W. Bao, K. Bowers, D. K. Tobias, F. B. Hu, and C. Zhang, "Prepregnancy dietary protein intake, major dietary protein sources, and the risk of gestational diabetes mellitus: a prospective cohort study," *Diabetes Care*, vol. 36, no. 7, pp. 2001–2008, 2013.

[19] F. B. Hu, "Dietary pattern analysis: a new direction in nutritional epidemiology," *Current Opinion in Lipidology*, vol. 13, no. 1, pp. 3–9, 2002.

[20] F. Jinlin, W. Binyou, and C. Terry, "A new approach to the study of diet and risk of type 2 diabetes," *Journal of Postgraduate Medicine*, vol. 53, no. 2, pp. 139–143, 2007.

[21] D. A. Schoenaker, G. D. Mishra, L. K. Callaway, and S. S. Soedamah-Muthu, "The role of energy, nutrients, foods, and dietary patterns in the development of gestational diabetes mellitus: a systematic review of observational studies," *Diabetes Care*, vol. 39, no. 1, pp. 16–23, 2016.

[22] D. K. Tobias, C. Zhang, J. Chavarro et al., "Prepregnancy adherence to dietary patterns and lower risk of gestational diabetes mellitus," *The American Journal of Clinical Nutrition*, vol. 96, no. 2, pp. 289–295, 2012.

[23] W. Bao, K. Bowers, D. K. Tobias et al., "Prepregnancy low-carbohydrate dietary pattern and risk of gestational diabetes mellitus: a prospective cohort study," *The American Journal of Clinical Nutrition*, vol. 99, no. 6, pp. 1378–1384, 2014.

[24] J. de Seymour, A. Chia, M. Colega et al., "Maternal dietary patterns and gestational diabetes mellitus in a multi-ethnic Asian cohort: the GUSTO study," *Nutrients*, vol. 8, no. 10, 2016.

[25] J. R. He, M. Y. Yuan, N. N. Chen et al., "Maternal dietary patterns and gestational diabetes mellitus: a large prospective cohort study in China," *British Journal of Nutrition*, vol. 113, no. 08, pp. 1292–1300, 2015.

[26] H. Berger, J. Crane, D. Farine et al., "Screening for gestational diabetes mellitus," *Journal of Obstetrics and Gynaecology Canada*, vol. 24, no. 11, pp. 894–912, 2002.

[27] P. Mirmiran, F. H. Esfahani, Y. Mehrabi, M. Hedayati, and F. Azizi, "Reliability and relative validity of an FFQ for nutrients in the Tehran lipid and glucose study," *Public Health Nutrition*, vol. 13, no. 05, pp. 654–662, 2010.

[28] M. Ghaffarpour, A. Houshiar-Rad, and H. Kianfar, "The manual for household measures, cooking yields factors and edible portion of foods," *Tehran: Tehran: Nashre Olume Keshavarzy*, pp. 1–40, 1999.

[29] M. Aadahl and T. Jorgensen, "Validation of a new self-report instrument for measuring physical activity," *Medicine and Science in Sports and Exercise*, vol. 35, no. 7, pp. 1196–1202, 2003.

[30] C. Zhang, S. Liu, C. G. Solomon, and F. B. Hu, "Dietary fiber intake, dietary glycemic load, and the risk for gestational diabetes mellitus," *Diabetes Care*, vol. 29, no. 10, pp. 2223–2230, 2006.

[31] T. T. Fung, E. B. Rimm, D. Spiegelman et al., "Association between dietary patterns and plasma biomarkers of obesity and cardiovascular disease risk," *The American Journal of Clinical Nutrition*, vol. 73, no. 1, pp. 61–67, 2001.

[32] M. Tong, L. Longato, and S. M. de la Monte, "Early limited nitrosamine exposures exacerbate high fat diet-mediated type 2 diabetes and neurodegeneration," *BMC Endocrine Disorders*, vol. 10, no. 1, p. 4, 2010.

[33] M. Tong, A. Neusner, L. Longato, M. Lawton, J. R. Wands, and S. M. de la Monte, "Nitrosamine exposure causes insulin resistance diseases: relevance to type 2 diabetes mellitus, non-alcoholic steatohepatitis, and Alzheimer's disease," *Journal of Alzheimer's Disease*, vol. 17, no. 4, pp. 827–844, 2009.

[34] S. M. Hofmann, H.-J. Dong, Z. Li et al., "Improved insulin sensitivity is associated with restricted intake of dietary glycoxidation products in the db/db mouse," *Diabetes*, vol. 51, no. 7, pp. 2082–2089, 2002.

[35] H. Ying and D. F. Wang, "Effects of dietary fat on onset of gestational diabetes mellitus," *Zhonghua Fu Chan Ke Za Zhi*, vol. 41, no. 11, pp. 729–731, 2006.

[36] H. Ghassemi, G. Harrison, and K. Mohammad, "An accelerated nutrition transition in Iran," *Public Health Nutrition*, vol. 5, no. 1A, pp. 149–155, 2002.

[37] W. Willett, *Nutritional Epidemiology*, Oxford University Press, New York, NY, USA, 2nd edition, 1998.

[38] M. E. Martinez, J. R. Marshall, and L. Sechrest, "Invited commentary: factor analysis and the search for objectivity," *American Journal of Epidemiology*, vol. 148, no. 1, pp. 17–19, 1998.

3

To Predict the Requirement of Pharmacotherapy by OGTT Glucose Levels in Women with GDM Classified by the IADPSG Criteria

Gülen Yerlikaya,[1] Veronica Falcone,[1] Tina Stopp,[1] Martina Mittlböck,[2] Andrea Tura ,[3] Peter Husslein,[1] Wolfgang Eppel,[1] and Christian S. Göbl [1]

[1]*Department of Obstetrics and Gynecology, Division of Obstetrics and Feto-Naternal Medicine, Medical University of Vienna, Vienna, Austria*
[2]*Center of Medical Statistics, Informatics, and Intelligent Systems, Section for Clinical Biometrics, Medical University of Vienna, Vienna, Austria*
[3]*Metabolic Unit, Institute of Neuroscience, National Research Council, Padova, Italy*

Correspondence should be addressed to Christian S. Göbl; christian.goebl@meduniwien.ac.at

Academic Editor: Kazuya Yamagata

The aim of this study was to assess the association between OGTT glucose levels and requirement of pharmacotherapy in GDM patients classified by the IADPSG criteria. This study included 203 GDM patients (108 managed with lifestyle modification and 95 requiring pharmacotherapy). Clinical risk factors and OGTT glucose concentrations at 0 (G0), 60 (G60), and 120 min (G120) were collected. OGTT glucose levels were significantly associated with the later requirement of pharmacotherapy (ROC-AUC: 71.1, 95% CI: 63.8–78.3). Also, the combination of clinical risk factors (age, BMI, parity, and pharmacotherapy in previous gestation) showed an acceptable predictive accuracy (ROC-AUC: 72.1, 95% CI: 65.0–79.2), which was further improved when glycemic parameters were added (ROC-AUC: 77.5, 95% CI: 71.5–83.9). Random forest analysis revealed the highest variable importance for G0, G60, and age. OGTT glucose measures in addition to clinical risk factors showed promising properties for risk stratification in GDM patients classified by the recently established IADPSG criteria.

1. Introduction

The International Associations for Diabetes in Pregnancy Study Groups (IADPSG) guidelines for gestational diabetes mellitus (GDM) classification recommends a primary testing until the early third trimester by a 2 h-75 g oral glucose tolerance test (OGTT) [1, 2]. However, it was found that these recommendations resulted in a markedly increased number of GDM cases [3] containing a heterogenic group of pregnant women on the wide range of disturbed glucose metabolism. Therefore, most patients achieve adequate glycemic control with lifestyle modification while others need intensified pharmacologic therapy.

An early stratification into low- and high-risk patients could markedly improve the efficiency of treatment. Within the last years, different risk factors were identified which are associated with the requirement of glucose-lowering medications in women with GDM. These include age, pre-pregnancy BMI, history of GDM in previous pregnancy, and others [4–7]. Although previous studies indicated that increased OGTT glucose concentrations were related to adverse gestational and fetal outcome [8, 9], their specific performance for the prediction of pharmacotherapy in patients meeting the IADPSG criteria is less well investigated.

Therefore, this study aims to examine the ability of OGTT glucose levels to distinguish between low- (achieving glycemic targets with lifestyle modification) and high-risk (requiring pharmacotherapy) GDM patients diagnosed by the IADPSG criteria. Moreover, their contribution to discriminate low- and high-risk patients additional to more common and routinely documented risk factors should be assessed.

2. Materials and Methods

In this retrospective case-control study, we included 203 pregnant women diagnosed with GDM (108 managed with lifestyle modification and 95 requiring pharmacotherapy with insulin ($n = 80$), metformin ($n = 11$), or both ($n = 4$)), who attended our outpatient clinic between May 2015 and January 2017. GDM was diagnosed via universal testing by a 75 g-OGTT at 24–28 weeks of gestation, according to the IADPSG recommendations [1, 2]. Intensified lifestyle modification (ILS) including medical nutrition therapy was used as the first line intervention. All patients were instructed for capillary blood glucose monitoring and informed about glycemic treatment targets. Follow-ups in two to three weeks' time were scheduled, and blood glucose levels were reviewed during each appointment. The pharmacologic intervention was started at any time point when blood glucose targets were not achieved (i.e., <95 mg/dl at fasting or <140 mg/dl one hour after each meal) according to the current guidelines [10]. The following variables were collected from the medical records: age,gravidity, parity, prepregnancy BMI, history of GDM, first-degree relative with diabetes, and OGTT results at 0 min (G0), 60 min (G60), and 120 min (G120). Patients with preexisting diabetes as well as multiple pregnancies or those with missing OGTT glucose values were excluded. The study was approved by the Ethics Committee of the Medical University of Vienna and performed in accordance with the Declaration of Helsinki.

2.1. Statistical Analysis. Continuous and categorical variables were summarized as the means ± SD or median (IQR) and counts and percentages and compared by Student's *t*-test (or the Wilcoxon rank sum test for skewed distributed variables) and Pearson's chi-square test. Binary logistic regression was used to assess the probability of initiation of pharmacotherapy by OGTT glucose levels and risk factors such as age, prepregnancy BMI, parity, and history of GDM and others. Thereby, the predictive accuracy of the models was expressed as the area under the receiver operating characteristic curves (ROC-AUC). Unbiased recursive partitioning was performed, whereby decision trees were created by the conditional inference (Ctree) framework [11]. Thereby, random decision forests with ntree = 5000 were created to derive measures of variable importance (i.e., the average difference in predictive accuracy before and after permutation of a predictor variable over all 5000 trees). As supporting time-to-event analysis, the competing risk model of Fine and Gray [12] was conducted where preterm delivery (before 38 + 0 weeks of gestation) is considered a competing event to the start of pharmacotherapy. As single observations were missing at random for some covariables (G0: 1.5%; G60: 7.4%; G120: 8.4%; BMIPK: 1.0%; and history of GDM: 10.8%), multivariate imputations by chained equations were performed to estimate missing observations by the median value of 50 complete data sets. These imputations were used in logistic and proportional hazard regression models in order to achieve a maximum of information from our data. Group-specific comparisons of raw data are provided in Table 1. Statistical analysis was performed with R (version 3.4.1) and contributed packages ("mice" for data imputations as well as "pROC," "party," and "cmprsk" for data analysis) [13]. A two-sided p value ≤ 0.05 was considered statistically significant. p values were interpreted in an explorative manner aiming to generate new hypotheses, and no adjustment for multiple statistical testing was used if not otherwise indicated.

3. Results

A descriptive comparison of the data is provided in Table 1. It was found that mothers requiring pharmacotherapy were older, had higher BMI, and reached higher plasma glucose concentrations during the OGTT. Although univariable analysis revealed significant associations between plasma glucose levels and risk for pharmacologic intervention, the relative contribution of each glucose measure including their mean value was only modest to fair (ROC-AUC ranged between 60.2 and 65.6% as provided in Figure 1(a)–1(c)). The predictive performance was, however, markedly improved when the information of all three OGTT glucose measurements was combined by multiple logistic regression (model 1: ROC-AUC: 71.1, Figure 1(d)). Also, the combination of clinical variables (age, pregestational BMI, parity, history of GDM in previous gestation, family history with type 2 diabetes, and time of diagnosis) showed an acceptable discrimination between low- and high-risk patients (model 2: ROC-AUC: 72.1, Figure 1(e); $p = 0.834$ versus model 1), which was further improved when OGTT glucose levels were included as additional predictors (model 3: ROC-AUC: 77.5, Figure 1(f); $p = 0.030$ versus model 1 and $p = 0.033$ versus model 2). Random forest analysis revealed the highest variable importance for G0 (1.11×10^{-2}), G60 (0.96×10^{-2}), and age (0.80×10^{-2}), while the importance of the remaining predictors was shown to be inferior (G120: 0.24×10^{-2}, BMI: 0.40×10^{-2}, parity: 0.05×10^{-2}, history of GDM: 0.31×10^{-2}, family history with type 2 diabetes: -0.17×10^{-2}, and time of diagnosis: 0.13×10^{-2}). An exemplary decision tree with possible cut-off values for G0, G60, and age is also provided. A very low risk for pharmacotherapy was observed for patients with G0 ≤ 81 mg/dl, whereas patients with G0 > 81 and G60 > 212 had a very high risk for pharmacologic intervention (Figure 2). Pharmacotherapy was initiated at a median time of 31.1 weeks of gestation. G0 (HR: 1.12, 95% CI: 1.01–1.24, for an increase of 10 mg/dl), G60 (HR: 1.14, 95% CI: 1.05–1.24, for an increase of 10 mg/dl), and age (HR: 1.25, 95% CI: 1.04–1.51, for an increase of 5 years) were also found to be independent predictors for pharmacologic intervention by time-to-event analysis, accounting for preterm delivery (before 38 + 0 weeks). Moreover, the combined information of G0, G60, and age showed a fair discrimination when included in a logistic regression model to predict the probability for delivering LGA offspring (ROC-AUC: 64.7%, 95% CI: 54.1–75.3). However, only G0 reached a significance in this model ($p = 0.012$).

Table 1: Characteristics of the study population.

	n	GDM-LSI ($n = 108$)	n	GDM-PT ($n = 95$)	p value
Age (years)	108	31.5 ± 5.9	95	34.6 ± 5.9	<0.001
BMI (kg/m^2)	107	27.8 ± 6.4	94	30.1 ± 6.9	0.014
Fertility treatment	108	6 (5.6%)	95	8 (8.4%)	0.421
Gravidity (count)	108	3.0 (2.0–4.0)	95	3.0 (2.0–5.0)	0.029
Gravidity (>1)	108	87 (80.6%)	95	83 (87.4%)	0.189
Parity (count)	108	1.0 (0.0–2.0)	95	1.0 (1.0–2.5)	0.054
Parity (≥1)	108	73 (67.6%)	95	74 (77.9%)	0.101
pGDM	102	19 (18.6%)	87	34 (39.0%)	0.002
G0 (mg/dl)	105	90.0 ± 10.8	95	98.8 ± 19.2	<0.001
G60 (mg/dl)	101	173.2 ± 29.5	87	189.0 ± 30.8	<0.001
G120 (mg/dl)	98	129.7 ± 29.0	88	140.4 ± 33.9	0.021
Gmean (mg/dl)	98	130.6 ± 15.2	87	141.7 ± 20.3	<0.001
Week diagnosis	108	28.0 (26.4–30.3)	95	27.7 (25.6–29.4)	0.032
Week treatment start		—	95	31.1 (28.0–33.3)	
BW (pct)	108	50.5 (24.0–70.5)	95	50.0 (26.0–86.0)	0.427
LGA	108	12 (11.1%)	95	21 (22.1%)	0.034

Data are mean ± standard deviations or median and interquartile range (IQR) for pregnant women affected by GDM and treated with lifestyle modification (GDM-LSI) or requiring pharmacologic treatment (GDM-PT). BMI: pregestational body mass index; pGDM: previous pregnancy with gestational diabetes mellitus; G0: fasting plasma glucose; G60: plasma glucose 60 min after oral glucose load; G120: plasma glucose 120 min after oral glucose load; BW: birth weight; LGA: large for gestational age offspring.

4. Discussion

This study assessed the association between glucose measures derived from a diagnostic 75 g-OGTT and future requirement of pharmacotherapy in women classified with GDM according to the IADPSG recommendations. Albeit the individual glucose measurements (G0, G60, and G120) were significantly associated with the risk of requiring glucose-lowering medication, their predictive performance was markedly improved when the information of all three OGTT glucose values was combined by multivariable logistic regression. The model discrimination of clinical risk factors was also improved when OGTT glucose measurements were added as further predictors. Thereby, G0 followed by G60 and age achieved the highest variable importance measures.

These findings are of clinical relevance: in 2010, the IADPSG recommended novel criteria for GDM classification based on one-step OGTT testing in all pregnant women [1]. These criteria were more recently adopted by the WHO and several local health care organizations [2]. However, it was criticized that this novel established strategy would substantially increase the number of GDM patients by additionally identifying very subtle alterations in disturbed glucose metabolism [14]. This limitation of the IADPSG approach emphasizes the need for accurate risk stratification early after diagnosis to separate low- from high-risk pregnancies, that is, patients who achieve adequate glycemic control with lifestyle modification and those who require more intensified treatment strategies. Although already previous research assessed a constellation of risk factors associated with antenatal insulin therapy, most of the available studies used earlier diagnostic algorithms (mostly two-step approaches) and therefore contain study populations with different risk profiles as compared to patients with GDM identified by the one-step IADPSG approach. While in accordance to our findings some of these previous studies also indicated a significant association between elevated fasting glucose levels and requirement of pharmacotherapy [4–7], more controversial results are reported for elevated post load OGTT glucose: Wong and Jalaludin found that G120 in addition to G0, BMI at booking, and gestational week at diagnosis was independently associated with insulin therapy [6], whereas in another study, which used a comparable diagnostic approach (two-step screening according to the Australasian Diabetes in Pregnancy Society (ADIPS)), the predictive performance of G120 lost its significance in multivariable regression [4]. A further Australian study identified several clinical determinants of antenatal insulin treatment including G0, G60, and HbA1c [5]. Nevertheless, these variables explained only a small amount of the variance and in accordance with others the authors concluded that antenatal factors including glycemic measures were insufficient to predict the attributable risk for intensified pharmacotherapy [5, 15]. This is in contrast to our finding in GDM patients identified by the one-step IADPSG approach, where aggregated information of glycemic as well as clinical risk factors showed an acceptable accuracy with an ROC-AUC ranging from 71.1% (glycemic parameters) to 77.5% (glycemic parameters and clinical risk factors). Only two further studies were identified using the IADPSG criteria for GDM classification: Bakiner et al. found that G0 (ROC-AUC: 73.4%) and HbA1c (ROC-AUC: 67.7%) were independently associated with antenatal insulin treatment in a retrospective study on 300 pregnancies [16]. However, dynamic OGTT glucose values were not reported in this study. Mitra et al. observed a significant association between G60 and antenatal insulin

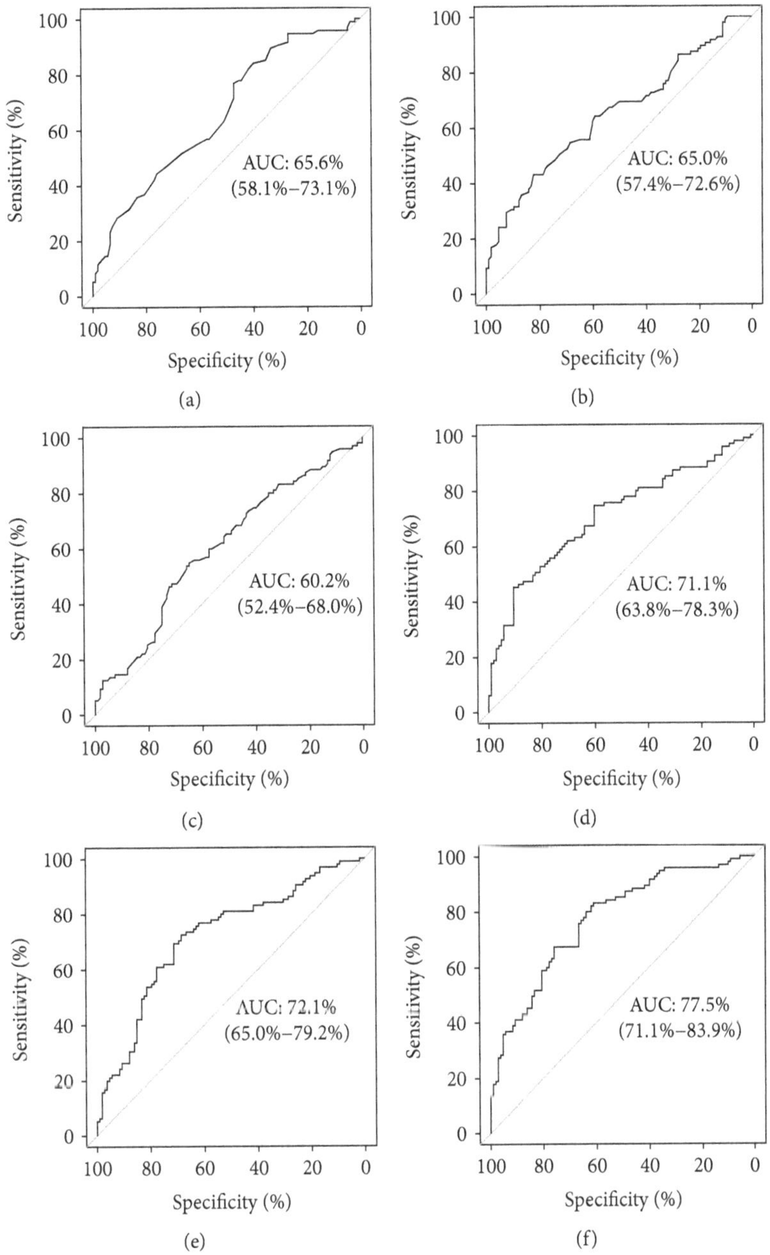

Figure 1: ROC curves for prediction of initiation of pharmacotherapy by OGTT glucose measurements at fasting (a), 60′(b), and 120′(c) after oral glucose load; combined information of OGTT glucose measurements (d); clinical predictors (age, pregestational BMI, parity, history of GDM, family history with type 2 diabetes, and time of diagnosis) (e); and OGTT glucose measurements and clinical predictors (f).

treatment with an ROC-AUC of 83.1% [17]. However, the sample size of this study was very small with 8 out of 83 patients requiring pharmacotherapy.

The importance of dynamic glucose measurements for risk stratification is also supported by previous research in nonpregnant patients indicating strong associations between elevated fasting and dynamic OGTT glucose measures with decreased insulin sensitivity and β-cell dysfunction [18]. Accordingly, a higher degree of insulin resistance and impaired insulin secretion was recently found to characterize patients with GDM requiring pharmacotherapy [19]. A standardized examination of HbA1c at the time of diagnosis was not available in our study, which could be seen as a limitation of this work. However, in contrast to dynamic measures of glucose levels, HbA1c is a weak surrogate of insulin sensitivity or secretion and gives almost no additive information to glycemic parameters assessed during the OGTT [20]. HbA1c is further subjected to pregnancy-specific changes [21, 22]. Although we provided an exemplary decision tree including the main predictors for intensified therapy identified by our study, this algorithm needs further validation. Of note, we were not able to assess lifestyle habits or several components of the "metabolic syndrome" due to the retrospective nature of this work. This data could be of additional importance and needs to be addressed in future prospective studies.

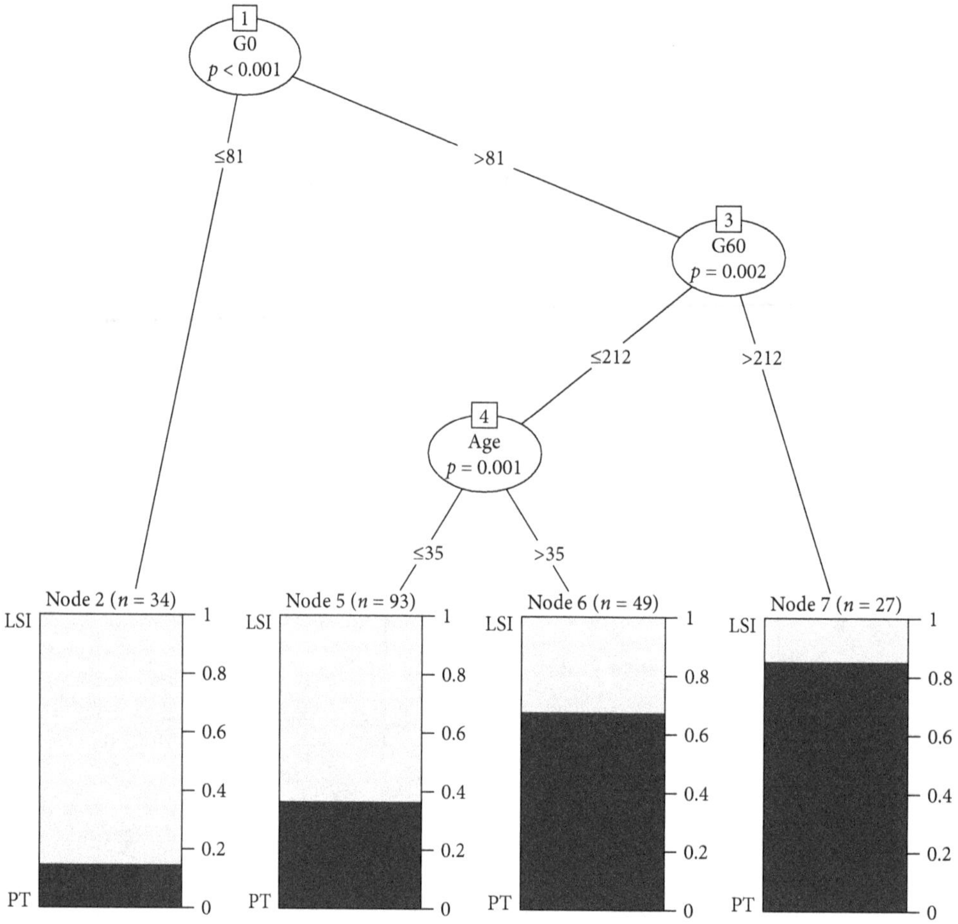

FIGURE 2: Example of a conditional inference tree for the prediction of intensified pharmacologic intervention in GDM patients. Bonferroni adjusted p values are given for each inner node, and the fraction of lifestyle intervention (LSI) and initiation of pharmacotherapy (PT) is provided at each terminal node.

5. Conclusions

In summary, we found that fasting and dynamic OGTT glucose measures in addition to clinical risk factors showed promising properties for risk stratification in GDM patients classified by the recently established IADPSG criteria. These findings should be considered in future studies to establish an accurate separation for the early treatment of high-risk patients.

Conflicts of Interest

The authors declare that there is no conflict of interest regarding the publication of this paper.

References

[1] International Association of Diabetes and Pregnancy Study Groups Consensus Panel, "International Association of Diabetes and Pregnancy Study Groups Recommendations on the Diagnosis and Classification of Hyperglycemia in Pregnancy," *Diabetes Care*, vol. 33, no. 3, pp. 676–682, 2010.

[2] World Health Organisation, *Diagnostic Criteria and Classification of Hyperglycaemia First Detected in Pregnancy*, WHO Press, World Health Organization, Geneva, Switzerland, 2013.

[3] D. A. Sacks, D. R. Hadden, M. Maresh et al., "Frequency of gestational diabetes mellitus at collaborating centers based on IADPSG Consensus Panel-Recommended Criteria: the Hyperglycemia and Adverse Pregnancy Outcome (HAPO) Study," *Diabetes Care*, vol. 35, no. 3, pp. 526–528, 2012.

[4] R. A. Barnes, T. Wong, G. P. Ross et al., "A novel validated model for the prediction of insulin therapy initiation and adverse perinatal outcomes in women with gestational diabetes mellitus," *Diabetologia*, vol. 59, no. 11, pp. 2331–2338, 2016.

[5] T. Pertot, L. Molyneaux, K. Tan, G. P. Ross, D. K. Yue, and J. Wong, "Can common clinical parameters be used to identify patients who will need insulin treatment in gestational diabetes mellitus?," *Diabetes Care*, vol. 34, no. 10, pp. 2214–2216, 2011.

[6] V. W. Wong and B. Jalaludin, "Gestational diabetes mellitus: who requires insulin therapy?," *Australian and New Zealand Journal of Obstetrics and Gynaecology*, vol. 51, no. 5, pp. 432–436, 2011.

[7] V. H. González-Quintero, N. B. Istwan, D. J. Rhea et al., "Antenatal factors predicting subsequent need for insulin treatment in women with gestational diabetes," *Journal of Women's Health*, vol. 17, no. 7, pp. 1183–1187, 2008.

[8] C. H. Lin, S. F. Wen, Y. H. Wu, and M. J. Huang, "Using the 100-g oral glucose tolerance test to predict fetal and maternal outcomes in women with gestational diabetes mellitus," *Chang Gung Medical Journal*, vol. 32, no. 3, pp. 283–289, 2009.

[9] HAPO Study Cooperative Research Group, B. E. Metzger, L. P. Lowe et al., "Hyperglycemia and adverse pregnancy outcomes," *New England Journal of Medicine*, vol. 358, no. 19, pp. 1991–2002, 2008.

[10] American Diabetes Association, "15. Diabetes advocacy:standards of medical care in diabetes—2018," *Diabetes Care*, vol. 41, Supplement 1, pp. S152–S153, 2017.

[11] T. Hothorn, K. Hornik, and A. Zeileis, "Unbiased recursive partitioning: a conditional inference framework," *Journal of Computational and Graphical Statistics*, vol. 15, no. 3, pp. 651–674, 2006.

[12] J. P. Fine and R. J. Gray, "A proportional hazards model for the subdistribution of a competing risk," *Journal of the American Statistical Association*, vol. 94, no. 446, pp. 496–509, 1999.

[13] R Core Team, *R: A Language and Environment for Statistical Computing*, R Foundation for Statistical Computing, Vienna, Austria, 2017.

[14] T. Cundy, E. Ackermann, and E. A. Ryan, "Gestational diabetes: new criteria may triple the prevalence but effect on outcomes is unclear," *BMJ*, vol. 348, article g1567, 2014.

[15] H. Mendez-Figueroa, J. Daley, V. V. Lopes, and D. R. Coustan, "Predicting the need for medical therapy in patients with mild gestational diabetes," *American Journal of Perinatology*, vol. 31, no. 2, pp. 105–112, 2014.

[16] O. Bakiner, E. Bozkirli, K. Ozsahin, C. Sariturk, and E. Ertorer, "Risk factors that can predict antenatal insulin need in gestational diabetes," *Journal of Clinical Medicine Research*, vol. 5, 2013.

[17] S. Mitra, P. K. Nayak, J. Sahoo et al., "Predictors for antenatal insulin requirement in gestational diabetes," *Gynecological Endocrinology*, vol. 30, no. 8, pp. 565–568, 2014.

[18] M. A. Abdul-Ghani, D. Tripathy, and R. A. DeFronzo, "Contributions of β-cell dysfunction and insulin resistance to the pathogenesis of impaired glucose tolerance and impaired fasting glucose," *Diabetes Care*, vol. 29, no. 5, pp. 1130–1139, 2006.

[19] K. Benhalima, K. Robyns, P. van Crombrugge et al., "Differences in pregnancy outcomes and characteristics between insulin- and diet-treated women with gestational diabetes," *BMC Pregnancy and Childbirth*, vol. 15, no. 1, p. 271, 2015.

[20] C. S. Göbl, L. Bozkurt, R. Yarragudi, A. Tura, G. Pacini, and A. Kautzky-Willer, "Is early postpartum HbA1c an appropriate risk predictor after pregnancy with gestational diabetes mellitus?," *Acta Diabetologica*, vol. 51, no. 5, pp. 715–722, 2014.

[21] K. Hashimoto, T. Osugi, S. Noguchi et al., "A1C but not serum glycated albumin is elevated because of iron deficiency in late pregnancy in diabetic women," *Diabetes Care*, vol. 33, no. 3, pp. 509–511, 2010.

[22] R. C. E. Hughes, J. Rowan, and C. M. Florkowski, "Is there a role for HbA1c in pregnancy?," *Current Diabetes Reports*, vol. 16, no. 1, p. 5, 2016.

4

Molecular Analysis of a Genetic Variants Panel Related to Nutrients and Metabolism: Association with Susceptibility to Gestational Diabetes and Cardiometabolic Risk in Affected Women

Marica Franzago,[1,2] Federica Fraticelli,[2,3] Antonio Nicolucci,[4] Claudio Celentano,[3] Marco Liberati,[3] Liborio Stuppia,[1,2] and Ester Vitacolonna[2,3]

[1]*Laboratory of Molecular Genetics, Department of Psychological, Health and Territorial Sciences, School of Medicine and Health Sciences, "G. d'Annunzio" University, Chieti-Pescara, Via dei Vestini 31, 66013 Chieti, Italy*
[2]*Ce.S.I-Met, "G. d'Annunzio" University, Chieti-Pescara, Via Colle dell'Ara No. 1, 66100 Chieti, Italy*
[3]*Department of Medicine and Aging, School of Medicine and Health Sciences, "G. d'Annunzio" University, Chieti-Pescara, Chieti, Italy*
[4]*Center for Outcomes Research and Clinical Epidemiology (CORE), Pescara, Italy*

Correspondence should be addressed to Ester Vitacolonna; e.vitacolonna@unich.it

Academic Editor: Emmanuel Cosson

Gestational diabetes mellitus (GDM) is the most frequent metabolic disorder in pregnancy. Women with a GDM history are at increased risk of developing diabetes and cardiovascular diseases. Studies have demonstrated a significant correlation between several genes involved in the metabolic pathway of insulin and environmental factors. The aim of this study was to investigate the relationship between clinical parameters in GDM and variants in genes involved with nutrients and metabolism. Several variants *PPARG2* rs1801282 (*C>G*); *PPARGC1A* rs8192678 (*C>T*); *TCF7L2* rs7903146 (*C>T*); *LDLR* rs2228671 (*C>T*); *MTHFR* rs1801133 (*C>T*); *APOA5* rs662799 (*T>C*); *GCKR* rs1260326 (*C>T*); *FTO* rs9939609 (*T>A*); *MC4R* rs17782313 (*T>C*) were genotyped in 168 pregnant Caucasian women with or without GDM by High Resolution Melting (HRM) analysis. A significant correlation was observed between TT genotype of *TCF7L2* gene and increased risk of GDM (OR 5.4 [95% CI 1.5–19.3]). Moreover, a significant correlation was observed between lipid parameters and genetic variations in additional genes, namely, *PPARG2* [$p = 0,02$], *APOA5* [$p = 0,02$], *MC4R* [$p = 0,03$], *LDLR* [$p = 0,01$], and *FTO* [$p = 0,02$]. Our findings support the association between *TCF7L2* rs7903146 variant and an increased GDM risk. Results about the investigated genetic variants provide important information about cardiometabolic risk in GDM and help to plan future prevention studies.

1. Introduction

Gestational diabetes mellitus (GDM) is defined as "diabetes diagnosed in the second or third trimester of pregnancy that is not clearly overt diabetes" [1].

GDM approximately affects 7% (range 2–18%) of all pregnancies [2] and may result in short- and long-term complications for both mother and foetus/infant [3], and GDM can be considered an unmasking of underlying and silent risk of diabetes and cardiovascular disease. Although the etiology of this disease has not been fully elucidated, overweight status before pregnancy, weight gain during pregnancy, ethnicity, and family history of diabetes play important roles in the development and progression of GDM [4]. Moreover, previous studies have demonstrated a significant correlation between polymorphisms of several genes involved in the metabolic pathway of insulin and increased risk for GDM [5, 6].

The recent advances in molecular technology have underscored the significant role of genetic factors in the development, treatment, and complications of diabetic pregnancy

[7]. However, so far the only example of genetic predisposition to GDM is represented by maturity onset diabetes of the young (MODY), a clinically heterogeneous autosomal dominant monogenic disease, accounting for up to 5% of diabetes and due to mutations in different genes such as *HNF4A*, *GCK*, *HNF1A*, *IPF1*, *HNF1B*, and *NEUROD1*. Common variants in MODY genes, especially in *HNF1A* and *GCK*, have been correlated with GDM and related traits [8–10].

The identification of additional genetic markers which could explain differences in susceptibility to GDM would represent a crucial point in order to set up a strategy for the prevention, early diagnosis, and treatment of this condition. In this regard, the aim of this study was to investigate the relationship between clinical parameters in GDM and variants in genes involved with nutrients and metabolism (namely, *TCF7L2*, *PPARG2*, *PPARGC1A*, carbohydrate metabolism; *FTO*, *MC4R*, *APOA5*, *LDLR*, *GCKR*, fat metabolism; *MTHFR*, folate metabolism). These variants were selected due to their correlation with lipid metabolism, glucose sensing, beta-cell function, and appetite control and are all adequately replicated by the literature. An additional aim was to identify an innovative tool for early prevention of cardiometabolic diseases after GDM. To the best of our knowledge, this is the first association study in GDM based on the use of a genetic panel able to identify variants related to the metabolism of both carbohydrates and lipids, in order to evaluate not only the susceptibility to GDM, but also the increase in cardiometabolic risk.

2. Materials and Methods

2.1. Study Design and Participants. From February 2015 to November 2015, one hundred and sixty eight Caucasian women attending the Diabetes and Metabolism Unit or the Obstetrics and Gynaecology Clinic at the Hospital of University "Gabriele d'Annunzio" in Chieti were recruited. Specifically, 102 consecutive women with GDM (mean age ± SD = 34.6 ± 5.4) and 66 nondiabetic pregnant consecutive control subjects (mean age ± SD = 31.9±5.1) were assessed. The diagnosis of GDM was based on an abnormal 75 g oral glucose tolerance test (OGTT) where either one or more blood glucose values were above the values of 5.1 mmol/L (92 mg/dL) at fasting, 10.0 mmol/L (180 mg/dL) at 1 h, and 8.5 mmol/L (153 mg/dL) at 2 h. [11]. The genetic analysis was conducted at the Laboratory *of Molecular Genetics, School of Medicine and Health Sciences,* "G. d'Annunzio" University of Chieti.

2.2. Methods. During the first visit (conducted at the Diabetes and Metabolism Unit or at the Obstetrics and Gynaecology Clinic) data on sociodemographic characteristics, anthropometric and clinical parameters were collected. In addition, clinical parameters, including prepregnancy body mass index (BMI), gestational weight gain, fasting insulin (FINS), blood glucose, total cholesterol (TC), high-density lipoprotein cholesterol (HDL-C), low-density lipoprotein cholesterol (LDL-C), triglycerides (TG), and blood pressure, were recorded. A blood sample was obtained from each patient and stored at 4°C before DNA extraction.

2.3. Inclusion and Exclusion Criteria. The inclusion criteria were pregnant women with ≥18 years of age. The exclusion criteria were women with type 1 or 2 prepregnancy diabetes, overt diabetes, or monogenic diabetes, specifically GCK diabetes, and women with other chronic diseases.

2.3.1. Women with GDM. The diagnostic criteria used for GDM were those proposed by the International Association of Diabetes and Pregnancy Study Groups (IADPSG) [11]. The GDM diagnosis was considered to be proved when established both at the 16–18th and the 24–28th weeks of gestation.

2.3.2. Women without GDM. Women, attending the Diabetes and Metabolism Unit and/or c/o the Department of Obstetrics and Gynaecology, that according to current recommendations [11] had no diagnosis of GDM, were included.

2.4. Genotyping. Nine single nucleotide polymorphisms (SNPs) from 9 genes were included in the analysis. Of the 9 genes, three (*TCF7L2*, *PPARG2*, and *PPARGC1A*) were related to carbohydrate metabolism, two (*APOA5*, *GCKR*) to triglycerides metabolism, one (*LDLR*) to cholesterol metabolism, one (*MTHFR*) to folate metabolism, and two (*FTO*, *MC4R*) to energy metabolism.

The SNPs rs1801282 (*C>G*) in *PPARG2*; rs8192678 (*C>T*) in *PPARGC1A*; rs7903146 (*C>T*) in *TCF7L2*; rs2228671 (*C>T*) in *LDLR;* rs1801133 (*C>T*) in *MTHFR* were genotyped. In addition rs662799 (*T>C*) in *APOA5*; rs1260326 (*C>T*) in *GCKR*; rs9939609 (*T>A*) in *FTO*; rs17782313 (*T>C*) near *MC4R* were genotyped. Genomic DNA was automatically isolated from peripheral blood lymphocytes using MagPurix 12s Automated Nucleic Acid Purification System (Zinexts Life Science Corp., Taiwan). SNPs were detected by High Resolution Melting (HRM) technique, according to the manufacturer's instructions. Primers were designed using Primer3 software to amplify a small fragment avoiding the presence of other sequence variations in the primers region. PCR amplification was performed under the same conditions in a 96-well plate in the PikoReal™ Real-Time PCR System (Thermo Scientific). Reaction volume was 10 μL: 1 μL of genomic DNA (10 ng/μL) was added to 9 μL of reaction master mix consisting of Luminaris Color HRM Master Mix (2x) containing chemically modified Hot Start Taq DNA Polymerase, EvaGreen™ fluorescent dye, dNTPs and $MgCl_2$ in an optimized PCR buffer with a blue dye, and 0.5 μM of forward and reverse primers. The PCR program started with an initial denaturation of 10 min at 95°C and continued with 40 cycles of 10 s at 95°C, 30 s at 60°C, and 30 s at 72°C: afterward one step for heteroduplex formation by heating to 95°C for 30 s and cooling down to 50°C for 30 s. Data were acquired over the 60–95°C range at the thermal transition rate of 0.2°C/s. Each sample was run in triplicate and each plate contained known controls. Genotypes were assigned by comparing sample curves with control curves. To evaluate the sensitivity of HRM, some of the results were randomly confirmed by direct sequencing.

Moreover, the promoter and the complete coding region for isoform 1 of *GCK* gene was sequenced in 13 pregnant women with suspect MODY2. In detail, fragments containing the promoter and ten exons were amplified by PCR using specific primers designed based on the reference gene sequence. PCR fragments were sequenced using the BigDye Terminator v3.1 and then analyzed on an automatic sequencing analyzer (ABI PRISM 3130XL).

2.5. Statistical Analysis. Statistical analysis was performed using the Statistical Package for Social Science (SPSS) program, version 17.0 software for Windows (SPSS, Chicago, IL, USA). p values < 0.05 were considered statistically significant. Fisher's exact test or the Chi-square test were used for categorical variables.

The association between gene variants and risk of GDM was assessed through logistic regression analysis with backward variable selection and gene variants: age and BMI tested as covariates. Results are expressed as odds ratios (ORs) with their 95% confidence intervals (95% CI). Comparisons among GDM group to test the effect of carrier/noncarrier and genotypes on TC, HDL-C, and LDL-C levels at 3rd trimester were performed through Mann–Whitney U Test and Kruskal-Wallis test, respectively. The association between carrier status and TC, HDL-C, and LDL-C levels at 3rd trimester was also explored through multiple regression adjusted for age and BMI and expressed as β parameters. Moreover, comparisons for both GDM and controls to test the effect of carrier/noncarrier and genotypes on BMI were performed through Mann–Whitney U Test and Kruskal-Wallis test, respectively. For each investigated locus, Hardy-Weinberg equilibrium was calculated.

3. Results

The study of *GCK* gene evidenced the presence in four patients of the variant −30 G>A in the promoter (two in homozygous and two in heterozygous). These cases were excluded from the study.

The characteristics of cases and controls are summarized in Table 1. GDM patients showed higher prepregnancy BMI, age, and lower diastolic blood pressure than control group. This could be because the women with GDM were followed up by the diabetes and nutrition team. All participants underwent OGTT, and mean glucose values according to GDM status are presented in Table 2. The genotype distributions of SNPs in the studies are shown in Supplementary Table 1 (see Supplementary Material available online.

Only one out of the nine investigated gene variants, namely, rs7903146 in the *TCF7L2* gene, showed a significant difference in the frequency between cases and controls (supplementary Table 1). In fact, the *TT* genotype was significantly more frequent among GDM patients as compared with healthy controls (27,5% versus 10,6%; p = 0.024) (supplementary Table 1). At analysis, the *TT* genotype was associated with a more than fivefold increased risk of GDM (OR 5.4 [95% CI 1.5–19.3]). Although the rs7903146 in the *TCF7L2* was the only variant associated with GDM, a significant relation was also found between *APOA5* −1131*T*>*C* polymorphism, and *MC4R* rs17782313 polymorphism with 3rd trimester HDL-C in women with GDM. Then, a significant correlation was observed between *PPARG2* rs1801282 and *LDLR* rs2228671 with 3rd trimester LDL-cholesterol levels. Finally, a significant correlation was observed between *FTO* rs9939609 and 3rd trimester LDL-cholesterol levels (Supplementary Tables 2-3). Our results show that the associations between SNPs and BMI are not statistically significant (Supplementary Tables 4-5).

TABLE 1: Characteristics of cases and controls.

Characteristics	GDM yes (N = 102)	GDM no (N = 66)	p^*
Age (years)[a]	34.6 ± 5.4	31.9 ± 5.1	<0.0001
Ethnicity[b]			0.56
Caucasian	99.0	97.0	
Other	1.0	3.0	
School education[b]			0.68
Low school	20.0	14.5	
High school	44.0	49.1	
University degree	36.0	36.4	
Employment[b]			0.11
Employed	56.9	53.6	
Unemployed	42.2	39.3	
Student	1.0	7.1	
Marital status[b]			0.24
Single	17.8	29.5	
Married	81.2	70.5	
Separated/divorced	1.0	0.0	
BMI (Kg/m^2) prepregnancy[a]	26.0 ± 8.4	21.3 ± 7.4	0.001
Systolic blood pressure (mmHg)[a]	114 ± 14	121 ± 14	0.10
Diastolic blood pressure (mmHg)[a]	72 ± 14	77 ± 15	0.03
Hypertension[b]	7.4	8.3	0.91
Smoking[b]			0.10
No	74.3	72.7	
Yes	2.0	9.1	
Ex	23.7	18.2	
Family history of DM (1st degree)[b]	33.3	17.6	0.09

*Mann–Whitney U Test or Chi-square test.
[a]Data are presented as means ± SD.
[b]Data are presented as percent (%).

After adjusting for age and BMI, the significant association was still present between *C* carrier in *APOA5* and HDL-C ($\beta = -8.6$; $p = 0{,}01$); *T* carrier in *LDLR* and LDL-C ($\beta = -43.0$; $p = 0{,}001$); *A* carrier in *FTO* and LDL-C ($\beta = 32.4$; $p = 0.017$), respectively.

All the investigated genotype frequencies were within the Hardy–Weinberg equilibrium (χ^2 test p value > 0.05) both in cases and in controls, except for *TCF7L2* rs7903146 (*C*<*T*) and *FTO* rs9939609 (*T*>*A*) in cases.

4. Discussion

In the present work, we evaluated the association between GDM and genetic variants involved with nutrients and

Table 2: OGTT values of cases and controls.

OGTT[a]	GDM yes	GDM no
T0	91,89 ± 8,77	79,50 ± 7,26
T60	160,86 ± 32,31	121,70 ± 25,63
T120	146,57 ± 35,42	107,87 ± 19,81

[a]Data are presented as means ± SD.

metabolism. Results support a significant association between the *TCF7L2* rs7903146 variant and GDM, since the risk was more than fivefold in the *TT* genotype.

The *TCF7L2* gene, located on chromosome 10q25.3, is an important, ubiquitously expressed transcription factor in the Wnt signaling pathway, involved in the proliferation of pancreatic β-cells, and controlling the production of incretins such as glucagon intestinal peptide (GIP) and glucagon-like peptide 1 (GLP-1) in intestinal endocrine cells.

The presence of the *TCF7L2 T* allele has been associated with an increased risk of T2DM. In fact, Grant et al. [12] reported that several SNPs within intronic regions of *TCF7L2*, including the rs7903146 (*C*>*T*), show significant associations with T2DM, and these findings have been replicated by numerous groups, demonstrating the rs7903146 (*C*>*T*) SNP as one of the most important T2DM susceptibility variants. Dahlgren et al. [13] suggested that the increased risk of T2DM in T allele carriers is associated with dysfunction in the production of insulin within the beta cells and Lyssenko et al. [14] showed that the presence of the *T* allele results in overexpression of *TCF7L2* in the pancreatic β cell, with a reduced insulin secretion in turn increasing hepatic glucose production. In addition, several studies previously observed a strong association between this variant and GDM in different ethnic groups [15–22]. Thus, our results confirm the association between rs7903146 (*C*>*T*) and GDM, previously reported by the literature. In addition, our results demonstrated that this association is not mediated by the presence of variants within other genes involved in food metabolism, among those selected, since no one of the other genes investigated in our study was associated with GDM. Future study will need to investigate the possible role of other genes in this condition.

Nevertheless, our study evidenced also a significant correlation between common genetic variations in several genes (*PPARG2*, *APOA5*, *MC4R*, *LDLR*, and *FTO*) and lipid parameters within the GDM women group.

In this regard, it has been demonstrated that higher level of LDL-C and lower level of HDL-C, as a result of a combination of genetic factors and gene-diet interaction, are directly associated to the risk of CAD or metabolic syndrome. The genetic variations underlying the link between lipids parameters and cardiometabolic traits have been analyzed by various studies but remain unclear. *PPARG2* rs1801282 polymorphism has been associated with impaired insulin sensitivity and was called indeed "insulin resistance locus" [23].

As to the *APOA5*-1131*T*>*C* variant, interestingly an Italian study based on 1,864 patients <45 years old suggested that this polymorphism may affect the risk of early-onset MI, with an odds ratio of 1.44 (CI: 1.23–1.69) per *C* allele [24]. Gene variants in *MC4R* and *FTO* are associated with severe obesity and metabolic impairment in Caucasians [25]. In the DPS, in men with Impaired Glucose Tolerance the *AA* genotype of rs9939609 in *FTO* was associated with 2.09-fold risk of CVD in men [26].

Regarding our results about the significant correlation observed between *TT* genotype of *LDLR* rs2228671 polymorphismand 3rd trimester LDL-cholesterol levels, it is interesting to note that a recent meta-analysis has established rs2228671 as a protective factor of CHD in Europeans [27].

All these findings are of great relevance and the presence of these gene variants in our panel could increase the use of genetic information in clinical practice for GDM patients: several data support the potential cardiometabolic risk in later life in patients with previous GDM. In fact, Mai et al. [28] demonstrated that GDM increases risk of developing cardiovascular (CV) diseases. Previously, Carr et al. [29] have analysed, in a large population-based retrospective study, the long-term adverse CV outcomes in women with prior GDM. Gestational diabetes is associated with a clustering of cardiovascular risk factors, but the mechanism remains unclear. In this view, the authors have proposed the necessity of new markers to be used to study the effect of GDM on cardiovascular risk during follow-up [29, 30]. Sokup et al. [31] showed that the TG/HDL-C ratio, an early marker of endothelial dysfunction and CV risk, was higher in GDM women one year after the pregnancy, as compared to controls. In this context, of particular relevance is the association found in the present study between, respectively, *APOA5*-1131*T*>*C* and *MC4R* rs17782313 with 3rd trimester HDL-C in GDM women. This result evokes the study [30] which has shown that an index of early vascular disease (*mean common carotid* IMT-CCIMT) was higher in subjects without diabetes but with previous GDM (pGDM) than in control subjects. In this study when these variables were introduced in a multiple regression analysis, only oxidized LDL (oxLDL) remained significantly associated with CC-IMT. The increased carotid IMT, a marker of preclinical atherosclerosis [32], shows that young women with pGDM have an early sign of vessel involvement, although within the upper limit of normal. These alterations were present in spite of the fact that no woman had diabetes [30].

Furthermore, Corella et al. [33] demonstrated that the *APOA5*-1131*T*>*C* SNP modulates the effects of macronutrient intake (total fat, carbohydrate, and protein) on BMI and obesity risk in both men and women. In fact, the presence of at least one *C* allele implicated less weight on a high fat diet than the presence of homozygosity for the *T* allele. Future studies are needed to evaluate this aspect and to predict increased cardiovascular events risk and diabetes in the mother and offspring [34].

As is known the diagnosis of GDM identifies a population at high risk for T2DM [35] and metabolic syndrome [30, 36]. The early identification of subjects who could benefit from preventive strategies is a priority for public health. The diagnosis of GDM increasingly represents an exceptional chance to alter the natural course of disease: it is important to have reliable predictive tools. Recently Köhler et al. [37] proposed a novel approach to calculate the diabetes risk in women with prior GDM. In the final predictive risk score were included several variables, as insulin treatment during pregnancy, family history of diabetes, BMI in early pregnancy, lactation, and maternal age at delivery [37]. However, this study did not evaluate metabolic measurements or genetic markers.

GDM represents an important opportunity in the era of "Precision Medicine." Further studies are required to examine whether incorporation of our panel genes into an algorithm including genetic, clinic, and metabolic variables will help further improving the identification of women with GDM at early risk of diabetes and CHD; this would allow a better allocation of resources and the implementation of effective and sustainable strategies of primary prevention. In the last decades, the nutrition science is taking off in the prevention of noncommunicable chronic diseases that account for more than 60% of global deaths annually [38] and the future goal is the development of personalized genomic medicine. It is necessary understanding the roles of the nutrition and lifestyle matching with genetic and clinic factors in the manifestation of the diseases and its complications. Furthermore, this approach could lead to a reduction in costs of the treatment of nutrition/lifestyle-related chronic diseases [39]. These results are promising, but other functional studies are needed to confirm their biological significance.

The present study has some limitations. First, the pooled sample size for the SNPs was relatively small. Future genome-wide studies with larger sample size are still required to identify genes with smaller allele effects and possibly GDM specific risk variants: this to understand the role of these variants of genes involved with nutrients and metabolism, in the aetiology and progression of GDM. Second, our results show the role of lipids only in GDM because in control group they were unavailable: our study suggests that in the future these parameters should be considered at least during 3rd trimester of pregnancy.

Third, additional analyses, such as epigenetic studies, will also be required to elucidate the role of the molecular mechanisms to the disease susceptibility. In fact, as is known, the development of noncommunicable chronic diseases is determined not only by genetic variants but also by epigenetic changes as DNA methylation and histone modifications, in response to diet and environmental conditions. It has become clear that adverse epigenetic effects might also influence the foetus during pregnancy and postnatal early life increasing the susceptibility to chronic diseases such as obesity, T2DM, cardiovascular disease, or clinically relevant phenotypic traits.

Fourth, we recruited a larger sample of women with GDM compared to the control group. This limit is because the recruitment was conducted primarily at the Diabetes and Metabolism Unit.

Therefore, future studies are warranted for better understanding the GDM pathogenesis considering gene-gene and gene-environmental interactions.

Abbreviations

CVD: Cardiovascular diseases
CHD: Coronary heart disease
GDM: Gestational diabetes mellitus
GIP: Glucagon intestinal peptide
GLP: Glucagon-like peptide 1
IADPSG: International association of diabetes and pregnancy study groups
MODY: Maturity onset diabetes of the young
ORs: Odds ratios
OXLDL: Oxidized LDL
SNPs: Single nucleotide polymorphisms
T2DM: Type 2 diabetes mellitus
TG: Triglycerides.

Competing Interests

The authors declare that there is no conflict of interests associated with this manuscript.

Authors' Contributions

The study was designed by Liborio Stuppia and Ester Vitacolonna. Claudio Celentano and Marco Liberati contributed to clinical evaluation and support to the recruitment of patients. Marica Franzago and Federica Fraticelli contributed to data acquisition, analysis, and interpretation. The experiments were performed by Marica Franzago. The manuscript was drafted by Ester Vitacolonna and Marica Franzago. Antonio Nicolucci was the statistician for the case-control study, supervised the statistical analyses, and helped in the drafting and editing of the article. All authors were involved in critical revision and approved the final version of the manuscript before submission. Ester Vitacolonna and Liborio Stuppia are the guarantors of this work and, as such, had full access to all the data in the study and take responsibility for the integrity of the data and the accuracy of the data analysis.

References

[1] American Diabetes Association (ADA), "Standards of medical care in diabetes-2016," *Diabetes Care*, vol. 39, supplement 1, pp. S13–S22, 2016.

[2] H. Alptekin, A. Çizmecioğlu, H. Işık, T. Cengiz, M. Yildiz, and M. S. Iyisoy, "Predicting gestational diabetes mellitus during the first trimester using anthropometric measurements and HOMA-IR," *Journal of Endocrinological Investigation*, vol. 39, no. 5, pp. 577–583, 2016.

[3] E. Sobngwi, P. Boudou, F. Mauvais-Jarvis et al., "Effect of a diabetic environment in utero on predisposition to type 2 diabetes," *The Lancet*, vol. 361, no. 9372, pp. 1861–1865, 2003.

[4] M. M. Hedderson, E. P. Gunderson, and A. Ferrara, "Gestational weight gain and risk of gestational diabetes mellitus," *Obstetrics & Gynecology*, vol. 115, no. 3, pp. 597–604, 2010.

[5] S. Aslani, A. Hossein-Nezhad, K. Mirzaei, Z. Maghbooli, A. N. Afshar, and F. Karimi, "VDR FokI polymorphism and its potential role in the pathogenesis of gestational diabetes mellitus and its complications," *Gynecological Endocrinology*, vol. 27, no. 12, pp. 1055–1060, 2011.

[6] C. Zhang, W. Bao, Y. Rong et al., "Genetic variants and the risk

of gestational diabetes mellitus: a systematic review," *Human Reproduction Update*, vol. 19, no. 4, pp. 376–390, 2013.

[7] K. Bajaj and S. J. Gross, "The genetics of diabetic pregnancy," *Best Practice & Research: Clinical Obstetrics & Gynaecology*, vol. 29, no. 1, article 1417, pp. 102–109, 2015.

[8] M. Lehto, T. Tuomi, M. M. Mahtani et al., "Characterization of the MODY3 phenotype. Early-onset diabetes caused by an insulin secretion defect," *The Journal of Clinical Investigation*, vol. 99, no. 4, pp. 582–591, 1997.

[9] S. Ellard, F. Beards, L. I. S. Allen et al., "A high prevalence of glucokinase mutations in gestational diabetic subjects selected by clinical criteria," *Diabetologia*, vol. 43, no. 2, pp. 250–253, 2000.

[10] K. L. Thomson, A. L. Gloyn, K. Colclough et al., "Identification of 21 novel glucokinase (GCK) mutations in UK and European Caucasians with maturity-onset diabetes of the young (MODY)," *Human Mutation*, vol. 22, no. 5, article 417, 2003.

[11] International Association of Diabetes and Pregnancy Study Groups Consensus Panel, B. E. Metzger, S. G. Gabbe et al., "International association of diabetes and pregnancy study groups recommendations on the diagnosis and classification of hyperglycemia in pregnancy," *Diabetes Care*, vol. 33, no. 3, pp. 676–682, 2010.

[12] S. F. A. Grant, G. Thorleifsson, I. Reynisdottir et al., "Variant of transcription factor 7-like 2 (TCF7L2) gene confers risk of type 2 diabetes," *Nature Genetics*, vol. 38, no. 3, pp. 320–323, 2006.

[13] A. Dahlgren, B. Zethelius, K. Jensevik, A.-C. Syvänen, and C. Berne, "Variants of the TCF7L2 gene are associated with beta cell dysfunction and confer an increased risk of type 2 diabetes mellitus in the ULSAM cohort of Swedish elderly men," *Diabetologia*, vol. 50, no. 9, pp. 1852–1857, 2007.

[14] V. Lyssenko, R. Lupi, P. Marchetti et al., "Mechanisms by which common variants in the TCF7L2 gene increase risk of type 2 diabetes," *Journal of Clinical Investigation*, vol. 117, no. 8, pp. 2155–2163, 2007.

[15] N. Shaat, Å. Lernmark, E. Karlsson et al., "A variant in the transcription factor 7 like 2 (TCF7L2) gene is associated with an increased risk of gestational diabetes mellitus," *Diabetologia*, vol. 50, no. 5, pp. 972–979, 2007.

[16] Y. M. Cho, T. H. Kim, S. Lim et al., "Type 2 diabetes-associated genetic variants discovered in the recent genome-wide association studies are related to gestational diabetes mellitus in the Korean population," *Diabetologia*, vol. 52, no. 2, pp. 253–261, 2009.

[17] J. Lauenborg, N. Grarup, P. Damm et al., "Common type 2 diabetes risk gene variants associate with gestational diabetes," *The Journal of Clinical Endocrinology & Metabolism*, vol. 94, no. 1, pp. 145–150, 2009.

[18] R. M. Freathy, M. G. Hayes, M. Urbanek et al., "Hyperglycemia and Adverse Pregnancy Outcome (HAPO) study: common genetic variants in GCK and TCF7L2 are associated with fasting and postchallenge glucose levels in pregnancy and with the new consensus definition of gestational diabetes mellitus from the International Association of Diabetes and Pregnancy Study Groups," *Diabetes*, vol. 59, no. 10, pp. 2682–2689, 2010.

[19] K. I. Pappa, M. Gazouli, K. Economou et al., "Gestational diabetes mellitus shares polymorphisms of genes associated with insulin resistance and type 2 diabetes in the Greek population," *Gynecological Endocrinology*, vol. 27, no. 4, pp. 267–272, 2011.

[20] A. Papadopoulou, K. F. Lynch, N. Shaat et al., "Gestational diabetes mellitus is associated with TCF7L2 gene polymorphisms independent of HLA-DQB1*0602 genotypes and islet cell autoantibodies," *Diabetic Medicine*, vol. 28, no. 9, pp. 1018–1027, 2011.

[21] S. H. Kwak, S.-H. Kim, Y. M. Cho et al., "A genome-wide association study of gestational diabetes mellitus in Korean women," *Diabetes*, vol. 61, no. 2, pp. 531–541, 2012.

[22] J. Vcelak, D. Vejrazkova, M. Vankova et al., "T2D risk haplotypes of the TCF7L2 gene in the Czech population sample: the association with FFAs composition," *Physiological Research*, vol. 61, no. 2, pp. 229–240, 2012.

[23] M. Trombetta, S. Bonetti, M. L. Boselli et al., "PPARG2 Pro12Ala and ADAMTS9 rs4607103 as 'insulin resistance loci' and 'insulin secretion loci' in Italian individuals. the GENFIEV study and the Verona Newly Diagnosed Type 2 Diabetes Study (VNDS) 4," *Acta Diabetologica*, vol. 50, no. 3, pp. 401–408, 2013.

[24] R. De Caterina, P. J. Talmud, P. A. Merlini et al., "Strong association of the APOA5-1131T>C gene variant and early-onset acute myocardial infarction," *Atherosclerosis*, vol. 214, no. 2, pp. 397–403, 2011.

[25] R. Liguori, G. Labruna, A. Alfieri et al., "The FTO gene polymorphism (rs9939609) is associated with metabolic syndrome in morbidly obese subjects from southern Italy," *Molecular and Cellular Probes*, vol. 28, no. 4, pp. 195–199, 2014.

[26] T. Lappalainen, M. Kolehmainen, U. S. Schwab et al., "Association of the FTO gene variant (rs9939609) with cardiovascular disease in men with abnormal glucose metabolism—the Finnish Diabetes Prevention Study," *Nutrition, Metabolism and Cardiovascular Diseases*, vol. 21, no. 9, pp. 691–698, 2011.

[27] H. Ye, Q. Zhao, Y. Huang et al., "Meta-analysis of low density lipoprotein receptor (*LDLR*) rs2228671 polymorphism and coronary heart disease," *BioMed Research International*, vol. 2014, Article ID 564940, 6 pages, 2014.

[28] C. Mai, M. Hou, R. Chen et al., "Cardiovascular risk factors in Chinese women with a history of gestational diabetes mellitus," *International Journal of Clinical and Experimental Medicine*, vol. 8, no. 11, pp. 21694–21698, 2015.

[29] D. B. Carr, K. M. Utzschneider, R. L. Hull et al., "Gestational diabetes mellitus increases the risk of cardiovascular disease in women with a family history of type 2 diabetes," *Diabetes Care*, vol. 29, no. 9, pp. 2078–2083, 2006.

[30] L. Volpe, I. Cuccuru, C. Lencioni et al., "Early subclinical atherosclerosis in women with previous gestational diabetes mellitus," *Diabetes Care*, vol. 31, no. 5, p. e32, 2008.

[31] A. Sokup, B. Ruszkowska, B. Góralczyk et al., "Elevation of sE-selectin levels 2-24 months following gestational diabetes is associated with early cardiometabolic risk in nondiabetic women," *International Journal of Endocrinology*, vol. 2012, Article ID 278050, 6 pages, 2012.

[32] L. Bokemark, J. Wikstrand, S. Attvall, J. Hulthe, H. Wedel, and B. Fagerberg, "Insulin resistance and intima-media thickness in the carotid and femoral arteries of clinically healthy 58-year-old men. The Atherosclerosis and Insulin Resistance Study (AIR)," *Journal of Internal Medicine*, vol. 249, no. 1, pp. 59–67, 2001.

[33] D. Corella, C.-Q. Lai, S. Demissie et al., "APOA5 gene variation modulates the effects of dietary fat intake on body mass index and obesity risk in the Framingham Heart Study," *Journal of Molecular Medicine*, vol. 85, no. 2, pp. 119–128, 2007.

[34] J. Harreiter, G. Dovjak, and A. Kautzky-Willer, "Gestational diabetes mellitus and cardiovascular risk after pregnancy," *Women's Health*, vol. 10, no. 1, pp. 91–108, 2014.

[35] L. Bellamy, J.-P. Casas, A. D. Hingorani, and D. Williams, "Type 2 diabetes mellitus after gestational diabetes: a systematic review and meta-analysis," *The Lancet*, vol. 373, no. 9677, pp. 1773–1779, 2009.

[36] J. L. Kitzmiller, L. Dang-Kilduff, and M. M. Taslimi, "Gestational diabetes after delivery: short-term management and long-term risks," *Diabetes Care*, vol. 30, no. 2, pp. S225–S235, 2007.

[37] M. Köhler, A. G. Ziegler, and A. Beyerlein, "Development of a simple tool to predict the risk of postpartum diabetes in women with gestational diabetes mellitus," *Acta Diabetologica*, vol. 53, no. 3, pp. 433–437, 2016.

[38] World Health Organization, *Global Action Plan for the Prevention and Control of Non Communicable Diseases 2013–2020*, World Health Organization, Geneva, Switzerland, 2012.

[39] B. Maire, S. Lioret, A. Gartner, and F. Delpeuch, "Nutritional transition and non-communicable diet-related chronic diseases in developing countries," *Sante*, vol. 12, no. 1, pp. 45–55, 2002.

5

Osteocalcin Serum Levels in Gestational Diabetes Mellitus and Their Intrinsic and Extrinsic Determinants

Raigam J. Martinez-Portilla,[1,2] Jose R. Villafan-Bernal,[3,4,5] Diana L. Lip-Sosa,[1] Eva Meler,[1] Jordi Clotet,[1] Francisco J. Serna-Vela,[5] Sergio Velazquez-Garcia,[6] Leopoldo C. Serrano-Diaz,[7] and Francesc Figueras[1,8]

[1]*Fetal i+D Fetal Medicine Research Center, BCNatal-Barcelona Center for Maternal-Fetal and Neonatal Medicine (Hospital Clínic and Hospital Sant Joan de Déu), IDIBAPS, University of Barcelona, Spain*
[2]*Maternal-Fetal Medicine and Therapy Research Center Mexico in behalf of the Iberoamerican Research Network in Translational, Molecular and Maternal-Fetal Medicine, Mexico*
[3]*Mexican Consortium of Biomedicine, Biotechnology and Health Dissemination-Consortium BIO2-DIS, Mexico*
[4]*CONACYT Researcher at the Department of Surgery, Health Science Center, Autonomous University of Aguascalientes, Mexico*
[5]*Center for Health Sciences, Autonomous University of Aguascalientes, Mexico*
[6]*CIMeTA Research Unit-ISSEA, Mexico*
[7]*Women's Hospital of the State of Aguascalientes-ISSEA, Mexico*
[8]*Center for Biomedical Research on Rare Diseases (CIBER-ER), Madrid, Spain*

Correspondence should be addressed to Francesc Figueras; ffiguera@clinic.ub.es

Academic Editor: Michaelangela Barbieri

Background. Undercarboxylated osteocalcin (ucOC) increases insulin release and insulin resistance in mice. In humans, evidence is scarce but a correlation of ucOC and total osteocalcin (tOC) with glycemic status markers has been demonstrated. The relationship of ucOC and tOC with gestational diabetes mellitus (GDM) has been even less characterized. *Objective.* To assess the mean difference of tOC and ucOC serum concentrations among nondiabetic pregnant women and women diagnosed as GDM in the second trimester of pregnancy and to determine the possible intrinsic and extrinsic contributors to this difference. *Methods.* A systematic search was performed to identify relevant studies published in English and Spanish using PubMed, SCOPUS, ISI Web of Knowledge, and PROSPERO database for meta-analysis. Observational studies measuring mean serum levels of osteocalcin among GDM, with at least 10 subjects analyzed in each group were selected. Mean difference (MD) by random effects model was used. Heterogeneity between studies was assessed using Cochran's Q, H, and I^2 statistics. *Results.* From 38 selected studies, 5 were retained for analysis for a total of 1119 pregnant women. Serum concentrations of tOC were not significantly different among women with GDM and nondiabetic pregnant controls (MD: 1.56; 95% CI: −0.70 to 3.82; $p = 0.175$). Meanwhile, ucOC serum levels were significantly higher among women with GDM (MD: 1.17; 95% CI: 0.24 to 2.11; $p = 0.013$). The only factor influencing tOC was the UV index, showing a reduction in mean difference between GDM and controls when exposed to higher concentrations of UV rays. *Conclusions.* This meta-analysis provides evidence to support the use of ucOC as a potential marker for GDM rather than tOC, yielding very little variability among studies and no difference among methods or brands used for its analysis.

1. Introduction

Gestational diabetes mellitus (GDM) is defined as any glucose impairment with first onset or recognition during pregnancy [1]. With a prevalence within 2 to 6%, which is increasing worldwide, this condition represents a leading cause of adverse perinatal outcomes [2], with delayed effects both for women and children [3, 4]. Diagnosis of GDM usually happens in an advanced gestational age, limiting preventive strategies. Development of prediction models for GDM is a challenge to contemporary fetal-maternal medicine.

Osteocalcin (OC) is a bone-derived protein that takes part in bone metabolism [5]. About 10% to 30% of osteocalcin is released into the main circulation, which is later cleared by the liver and kidney [6–8]. The three primary forms of OC are carboxylated (cOC), undercarboxylated (ucOC), and total osteocalcin (tOC) [9]; these three biochemical markers can be separately measured in blood by different methods such as RIA (radioimmunoassay), IRMA (immunoradiometric assay), ELISA (enzyme-linked immunoassay), or electrochemiluminescence immunoassay (ECLIA).

From a clinical point of view, tOC and ucOC serum levels are lower among patients with type 1 and type 2 diabetes [10–27], while only a few studies have assessed the mean concentration of cOC suggesting increased levels in individuals with type 2 diabetes [26]. Some studies have shown that ucOC increases insulin secretion and proliferation of pancreatic beta-cells. It also increases adiponectin secretion from adipose tissue, reducing fat mass and increasing energy expenditure by increasing the expression of genes involved in beta-oxidation [28]. Nonetheless, gestational diabetes mellitus (GDM) is a different entity defined as glucose intolerance resulting in hyperglycemia of variable severity with onset or first recognition during pregnancy [1]. Maternal physiological changes during pregnancy lead to a decrease in fasting glucose at early pregnancy and continuously during gestation, together with a marked decline in insulin sensitivity during second and third trimester [29, 30]. One study performed in pregnant women demonstrated that tOC serum levels are higher during the first trimester of pregnancy in women subsequently developing GDM when compared to controls [31]. However, studies measuring tOC and ucOC during second trimester in nonprevious diabetic women have yielded controversial results [32, 33].

Defining the changes in serum levels of proteins or hormones related to insulin resistance or glucose tolerance such as tOC and ucOC among women developing GDM is vital for adequate future prediction models aimed to determine which women are at risk for developing this disease [34]. Indeed, a model combining maternal characteristics plus insulin-resistance-related proteins could lead to effective predictive algorithms for GDM [35].

The aim of this systematic review and meta-analysis is to quantify the changes of tOC and ucOC serum concentrations in women diagnosed with GDM in the second trimester of pregnancy and to determine the possible intrinsic and extrinsic determinants of these changes.

2. Methods

2.1. Protocol Registration. Before data extraction, the project was registered in the PROSPERO international prospective register of systematic reviews (registration number: CRD42018091727).

2.2. Eligibility Criteria, Information Sources, and Search Strategy. A systematic search was performed using PubMed, EBSCO, ISI Web of Science, and PROSPERO database for meta-analysis to identify relevant studies published in English or Spanish, without publication time restrictions. Institutional review board approval is not required for systematic reviews in our institution. References of relevant publications were manually searched for additional potentially relevant studies. The first search was run on May 20, 2017. Afterward, an update was extended until March 23, 2018.

This review was carried out adhering to the Meta-analysis of Observational Studies in Epidemiology (MOOSE) guidelines [36] and the Preferred Reporting Items for Systematic Reviews and Meta-Analyses (PRISMA) guidelines for systematic reviews and meta-analysis [37, 38]. Two independent evaluators (R.M. and R.V.) assessed abstracts identified as relevant, both blinded to authorship, authors' institutional affiliation, and study results. If the abstract fulfilled inclusion criteria, full-text articles were then reviewed. A third investigator (F.F.) independently settled any disagreement between evaluators. In case of relevant studies with missing information, corresponding authors were reached by e-mail to request such data. Annex 1 of supplemental material details the search strategy and query syntaxes.

2.3. Study Selection. The inclusion criteria for this systematic review were observational studies (prospective or retrospective) on women diagnosed with GDM between 24 and 28 weeks of gestation and their respective nondiabetic pregnant controls, with at least ten women in each group and reporting serum levels of OC.

2.4. Data Extraction. The following information was extracted on a datasheet based on Cochrane Consumers and Communication Review Group's data extraction template [39]: author, year of publication, country where the study was conducted, study period, type of study, original inclusion and exclusion criteria, total number of patients included in the study, number of participants with GDM, number of nondiabetic pregnant women, osteocalcin quantification method, form of osteocalcin determined, mean maternal age at analysis, mean maternal body mass index (BMI), mean gestational age at measurement of OC, method of quantification, brand of the kit used for the measurement, and mean UV index as a surrogate of sun exposure.

2.5. Assessment of Risk of Bias. Two reviewers (R.M. and D.L.) independently assessed the quality of the selected studies. Quality assessment of observational studies was carried out using the Newcastle-Ottawa scale for case-control studies and cohort studies. Each study was judged on three dimensions: the selection of the study groups, the comparability of the groups, and the ascertainment of the exposure. One star was given for each signaling question among each dimension. For a total of 9 possible stars, studies with 7 or more stars were considered as high quality [40].

2.6. Data Analysis. Extracted results were pooled in the meta-analysis. Data analysis was performed as recommended by the Cochrane handbook in the following manner: tOC and ucOC within the comparison of GDM and nondiabetic pregnant controls. The effect size was expressed as mean difference (MD) by random effects models (REM) weighting by the inverse of the variance since all studies used randomly sampled [41].

Results are presented using forest plots including the MDs for the main groups (cases and controls). For subgroup analysis, a mixed effects model (MEM) was employed [42].

Between-study variability was assessed using the τ^2 and Cochran's Q and I^2 statistics [43]. The contribution of individual-study heterogeneity was visually assessed by Baujat plots [44].

Multiple metaregressions were performed to add another approach for unexplained heterogeneity and to determine which variables influenced tOC and ucOC serum levels. When enough information was available, we used the following covariates: mean gestational age at inclusion; mean maternal age; body mass index; mean weight gain at inclusion; mean serum levels of triglycerides; mean serum levels of fasting glucose; mean serum levels of fasting insulin; mean latitude; mean altitude; and UV where the study was conducted. The UV index was classified as follows: 1–2 low, 3–5 moderate, 6–7 high, 8–10 very high, and ≥11 extremely high. I^2 and R^2 values were reported to present residual heterogeneity and the amount of heterogeneity explained by each variable, respectively.

Publication bias was visually assessed by contour-enhanced funnel plots and quantified by Egger method. Also, in order to assess "small-study effect" defined as the chance of finding a trend towards a larger effect due to the higher probability of a small study of being published when a more "significant" result is found, a cumulative analysis was performed and presented as a forest plot [45, 46]. A sensitivity analysis was performed to assess the pooled estimates according to study quality. Statistical analysis was conducted using R studio v1.0.136 (The R Foundation for Statistical Computing) [package "meta v4.2"] [47].

3. Results

3.1. Study Selection and Study Characteristics. A total of 38 studies were identified by database searching, with one additional study included manually. Of them, eight studies were eligible for full-text review. After review, five studies [32, 33, 48–50] were retained for the systematic review and meta-analysis. Figure 1 depicts the review flow diagram.

Reasons for excluding three full-text studies were as follows: one of them used the same cohort of another included study in our analysis [51], while the second one performed the diagnostic tests for GDM from 24 to 32 weeks of gestation [52]. The last excluded study was due to inclusion of women with a diagnosis of diabetes before pregnancy [53]. The following authors were reached by mail and they provided aggregated data on their published studies: Tabatabaei et al. [49], Saucedo et al. [33], and Srichomkwun et al. [50]. Annex 2 in the supplemental material details the shared information. Also, the characteristics of the included articles are described in Table 1.

We used the Newcastle-Ottawa scale for study-quality assessment in observational studies. From a total of 9 possible rating points, three studies [32, 48, 50] presented 6 points mainly due to lack of representativeness of the cases, lack of nonresponse rate description, or no description for control selection. Two studies [33, 49] had 7 points or more due to the representativeness of the cases, study controls for each additional outcome, or lack of nonresponse rate description. Tables 2 and 3 show the full Newcastle-Ottawa scale assessment. From the five included studies [32, 33, 48–50], a total of 1119 pregnant women underwent assessment for OC serum concentrations; from these, 23% (259/1119) were diagnosed as GDM. The mean reported maternal age among studies was 30.5 (SD 2.3) years. Also, the mean BMI was 27.3 (SD 3) kg/m^2 with a weight gain of 11.7 (SD 3.7) kg. Mean gestational age at diagnosis of GDM was 26.6 (SD 1.5) weeks; this was also the gestational age at enrollment and measurement of OC.

3.2. Total Osteocalcin among Gestational Diabetes Mellitus. Three studies [32, 33, 50] had information regarding tOC concentrations among GDM. There was no statistically significant mean difference between women with GDM and nondiabetic pregnant controls (2.28; 95% CI: −0.43 to 5.00; $p = 0.099$). A Q value of 4.42 with 2 degrees of freedom and $p < 0.01$ provides evidence that the effect size varies across studies. I^2 indicates that 88% of the variation can be attributed to true effect rather than random error (Figure 2).

Baujat plot showed that the study from Hossein-nezhad et al. [32] contributed the most to the overall heterogeneity and influenced the most to the overall results (Figure 3).

Contour-enhanced funnel plot showed no significant publication bias (Figure 4), also quantified by Egger method (estimate: −0.670; $p = 0.119$).

According to the cumulative analysis, there was no trend towards more significant results in smaller studies, reducing the probability of publication bias (Figure 5).

3.3. Subgroup Analysis for tOC. Formal assessment of heterogeneity could not be performed by subgroup analysis since all studies differed among solar exposition, brand, and method for OC measurement.

3.4. Metaregressions for tOC. Several covariates were used to assess their influence on the mean serum concentrations of OC. Mean UV index was the only variable significantly influencing serum levels of OC; the higher the UV index, the lower the mean difference of tOC between women with GDM and pregnant controls (estimate: −0.812; 95% CI: −1.22 to −0.39; $p < 0.001$). The effect of UV index accounted for 100% of the heterogeneity in this sample ($R^2 = 1.0$), leaving no residual heterogeneity ($I^2 = 0\%$). Figure 6 shows the metaregression for mean UV index.

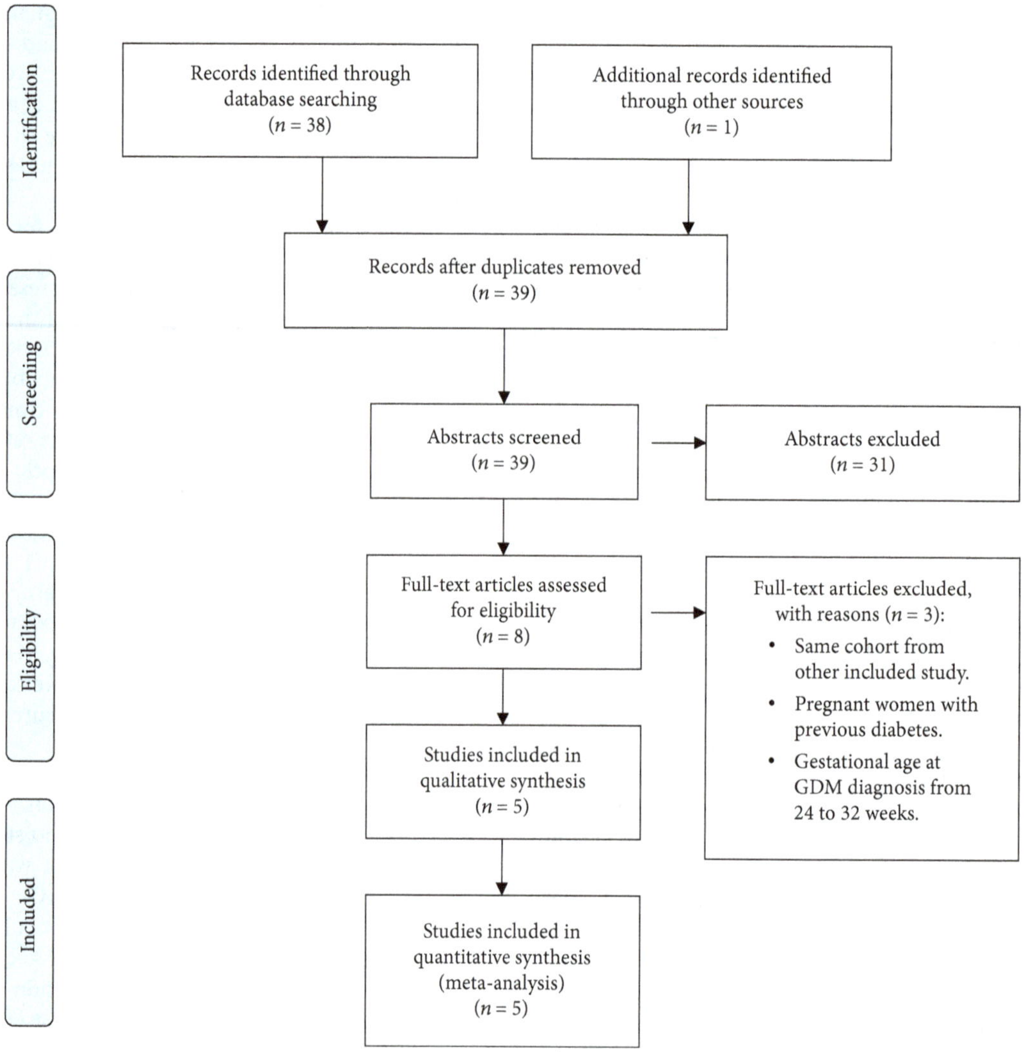

FIGURE 1: PRISMA flow diagram of included studies.

3.5. Undercarboxylated Osteocalcin among Gestational Diabetes Mellitus. Four studies [33, 48–50] had information regarding ucOC concentrations among GDM. Mean serum levels of ucOC were significantly higher in women with GDM when compared to nondiabetic pregnant women (1.17; 95% CI: 0.24 to 2.11; $p = 0.013$). Q value of 2.64 with 3 degrees of freedom and $p = 0.45$ provides evidence that the true-effect size does not significantly vary across studies. I^2 also depicts this true-effect variability to be 0% (Figure 7).

Prediction interval from −0.88 to 3.22 shows the probability of a future ucOC measurements to lie within this range. Baujat plot showed that the study from Winhofer et al. [48] contributed the most to the overall heterogeneity among studies, while the study from Srichomkwu et al. [50] influenced the most to the overall results (Figure 8).

Contour-enhanced funnel plot showed no significant publication bias (Figure 9), also quantified by Egger method (estimate: −0.670; $p = 0.119$).

According to the cumulative analysis, there was a trend towards more significant results in smaller studies, increasing the probability of publication bias (Figure 10).

3.6. Subgroup Analysis for ucOC. Formal assessment of heterogeneity showed that the use of ELISA as the method for ucOC analysis depicted similar results between studies. No added variability was found in this subgroup ($I^2 = 0\%$). Figure 11 shows the forest plot for method analysis. Also, no covariate significantly influenced the pooled mean difference for ucOC.

4. Discussion

4.1. Main Findings. There are some crucial points elucidated by the present study. (1) There is no significant difference in tOC concentrations among women with GDM and nondiabetic pregnant controls during the second trimester (at time of GDM screening). (2) Serum concentrations of ucOC are significantly higher in women with GDM when compared to nondiabetic controls. (3) The only extrinsic factor influencing the serum concentrations of tOC is the UV index, showing an inverse correlation between the mean difference in tOC and the level of exposition to UV rays. (4) There was no intrinsic factor such as maternal age, BMI, fasting

Table 1: Characteristics of included studies.

Study	Year	Country	Type of study	Inclusion criteria	Exclusion criteria	Diagnostic criteria for GDM	Type of osteocalcin	Analysis method	Study participants	Number of nondiabetic women	Number of diabetic women
Winhofer	2010	Iran	Case control	Healthy pregnant women, who were referred from the department of obstetrics and gynecology to the outpatient clinic for routine glucose tolerance testing between the 24th and 28th gestational weeks	History of GDM or obstetric complications in a previous pregnancy, any history of impaired glucose tolerance, or signs of fetal macrosomia. Previous OGTT during pregnancy	One-step: 75 g of glucose (5.5, 10.0, and 7.8 mmol/l cutoff at 0, 1, and 2 h)	ucOC	ELISA for tOC	78	52	26
Hossein-nezhad	2010	Iran	Case control	Pregnant women without previous history of diabetes mellitus who referred to the clinics for prenatal care during the first half of the pregnancy	None	Two-step: 50 g if >7.2 mmol/L, 100 g	tOC	ELISA	695	644	51
Tabatabaei	2014	Canada	Cohort	Healthy pregnant Caucasian women and women with GDM having singleton and term pregnancies with gestation duration of 37 to 42 weeks. With high risk of GDM (obesity and previous history of GDM)	History or new diagnosis of corticosteroid-treated asthma, liver disease, renal disease, Crohn's disease, ulcerative colitis, celiac disease, medication known to affect bone metabolism, and history of type 1 diabetes or type 2 diabetes	Two-step: 50 g if >7.2 mmol/L, 100 g	ucOC	ELISA	96	48	48
Saucedo	2015	Mexico	Case control	Nongestational diabetic women and gestational diabetic women screened at 24–28 weeks	History of arterial hypertension, renal disease, liver disease, thyroid disorders, and other endocrine or chronic diseases	Two-step: 50 g if >7.2 mmol/L, 100 g	tOC & ucOC	IRA for tOC & ELISA for ucOC	120	60	60
Srichomkwun	2015	Thailand	Case control	Pregnant women without risk of gestational diabetes mellitus	History of DM before pregnancy, twin or multiple pregnancy, or significant medical problem, such as cardiovascular, liver, or renal disease	Two-step: 50 g if >7.2 mmol/L, 100 g (cutoff Carpenter Coustan 5.3, 10.0, 9.2, and 8.1 mmol/L at 0, 1, 2, and 3 h	tOC & ucOC	ELISA	130	56	74

tOC: total osteocalcin; ucOC: undercarboxylated osteocalcin; ELISA: electrochemiluminescence immunoassay; IRA: immunoradiometric assay; GDM: gestational diabetes mellitus.

Table 2: Newcastle-Ottawa scale for case-control studies.

Study		Selection				Comparability		Exposure		
Author	Year	Is the case definition adequate?	Representativeness of the cases	Selection of controls	Definition of controls	Study controls for main outcome	Study controls for additional outcomes	Ascertainment of exposure	Same method of ascertainment for cases and controls	Nonresponse rate	Stars
Winhofer	2010	*		*	*	*		*	*		6
Saucedo	2015	*		*	*	*		*	*	*	7
Tabatabaei	2014	*	*	*	*	*		*	*		7
Srichomkwun	2015	*	*			*		*	*	*	6

Table 3: Newcastle-Ottawa scale for cohort studies.

Study		Selection				Comparability		Exposure			
Author	Year	Representativeness of the exposed cohort	Selection of the nonexposed cohort	Ascertainment of exposure	Demonstration that outcome of interest was not present at start of study	Study controls for main outcome	Study controls for additional outcomes	Ascertainment of outcome	Was follow-up enough for outcomes to occur	Adequacy of follow-up cohorts	Stars
Hossein-nezhad	2010	*	*	*	*	*		*			6

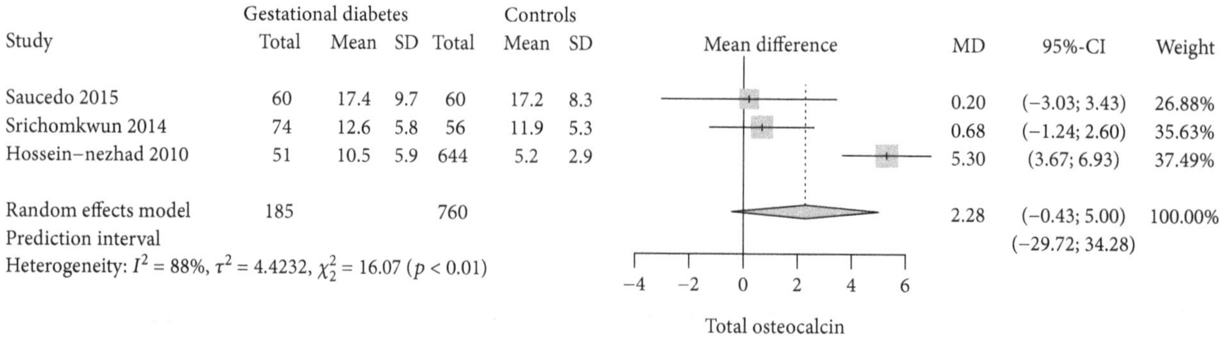

FIGURE 2: Forest plot on the mean difference of tOC among GDM and nondiabetic pregnant controls.

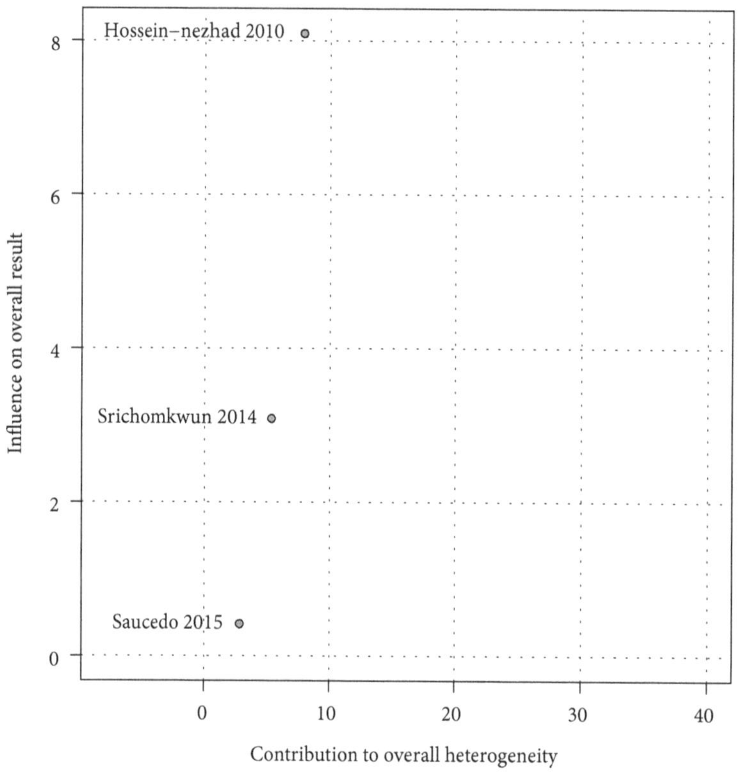

FIGURE 3: Baujat plot for the mean difference and contribution to heterogeneity among studies measuring tOC.

insulin, fasting glucose, triglycerides, or gain weight during pregnancy, significantly influencing the mean difference of ucOC or tOC. Finally, (5) ELISA as a method for measuring ucOC was the only one comparable among studies, showing no heterogeneity and yielding similar results.

The molecular mechanisms underlying OC differences among pregnant and nonpregnant women have not been yet described. One of the reasons why OC may be higher among women with GDM is the fact that placental-induced insulin resistance reaches its peak between 24 and 28 weeks of gestation. This insulin resistance leads to an increase in insulin secretion by pancreatic B-cells as a compensatory mechanism that derives in an increased anabolic feature on bone metabolism via IGF-1, therefore, influencing OC concentrations especially during the second trimester of pregnancy as described by Winhofer et al. [48].

Similar to our results, the study of Telejko et al. [52] showed no significant difference in tOC levels among women with and without GDM. This study was excluded due to the inclusion of women after 28 weeks of gestation as defined previously. The study conducted by Martinez et al. [53] showed an increase of tOC concentrations among women with diabetes, which was also discarded from our meta-analysis due to the inclusion of prediabetic patients.

4.2. Clinical Implications. Because GDM is usually diagnosed late in pregnancy, early preventive strategies are precluded. Indeed, there is good evidence that timely diagnosis and treatment of GDM by dietary advice, blood glucose monitoring, and insulin therapy when needed significantly reduce perinatal complications such as preeclampsia or macrosomia [54, 55]. Furthermore, there is mounting evidence that

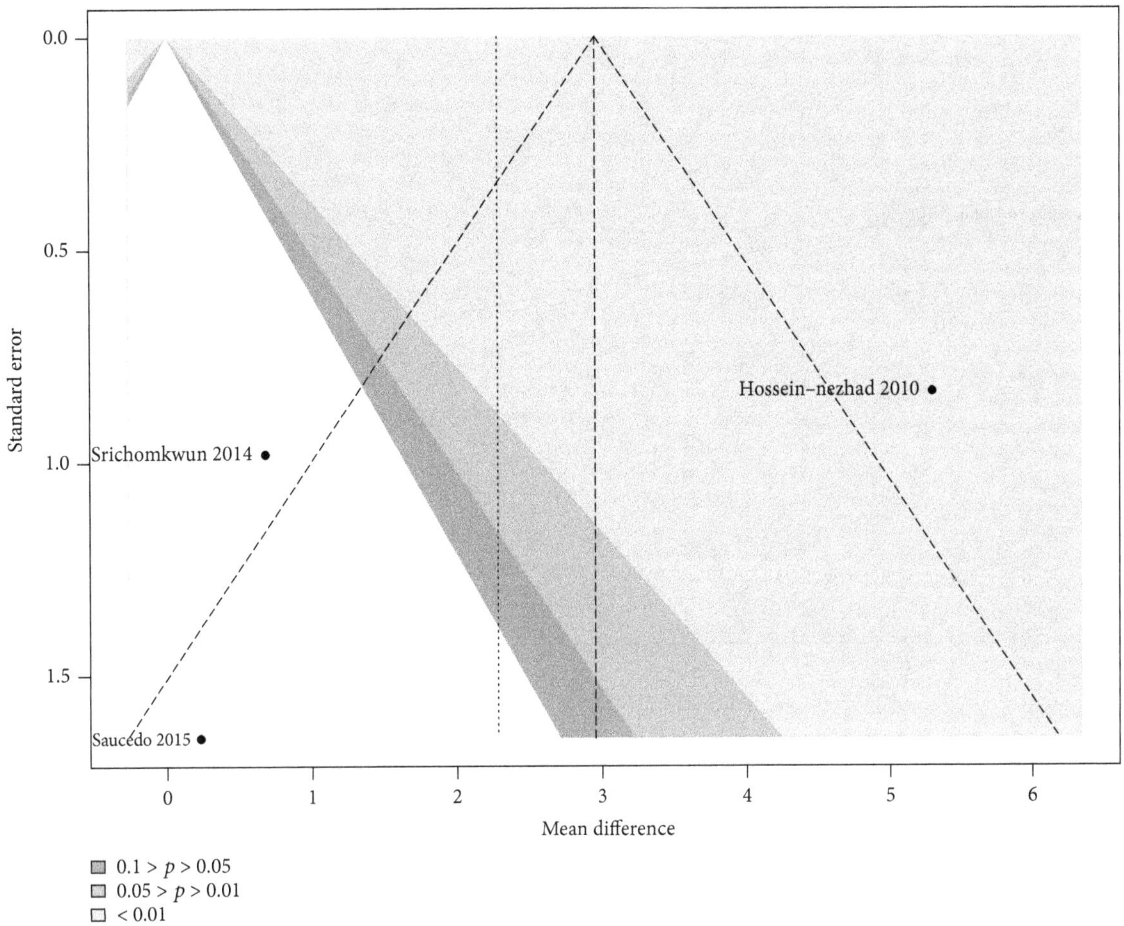

Figure 4: Funnel plot for publication bias assessment among studies measuring tOC.

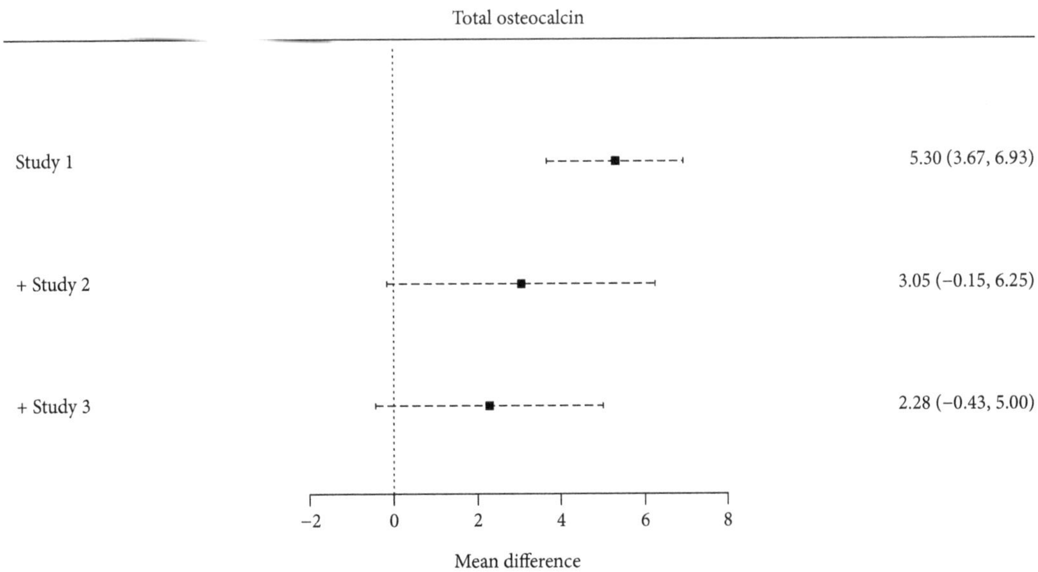

Figure 5: Cumulative forest plot among studies measuring tOC.

lifestyle interventions early in pregnancy in high-risk women reduce the risk of developing GDM and its associated complications [56, 57]. Thus, developing predictive models for GDM is a challenge in contemporary fetal-maternal medicine. However, the models described so far have limited predictive capacity. At least five predictive models are aiming

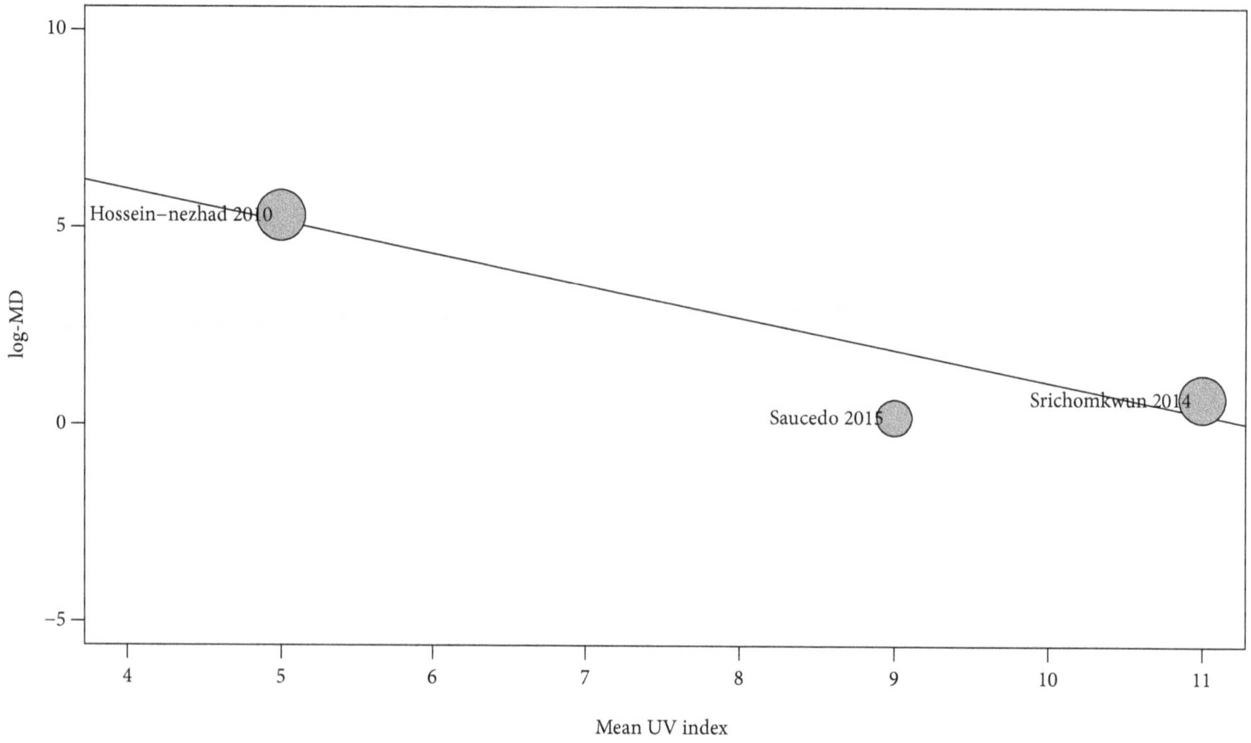

Figure 6: Metaregression on the pooled mean difference for tOC and the mean UV index.

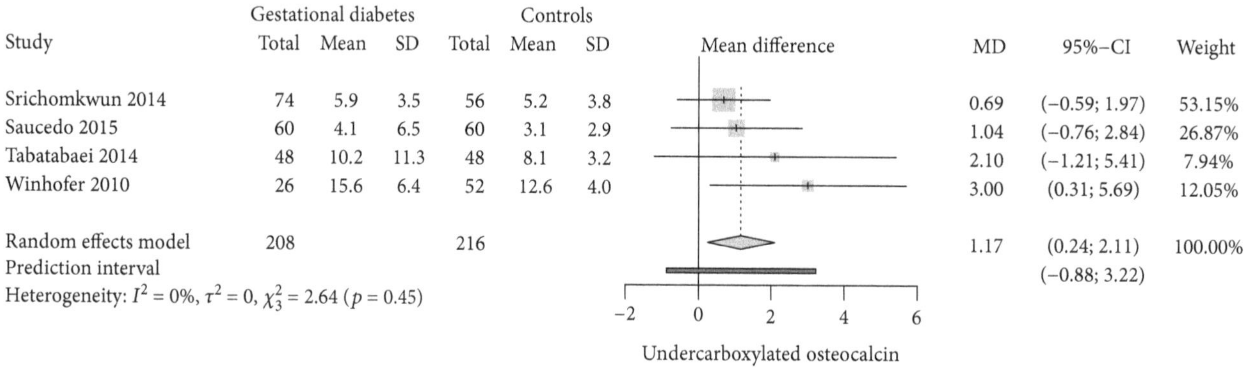

Figure 7: Forest plot on the mean difference of ucOC among GDM and nondiabetic pregnant controls.

to assess the predictive performance for GDM during the first trimester based on maternal characteristics, but none of them have found more than 55% prediction based on these variables. Also, their described AUC ranged from 0.703 to 0.832 [58–62], showing modest overall results. Our study suggests that OC levels may have the potential to improve current predictive strategies based on previous maternal characteristic models.

4.3. Strengths and Limitations. There are two main strengths of our study: firstly, we conducted a rigorous systematic review by independent reviewers and a third one for evaluation, assessment of bias, and database searching was also done by independent investigators all blinded to authorship and hospital where the study was conducted, allowing us to minimize bias when selecting publications for inclusion. Finally, an exhaustive analysis for assessment of intrinsic and extrinsic factors was performed to determine the influence that each one had on the mean difference between GDM and controls.

The main limitation of this study is the small number of publications found in the literature. This limitation is not due to the search strategy but to the real limited number of published papers aiming to measure OC in GDM. Also, there are other causes that may influence OC concentration among women with gestational diabetes such as thyroid diseases or smoking status, but due to the limited information of all possible causes described in each study, it was implausible for us to analyze other causes on individual basis.

4.4. Osteocalcin as a Predictive Protein for Gestational Diabetes Mellitus. As mentioned before, OC is implicated

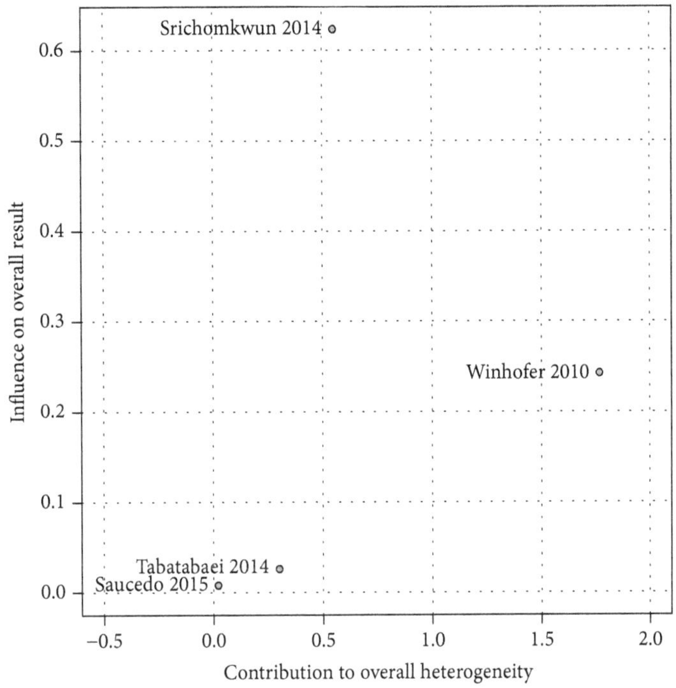

FIGURE 8: Baujat plot for the mean difference and contribution to heterogeneity among studies measuring ucOC.

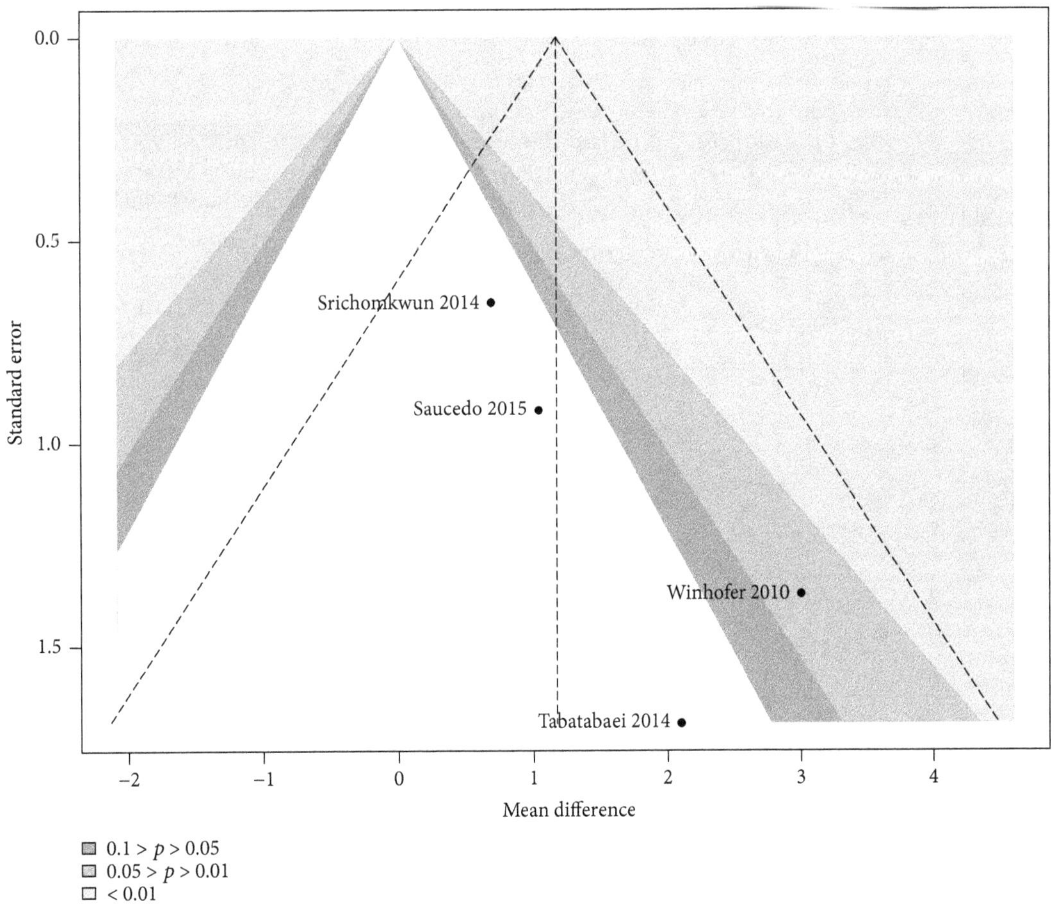

FIGURE 9: Funnel plot for publication bias assessment among studies measuring ucOC.

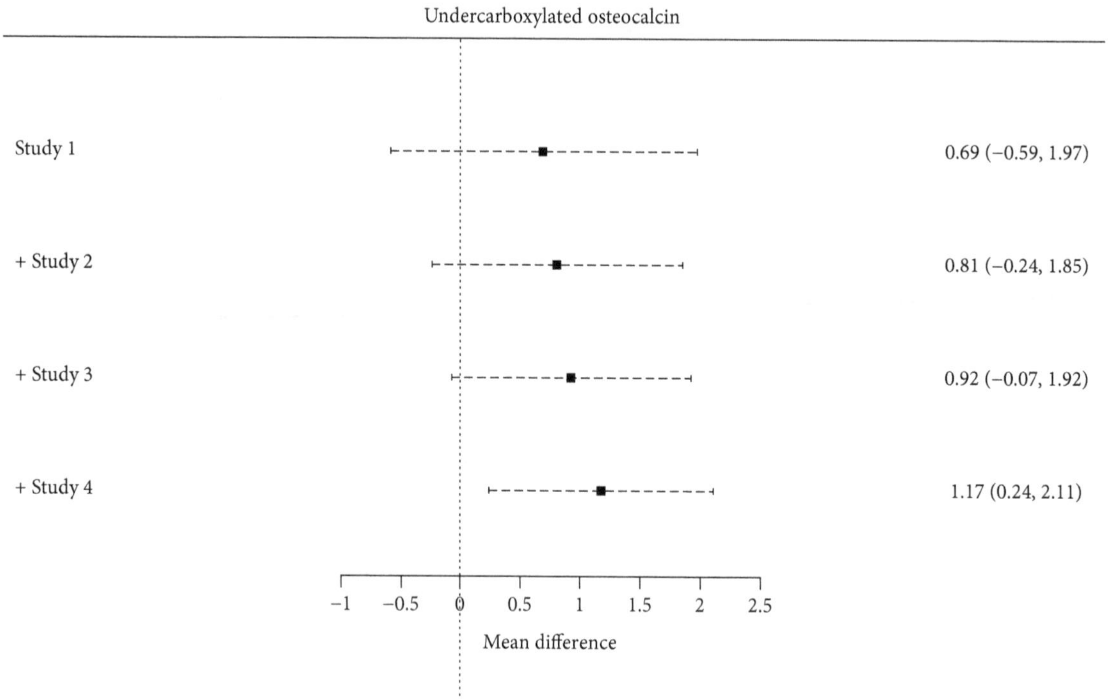

Figure 10: Cumulative forest plot among studies measuring ucOC.

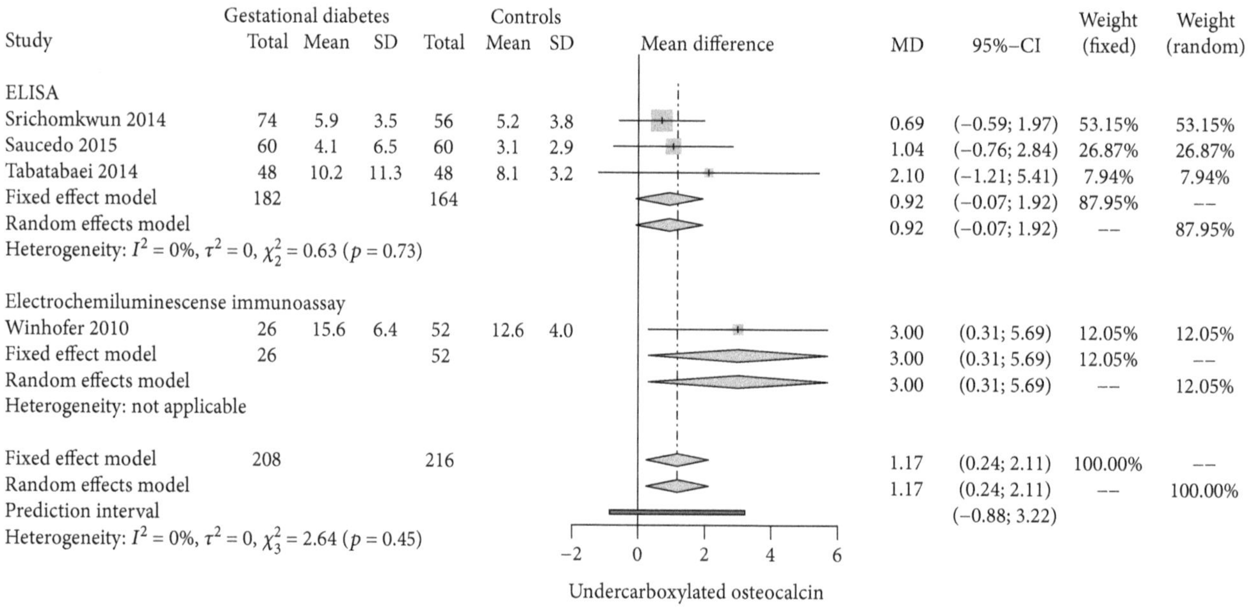

Figure 11: Forest plot for subgroup analysis on the methods used for measuring ucOC.

not only in bone metabolism but in the function of the whole body by exerting its effect when binding to the GPRC6A receptor [28, 63, 64]. The potential role for OC as a predictive protein for GDM comes from previous studies relating knockout mice for GPRAC6A (OC receptor) and later smaller pancreatic islet size, lower insulin content, lower pancreatic weight, lower number of islets, lower insulin mRNA expression, and lower insulin secretion in response to osteocalcin with glucose intolerance [65]. Also, the study of Papastefanou and colleagues [31] reported that an elevation of tOC serum levels in maternal serum during the first trimester of gestation is a significant predictor for GDM as a standalone parameter (AUC 0.61) or in combination with maternal and pregnancy characteristics (AUC 0.80). Our study adds to the current knowledge by showing that ucOC is the type of OC that has more pronounced changes in women with GDM. The next research step would be to assess if first-trimester ucOC adds to other existing algorithms in predicting GDM [35].

5. Conclusions and Implications

This meta-analysis provides evidence to support the use of ucOC as a potential marker for GDM rather than tOC, probably because the latter is more influenced by baseline UV exposure. In addition, our study also suggests that measuring ucOC during pregnancy also has the advantage of reduced variability, regardless of the platforms or methods used.

Additional Points

Condensation. This meta-analysis provides evidence to support the use of ucOC as a potential marker for GDM rather than tOC, yielding very little variability among studies and no difference among methods or brands used for its analysis.

Conflicts of Interest

The authors declare that they have no conflict of interest.

Authors' Contributions

Raigam J. Martinez-Portilla and Jose R. Villafan-Bernal are co-first authors.

Acknowledgments

We would like to acknowledge Dr. Hope Wiler, Dr. Renata Saucedo García, and Dr. Weerapan Khovidhunkit for sharing their original databases. Your willingness to contribute to our study enhances the world of research.

References

[1] B. E. Metzger, D. R. Coustan, and Organizing Committee, "Summary and recommendations of the fourth international workshop-conference on gestational diabetes mellitus," *Diabetes Care*, vol. 21, pp. B161–B167, 1998.

[2] J. Djelmis, M. Pavic, V. Mulliqi Kotori, I. Pavlic Renar, M. Ivanisevic, and S. Oreskovic, "Prevalence of gestational diabetes mellitus according to IADPSG and NICE criteria," *International Journal of Gynecology & Obstetrics*, vol. 135, no. 3, pp. 250–254, 2016.

[3] D. Farrar, M. Simmonds, M. Bryant et al., "Hyperglycaemia and risk of adverse perinatal outcomes: systematic review and meta-analysis," *BMJ*, vol. 354, article i4694, 2016.

[4] S. Burlina, M. G. Dalfrà, and A. Lapolla, "Short- and long-term consequences for offspring exposed to maternal diabetes: a review," *The Journal of Maternal-Fetal & Neonatal Medicine*, vol. 32, no. 4, pp. 687–694, 2017.

[5] P. V. Hauschka, J. B. Lian, D. E. Cole, and C. M. Gundberg, "Osteocalcin and matrix Gla protein: vitamin K-dependent proteins in bone," *Physiological Reviews*, vol. 69, no. 3, pp. 990–1047, 1989.

[6] M. J. Seibel, "Biochemical markers of bone turnover part I: biochemistry and variability," *Clinical Biochemist Reviews*, vol. 26, no. 4, pp. 97–122, 2005.

[7] P. D. Delmas, D. M. Wilson, K. G. Mann, and B. L. Riggs, "Effect of renal function on plasma levels of bone Gla-protein," *The Journal of Clinical Endocrinology & Metabolism*, vol. 57, no. 5, pp. 1028–1030, 1983.

[8] W. Farrugia and R. A. Melick, "Metabolism of osteocalcin," *Calcified Tissue International*, vol. 39, no. 4, pp. 234–238, 1986.

[9] J. R. Villafán-Bernal, S. Sánchez-Enriquez, and M.-V. J. Francisco, "Molecular modulation of osteocalcin and its relevance in diabetes (review)," *International Journal of Molecular Medicine*, vol. 28, no. 3, pp. 283–293, 2011.

[10] Z. Berberoglu, A. Gursoy, N. Bayraktar, A. C. Yazici, N. Bascil Tutuncu, and N. Guvener Demirag, "Rosiglitazone decreases serum bone-specific alkaline phosphatase activity in postmenopausal diabetic women," *The Journal of Clinical Endocrinology & Metabolism*, vol. 92, no. 9, pp. 3523–3530, 2007.

[11] A. B. Choudhury, P. D. Sarkar, D. K. Sakalley, and S. B. Petkar, "Role of adiponectin in mediating the association of osteocalcin with insulin resistance and type 2 diabetes: a cross sectional study in pre- and post-menopausal women," *Archives of Physiology and Biochemistry*, vol. 120, no. 2, pp. 73–79, 2014.

[12] D. M. S. L. Cutrim, F. A. Pereira, F. J. A. Paula, and M. C. Foss, "Lack of relationship between glycemic control and bone mineral density in type 2 diabetes mellitus," *Brazilian Journal of Medical and Biological Research*, vol. 40, no. 2, pp. 221–227, 2007.

[13] K. K. Danielson, M. E. Elliott, T. LeCaire, N. Binkley, and M. Palta, "Poor glycemic control is associated with low BMD detected in premenopausal women with type 1 diabetes," *Osteoporosis International*, vol. 20, no. 6, pp. 923–933, 2009.

[14] D. Gogas Yavuz, L. Keskin, S. Kıyıcı et al., "Vitamin D receptor gene BsmI, FokI, ApaI, TaqI polymorphisms and bone mineral density in a group of Turkish type 1 diabetic patients," *Acta Diabetologica*, vol. 48, no. 4, pp. 329–336, 2011.

[15] R. M. Hussein, "Biochemical relationships between bone turnover markers and blood glucose in patients with type 2 diabetes mellitus," *Diabetes & Metabolic Syndrome: Clinical Research & Reviews*, vol. 11, pp. S369–S372, 2017.

[16] E. Y. Liu, J. Wactawski-Wende, R. P. Donahue, J. Dmochowski, K. M. Hovey, and T. Quattrin, "Does low bone mineral density start in post-teenage years in women with type 1 diabetes?," *Diabetes Care*, vol. 26, no. 8, pp. 2365–2369, 2003.

[17] L. D. Mastrandrea, J. Wactawski-Wende, R. P. Donahue, K. M. Hovey, A. Clark, and T. Quattrin, "Young women with type 1 diabetes have lower bone mineral density that persists over time," *Diabetes Care*, vol. 31, no. 9, pp. 1729–1735, 2008.

[18] T. Neumann, S. Lodes, B. Kästner et al., "Osteocalcin, adipokines and their associations with glucose metabolism in type 1 diabetes," *Bone*, vol. 82, pp. 50–55, 2016.

[19] J. M. Olmos, J. L. Pérez-Castrillón, M. T. García, J. C. Garrido, J. A. Amado, and J. González-Macías, "Bone densitometry and biochemical bone remodeling markers in type 1 diabetes mellitus," *Bone and Mineral*, vol. 26, no. 1, pp. 1–8, 1994.

[20] S. Sanchez-Enriquez, I. T. Ballesteros-Gonzalez, J. R. Villafán-Bernal et al., "Serum levels of undercarboxylated osteocalcin

are related to cardiovascular risk factors in patients with type 2 diabetes mellitus and healthy subjects," *World Journal of Diabetes*, vol. 8, no. 1, pp. 11–17, 2017.

[21] P. D. Sarkar and A. B. Choudhury, "Relationship of serum osteocalcin levels with blood glucose, insulin resistance and lipid profile in central Indian men with type 2 diabetes," *Archives of Physiology and Biochemistry*, vol. 118, no. 5, pp. 260–264, 2012.

[22] P. D. Sarkar and A. B. Choudhury, "Relationships between serum osteocalcin levels versus blood glucose, insulin resistance and markers of systemic inflammation in central Indian type 2 diabetic patients," *European Review for Medical and Pharmacological Sciences*, vol. 17, no. 12, pp. 1631–1635, 2013.

[23] K. Suzuki, T. Kurose, M. Takizawa et al., "Osteoclastic function is accelerated in male patients with type 2 diabetes mellitus: the preventive role of osteoclastogenesis inhibitory factor/osteoprotegerin (OCIF/OPG) on the decrease of bone mineral density," *Diabetes Research and Clinical Practice*, vol. 68, no. 2, pp. 117–125, 2005.

[24] M. Takizawa, K. Suzuki, T. Matsubayashi et al., "Increased bone resorption may play a crucial role in the occurrence of osteopenia in patients with type 2 diabetes: possible involvement of accelerated polyol pathway in its pathogenesis," *Diabetes Research and Clinical Practice*, vol. 82, no. 1, pp. 119–126, 2008.

[25] A. Verrotti, F. Basciani, F. Carle, G. Morgese, and F. Chiarelli, "Calcium metabolism in adolescents and young adults with type 1 diabetes mellitus without and with persistent microalbuminuria," *Journal of Endocrinological Investigation*, vol. 22, no. 3, pp. 198–202, 1999.

[26] J. R. Villafán-Bernal, M. A. Llamas-Covarrubias, J. F. Muñoz-Valle et al., "A cut-point value of uncarboxylated to carboxylated index is associated with glycemic status markers in type 2 diabetes," *Journal of Investigative Medicine*, vol. 62, no. 1, pp. 33–36, 2014.

[27] B. B. Yeap, H. Alfonso, S. A. P. Chubb et al., "Higher serum undercarboxylated osteocalcin and other bone turnover markers are associated with reduced diabetes risk and lower estradiol concentrations in older men," *The Journal of Clinical Endocrinology & Metabolism*, vol. 100, no. 1, pp. 63–71, 2015.

[28] N. K. Lee, H. Sowa, E. Hinoi et al., "Endocrine regulation of energy metabolism by the skeleton," *Cell*, vol. 130, no. 3, pp. 456–469, 2007.

[29] P. M. Catalano, E. D. Tyzbir, N. M. Roman, S. B. Amini, and E. A. H. Sims, "Longitudinal changes in insulin release and insulin resistance in nonobese pregnant women," *American Journal of Obstetrics & Gynecology*, vol. 165, no. 6, pp. 1667–1672, 1991.

[30] J. L. Mills, L. Jovanovic, R. Knopp et al., "Physiological reduction in fasting plasma glucose concentration in the first trimester of normal pregnancy: the diabetes in early pregnancy study," *Metabolism*, vol. 47, no. 9, pp. 1140–1144, 1998.

[31] I. Papastefanou, M. Eleftheriades, D. Kappou et al., "Maternal serum osteocalcin at 11-14 weeks of gestation in gestational diabetes mellitus," *European Journal of Clinical Investigation*, vol. 45, no. 10, pp. 1025–1031, 2015.

[32] A. Hossein-nezhad, Z. Maghbooli, K. Mirzaei, M. Rahmani, and B. Larijani, "Osteocalcin and cross laps status among women with gestational diabetes mellitus during pregnancy," *Journal of Diabetes and Metabolic Disorders*, vol. 9, pp. 1–7, 2010.

[33] R. Saucedo, G. Rico, G. Vega et al., "Osteocalcin, undercarboxylated osteocalcin and osteopontin are not associated with gestational diabetes mellitus but are inversely associated with leptin in non-diabetic women," *Journal of Endocrinological Investigation*, vol. 38, no. 5, pp. 519–526, 2015.

[34] A. M. Maged, G. A. F. Moety, W. A. Mostafa, and D. A. Hamed, "Comparative study between different biomarkers for early prediction of gestational diabetes mellitus," *The Journal of Maternal-Fetal & Neonatal Medicine*, vol. 27, no. 11, pp. 1108–1112, 2014.

[35] C. E. Powe, "Early pregnancy biochemical predictors of gestational diabetes mellitus," *Current Diabetes Reports*, vol. 17, no. 2, p. 12, 2017.

[36] D. F. Stroup, J. A. Berlin, S. C. Morton et al., "Meta-analysis of observational studies in epidemiology: a proposal for reporting," *JAMA*, vol. 283, no. 15, pp. 2008–2012, 2000.

[37] D. Moher, A. Liberati, J. Tetzlaff, D. G. Altman, and The PRISMA Group, "Preferred reporting items for systematic reviews and meta-analyses: the PRISMA statement," *PLoS Medicine*, vol. 6, no. 7, article e1000097, 2009.

[38] E. Stovold, D. Beecher, R. Foxlee, and A. Noel-Storr, "Study flow diagrams in Cochrane systematic review updates: an adapted PRISMA flow diagram," *Systematic Reviews*, vol. 3, no. 1, p. 54, 2014.

[39] J. P. T. Higgins and S. Green, *Cochrane Handbook for Systematic Reviews of Interventions Version 5.1.0 [Updated March 2011]*, The Cochrane Collaboration, 2011.

[40] A. Wells, B. Shea, D. O'Connell et al., "The Newcastle-Ottawa scale (NOS) for assessing the quality of nonrandomised studies in meta-analyses," http://www.ohri.ca/programs/clinical_epidemiology/oxford.asp.

[41] I. R. White and J. Thomas, "Standardized mean differences in individually-randomized and cluster-randomized trials, with applications to meta-analysis," *Clinical Trials: Journal of the Society for Clinical Trials*, vol. 2, no. 2, pp. 141–151, 2005.

[42] M. Borenstein, L. V. Hedges, J. P. T. Higgins, and H. R. Rothstein, "Fixed-effect versus random-effects models," in *Introduction to Meta-Analysis*, pp. 77–86, John Wiley & Sons, Ltd., 2009.

[43] M. Borenstein, J. P. T. Higgins, L. V. Hedges, and H. R. Rothstein, "Basics of meta-analysis: I^2 is not an absolute measure of heterogeneity," *Research Synthesis Methods*, vol. 8, no. 1, pp. 5–18, 2017.

[44] B. Baujat, C. Mahe, J. P. Pignon, and C. Hill, "A graphical method for exploring heterogeneity in meta-analyses: application to a meta-analysis of 65 trials," *Statistics in Medicine*, vol. 21, no. 18, pp. 2641–2652, 2002.

[45] J. Lau, C. H. Schmid, and T. C. Chalmers, "Cumulative meta-analysis of clinical trials builds evidence for exemplary medical care," *Journal of Clinical Epidemiology*, vol. 48, no. 1, pp. 45–57, 1995.

[46] M. Borenstein, L. V. Hedges, J. P. T. Higgins, and H. R. Rothstein, *Introduction to Meta-Analysis*, John Wiley & Sons, Ltd., 2009.

[47] G. Schwarzer, "Meta: an R package for meta-analysis," *R News*, vol. 7, no. 3, pp. 40–45, 2007.

[48] Y. Winhofer, A. Handisurya, A. Tura et al., "Osteocalcin is related to enhanced insulin secretion in gestational diabetes mellitus," *Diabetes Care*, vol. 33, no. 1, pp. 139–143, 2010.

[49] N. Tabatabaei, Y. Giguere, J. C. Forest, C. J. Rodd, R. Kremer, and H. A. Weiler, "Osteocalcin is higher across pregnancy in

Caucasian women with gestational diabetes mellitus," *Canadian Journal of Diabetes*, vol. 38, no. 5, pp. 307–313, 2014.

[50] P. Srichomkwun, N. Houngngam, S. Pasatrat, T. Tharavanij, L. Wattanachanya, and W. Khovidhunkit, "Undercarboxylated osteocalcin is associated with insulin resistance, but not adiponectin, during pregnancy," *Endocrine*, vol. 53, no. 1, pp. 129–135, 2016.

[51] Y. Winhofer, F. W. Kiefer, A. Handisurya et al., "CTX (crosslaps) rather than osteopontin is associated with disturbed glucose metabolism in gestational diabetes," *PLoS One*, vol. 7, no. 7, article e40947, 2012.

[52] B. Telejko, K. Kalejta, M. Kuzmicki et al., "The association of bone turnover markers with pro- and anti-inflammatory adipokines in patients with gestational diabetes," *Annals of Agricultural and Environmental Medicine*, vol. 22, no. 2, pp. 307–312, 2015.

[53] M. Martinez, P. Catalan, A. Lisbona et al., "Serum osteocalcin concentrations in diabetic pregnant women and their newborns," *Hormone and Metabolic Research*, vol. 26, no. 7, pp. 338–342, 1994.

[54] M. B. Landon, C. Y. Spong, E. Thom et al., "A multicenter, randomized trial of treatment for mild gestational diabetes," *The New England Journal of Medicine*, vol. 361, no. 14, pp. 1339–1348, 2009.

[55] C. A. Crowther, J. E. Hiller, J. R. Moss et al., "Effect of treatment of gestational diabetes mellitus on pregnancy outcomes," *The New England Journal of Medicine*, vol. 352, no. 24, pp. 2477–2486, 2005.

[56] N. Oostdam, M. N. M. van Poppel, M. G. A. J. Wouters, and W. van Mechelen, "Interventions for preventing gestational diabetes mellitus: a systematic review and meta-analysis," *Journal of Women's Health*, vol. 20, no. 10, pp. 1551–1563, 2011.

[57] S. Thangaratinam, E. Rogozinska, K. Jolly et al., "Effects of interventions in pregnancy on maternal weight and obstetric outcomes: meta-analysis of randomised evidence," *BMJ*, vol. 344, no. may16 4, p. e2088, 2012.

[58] E. Caliskan, F. Kayikcioglu, N. Ozturk, S. Koc, and A. Haberal, "A population-based risk factor scoring will decrease unnecessary testing for the diagnosis of gestational diabetes mellitus," *Acta Obstetricia et Gynecologica Scandinavica*, vol. 83, no. 6, pp. 524–530, 2004.

[59] S. Nanda, M. Savvidou, A. Syngelaki, R. Akolekar, and K. H. Nicolaides, "Prediction of gestational diabetes mellitus by maternal factors and biomarkers at 11 to 13 weeks," *Prenatal Diagnosis*, vol. 31, no. 2, pp. 135–141, 2011.

[60] C. D. Naylor, M. Sermer, E. Chen, and D. Farine, "Selective screening for gestational diabetes mellitus," *The New England Journal of Medicine*, vol. 337, no. 22, pp. 1591–1596, 1997.

[61] H. J. Teede, C. L. Harrison, W. T. Teh, E. Paul, and C. A. Allan, "Gestational diabetes: development of an early risk prediction tool to facilitate opportunities for prevention," *Australian and New Zealand Journal of Obstetrics and Gynaecology*, vol. 51, no. 6, pp. 499–504, 2011.

[62] M. van Leeuwen, B. C. Opmeer, E. J. K. Zweers et al., "Estimating the risk of gestational diabetes mellitus: a clinical prediction model based on patient characteristics and medical history," *BJOG: An International Journal of Obstetrics & Gynaecology*, vol. 117, no. 1, pp. 69–75, 2010.

[63] G. Karsenty and F. Oury, "Regulation of male fertility by the bone-derived hormone osteocalcin," *Molecular and Cellular Endocrinology*, vol. 382, no. 1, pp. 521–526, 2014.

[64] J. Wei, T. Hanna, N. Suda, G. Karsenty, and P. Ducy, "Osteocalcin promotes β-cell proliferation during development and adulthood through Gprc6a," *Diabetes*, vol. 63, no. 3, pp. 1021–1031, 2014.

[65] M. Pi, Y. Wu, and L. D. Quarles, "GPRC6A mediates responses to osteocalcin in β-cells in vitro and pancreas in vivo," *Journal of Bone and Mineral Research*, vol. 26, no. 7, pp. 1680–1683, 2011.

6

Views and Experiences of New Zealand Women with Gestational Diabetes in Achieving Glycaemic Control Targets

Ruth Martis, Julie Brown, and Caroline A. Crowther

Liggins Institute, The University of Auckland, Private Bag 92019, Auckland 1142, New Zealand

Correspondence should be addressed to Caroline A. Crowther; c.crowther@auckland.ac.nz

Academic Editor: Bernard Portha

Introduction. Optimal glycaemic control in women with gestational diabetes mellitus (GDM) reduces maternal and infant morbidity. *Method.* A survey was administered to women diagnosed with GDM to explore their views and experiences in achieving optimal glycaemic control. *Results.* Sixty women participated. Enablers included being taught to test capillary blood glucose in group settings where the health professional demonstrated this on themselves first (60, 100%); health professionals listening (41, 68%); being reminded to perform blood glucose testing (33, 55%); and being provided healthy meals by friends and family (28, 47%). Barriers included not having information in a woman's first language (33, 55%); being offered unhealthy food (19, 31%); not being believed by health professionals (13, 21%); receiving inconsistent information by health professionals (10, 16%); never being seen twice by the same health professional (8, 13%); and long waiting hours at clinics (7, 11%). Two-thirds of women (37, 62%) reported that food costs were not a barrier, but that they were always or frequently hungry. *Conclusion.* Optimising experiences for women with GDM for achieving glycaemic control and overcoming barriers, regardless of glycaemic targets, requires further focus on providing meaningful health literacy and support from health professionals, family, friends, and work colleagues.

1. Introduction

Globally, there are increasing rates of diabetes, including gestational diabetes mellitus (GDM) [1, 2]. The prevalence of GDM varies among populations but probably affects 10–25% of pregnancies [3–5].

Short- and long-term health risks for women with GDM include preeclampsia, induction of labour, caesarean section, and postnatal depression for the women [6–8]. For the baby, health risks include shoulder dystocia, nerve palsy, preterm birth, neonatal hypoglycaemia, respiratory distress syndrome, and the risk of developing obesity and type 2 diabetes (T2DM) in childhood [9–11].

Treatments for women with GDM that maintain glycaemic control within specified targets have a significant impact on short- and long-term health for the woman and her baby [12–14]. Treatments for GDM include dietary and exercise advice alone or combined with pharmacological therapy [15–19].

While some published studies have described women's experiences of developing gestational diabetes [20–25], little is known as to how women feel about achieving their glycaemic treatment targets. This nested study within the TARGET trial (Australian New Zealand Trial Registry: ACTRN12615000282583) aimed to explore women's views and experiences in achieving their recommended glycaemic treatment targets and to identify potential barriers and enablers.

2. Materials and Methods

2.1. Participant Selection. Women diagnosed with GDM were eligible to participate if they had a singleton pregnancy, could communicate in English, had been self-monitoring their

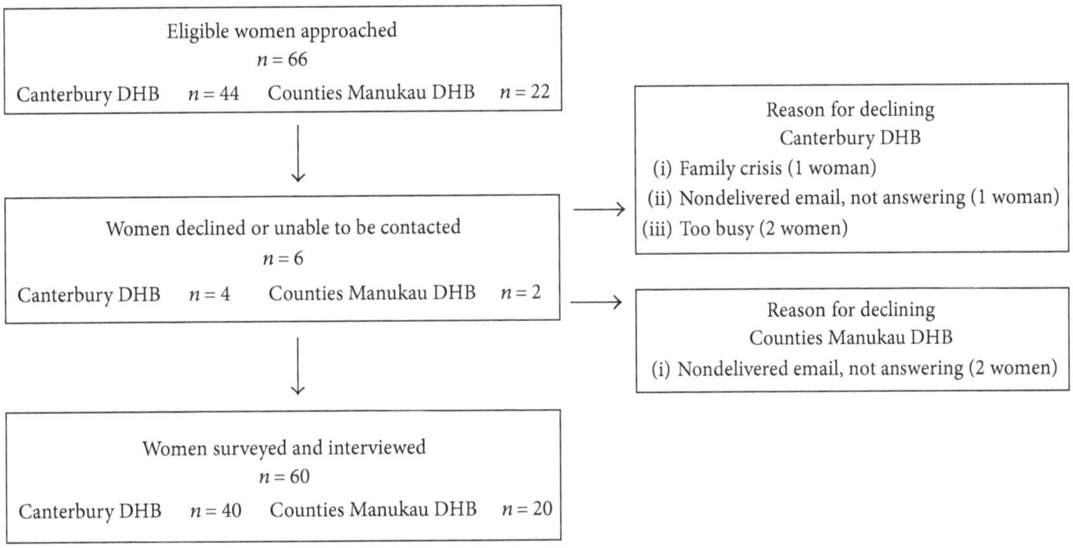

FIGURE 1: Flowchart of recruitment.

capillary blood glucose levels for at least two weeks, and provided written consent. Eligible women were sent an email invitation that included a participant information sheet and consent form. Women could choose to be interviewed face to face, or to be telephoned. Women were aware that the survey was not an assessment of their knowledge about GDM and advised that all their information would be kept confidential.

Hospital sites from two different geographical locations in New Zealand participated. Twenty women, recruited from Canterbury District Health Board (DHB) in the South Island, were using less tight glycaemic treatment targets (fasting blood glucose < 5.5 mmol/L, 1 hour postprandial < 8.0 mmol/L, and 2 hours postprandial < 7.0 mmol/L). Forty women were using tighter glycaemic treatment targets (fasting blood glucose ≤ 5.0 mmol/L, 1 hour postprandial ≤ 7.4 mmol/L, and 2 hours postprandial ≤ 6.7 mmol/L): twenty women recruited from Canterbury DHB in the South Island and twenty women recruited from Counties Manukau DHB in the North Island.

Local hospital policies differed for testing of capillary blood glucose. Canterbury DHB moved from initially less tight targets to tighter glycaemic treatment targets during the survey time. Women were asked to test their capillary blood glucose at one hour postprandial. Counties Manukau DHB was using tighter glycaemic treatment targets during the survey time. Women were asked to test their capillary blood glucose two hours postprandial.

2.2. The Survey. The survey comprised 45 questions. Twenty questions identified participant demographics and twenty-five their views and knowledge of their glycaemic treatment targets. Questions included identifying what had been helpful in learning how to self-monitor blood glucose levels; support received from family, friends, and health professionals; access to written information; costs associated with their GDM management and treatment; and experience of hunger. The survey was piloted with three women following which three questions were modified. There was an opportunity for women to provide additional information. All women answered all the survey questions.

2.3. Analysis. Data analysis was conducted using Pivot Tables in Microsoft Office Excel 2016 calculating frequency and corresponding percentage to describe the responses to the survey questions and included mean and standard deviation for normally distributed data. All analyses were undertaken in Microsoft Office Excel 2016, reporting descriptive statistics for baseline demographics and using simple numeric calculations for survey responses.

2.4. Ethical Approval. The Views Survey was nested within the TARGET trial approved by the New Zealand Health and Disability Ethics committee (HDEC) Ref. 14/NTA/163 and research registration number 1965.

3. Results

3.1. Participants. Sixty-six eligible women were approached and sixty women consented to participate in the survey. Six women did not participate because they were too busy, having a family crisis, or not responding to the invitations (Figure 1). Face-to-face surveys were conducted with 34 (57%) women and 26 (43%) of the women chose to be surveyed by telephone. The average age of the participating women was 33 years (standard deviation (SD) ± 4.5). Just under half of the women were primigravid and had a family history of diabetes (27, 45%), and two-thirds were classified as obese or overweight in early pregnancy (39, 65%) (Table 1). Most women were European (24, 40%) followed by Asian ethnicity (22, 37%). Women taking part were evenly distributed across the deprivation index: 18 (30%) women least deprived (levels 1–3) and 19 (32%) women (levels 4–6) and 22 (37%) women most deprived (levels 7–10)

(Table 1). The demographics of the participating women are reflective of a cross section of the demographics of New Zealand's pregnant population [26–28] (Table 1).

Women were diagnosed with GDM at a mean of 27.8 ± 2.0-week gestation. At the time of the survey, participants had been checking their daily capillary blood glucose for an average of 6.8 ± 2.3 weeks (Table 1), with just over half checking their blood glucose four times a day (32, 53%) and the other participants six times a day (28, 47%). Ten women (17%) reported having a diagnosis of GDM from a previous pregnancy. Almost a third of women (18, 30%) were treated with diet alone; the remainder received a combination of dietary advice and medications. Thirteen (22%) women were treated with subcutaneous insulin for their GDM, 17 (28%) women metformin, and 12 (20%) women were treated with insulin and metformin (Table 1).

3.2. Views and Experiences about Achieving Recommended Glycaemic Treatment Targets. The majority of women correctly identified their glycaemic treatment targets (59, 98%) and viewed it as very important or important to try to adhere to these targets (Table 2). Documenting the blood glucose results were viewed as less important (56, 93%) compared to viewing adherence to the targets because women knew the results could be downloaded from the glucometer. These findings were similar across participants regardless of their glycaemic treatment targets (Table 2).

Almost two-thirds of women (37, 62%) described achieving their morning fasting glycaemic treatment target as most difficult. These findings were similar across participants, regardless of their recommended glycaemic targets (12 (60%) for less tight targets and 25 (62.5%) for tighter targets) (Table 2). The next most frequent difficulty reported for women to achieve their recommended glycaemic targets was after their evening meal (11, 18%). Again, these findings were similar across participants regardless of their glycaemic treatment targets (Table 2). Almost two-thirds of women (37, 62%) experienced being always or frequently hungry (Table 3).

3.3. Enablers to Achieving Optimal Blood Glucose Control. Participants were asked to identify what helped them when learning to test their capillary blood glucose levels. All 60 (100%) women indicated that having a health professional to demonstrate the collection of capillary blood glucose on themselves and then watch the participant perform it was helpful (Table 3). Fifty-six (93%) women opted to comment further about other factors that they felt were helpful for learning self-monitoring of blood glucose. These related mainly to group or individual teaching. Forty-four (79%) of the women who commented further stated that they found group sessions helpful with some women explaining that they enjoyed talking to other women and recognising that they are not alone living with GDM. A smaller proportion of women (12, 21%) received additional one-to-one teaching sessions and enjoyed them as these enabled them to ask "stupid" questions, they could ask the teacher to slow down when English was their second language, or they felt less as though it was "mass produced" and liked to be treated more as an individual. Over a third of women (22, 37%) identified Google as a helpful tool. It is unclear which websites they visited and in which language.

Support from family, friends, and work colleagues was seen as enabling for achieving glycaemic control. Over half of the women (33, 55%) indicated that they found it helpful to be asked about their capillary blood glucose levels and to be reminded to do them by their partners, children, extended family members, and work colleagues. Having their meals cooked by either their partners or extended family members, who incorporated the GDM diet recommendations, was found to be helpful for nearly half of the women (28, 47%) (Table 4). Comments indicated that this enabled women to eat more vegetables and stopped them from buying confectionary or sugar-sweetened beverages (fizzy drinks). Further comments around supportive provision of food by others included colleagues organising healthy morning teas at work and friends providing healthy food choices for baby showers. While nearly two-thirds of women (37, 62%) indicated that the cost associated with the GDM diagnosis, such as food, petrol, or child care, stayed the same, some women (8, 13%) reported reduced food costs since being diagnosed with GDM as an enabler due to buying fewer take-away meals (fast foods) (Table 3).

All women attended Diabetes in Pregnancy Services where they saw a range of health professionals. Most women (47, 78%) attended the clinic fortnightly (Table 4). Support from health professionals was valued. Over two-thirds of the women (41, 68%) appreciated that health professionals took time to listen and explain (Table 3). One (1.7%) woman could email the endocrinologist for advice and appreciated their prompt response.

3.4. Barriers to Achieving Optimal Blood Glucose Control. All women received written information about GDM, which explained the importance of healthy eating and its effect on blood glucose levels and how to self-monitor capillary blood glucose levels. Barriers to this written information included feeling overwhelmed with the amount of written material and not being able to read it in their first language. Women requested to receive visual information (16, 27%) rather than words for food choices, food label reading, how to perform the finger pricks for capillary blood glucose collection, and how to give subcutaneous insulin injections (Table 4). Over half of the women (33, 55%) found it difficult that the written information was in English and wanted the health information in their first language for themselves and for their families to better understand what GDM is and what optimal blood glucose control meant (Table 4). Hindi was the language most frequently requested (9, 27% women), followed by Samoan (6, 18% women) and then Chinese and Māori each by 5 (15%) women. This reflects the ethnic diversity of this cohort of women (Table 1).

Over a third of women (23, 38%) reported being offered unhealthy food by family, friends, and work colleagues and their lack of understanding as barriers to achieving optimal glycaemic control.

When engaging with the Diabetes in Pregnancy Services women, just over a fifth of women (13, 22%) reported a

Table 1: Demographic characteristics of women who participated in the survey.

Characteristics	Women with less tight[1] glycaemic treatment targets $n = 20$ (% or ±20)	Women with tighter[2] glycaemic treatment targets $n = 40$ (% or ±40)	Women total $n = 60$ (% or ±60)
Age (years)[4]	34 (±4.3)	32 (±4.5)	33 (±4.5)
Primigravida (G_1P_0)[3]	9 (45)	18 (45)	27 (45)
BMI category[5,3]			
Normal	8 (40)	13 (32.5)	21 (35)
Overweight	5 (25)	6 (15)	11 (18.3)
Obese (class I)	2 (10)	9 (22.5)	11 (18.3)
Obese (class II)	2 (10)	6 (15)	8 (13.3)
Obese (class II)	3 (15)	6 (15)	9 (15)
Total obese	7 (35)	21 (52.5)	28 (46.6)
Ethnicity[6,3]			
European	12 (60)	12 (30)	24 (40)
Māori	—	6 (15)	6 (10)
Asian	7 (35)	15 (37.5)	22 (36.7)
Pacific Peoples	—	7 (17.5)	7 (11.6)
MELAA	1 (5)	—	1 (1.7)
Highest educational qualifications after leaving school[7,3]			
(1) No qualification	1 (5)	2 (5)	3 (5)
(2) Level 1 certificate	—	2 (5)	2 (3.3)
(3) Level 2 certificate	2 (10)	2 (5)	4 (6.7)
(4) Level 3 certificate	2 (10)	4 (10)	6 (10)
(5) Level 4 certificate	—	4 (10)	4 (6.7)
(6) Level 5 and level 6 diploma	4 (20)	9 (22.5)	13 (21.7)
(7) Bachelor degree and level 7 qualification	8 (40)	17 (42.5)	25 (41.6)
(8) Postgraduate and honours degree	1 (5)	—	1 (1.7)
(9) Master's degree	2 (10)	—	2 (3.3)
NZ deprivation index[8,3]			
1 (least deprived)	3 (15)	5 (12.5)	8 (13.5)
2	2 (10)	3 (7.5)	5 (8.4)
3	2 (10)	3 (7.5)	5 (8.4)
4	4 (20)	6 (15)	10 (16.7)
5	2 (10)	5 (12.5)	7 (11.8)
6	1 (5)	1 (1.7)	2 (3.4)
7	2 (10)	3 (7.5)	5 (8.5)
8	3 (15)	3 (7.5)	6 (10)
9	1 (5)	4 (10)	5 (8.7)
10 (most deprived)	—	6 (15)	6 (10)
Lead maternity carer (LMC)[9,3]			
Midwife	19 (95)	36 (90)	55 (91.7)
Obstetrician	1 (5)	—	1 (1.7)
Hospital team	—	4 (10)	4 (6.7)
Gestational age at GDM diagnosis[4] (weeks)	27.7 (±1.9)	27.9 (±2.0)	27.8 (±2.0)
Time of self-testing capillary blood glucose for (weeks)[4]	7.6 (±2.5)	6.4 (±2.1)	6.8 (±2.3)
Previous GDM[3]	4 (20)	6 (15)	10 (16.7)
Previous hypertension[3]	2 (10)	—	2 (3.3)
Current hypertension	—	3 (7.5)	3 (5)
Family history of hypertension[3]	8 (45)	16 (40)	24 (40)

Table 1: Continued.

Characteristics	Women with less tight[1] glycaemic treatment targets $n = 20$ (% or ±20)	Women with tighter[2] glycaemic treatment targets $n = 40$ (% or ±40)	Women total $n = 60$ (% or ±60)
Family history of diabetes[3]	7 (35)	20 (50)	27 (45)
Current smoker[3]	—	3 (7.5)	3 (15)
Current treatment[3]			
Diet only	7 (35)	11 (27.5)	18 (30)
Insulin and diet	2 (10)	11 (27.5)	13 (21.7)
Metformin and diet	5 (25)	12 (30)	17 (28.3)
Insulin, metformin, and diet	6 (30)	6 (15)	12 (20)

[1]Less tight glycaemic treatment targets for women with GDM: fasting blood glucose < 5.5 mmol/L, 1 hour postprandial < 8.0 mmol/L, and 2 hours postprandial < 7.0 mmol/L; [2]tighter glycaemic treatment targets for women with GDM: fasting blood glucose ≤ 5.0 mmol/L, 1 hour postprandial ≤ 7.4 mmol/L, and 2 hours postprandial ≤6.7 mmol/L; [3]figures are numbers and percentages; [4]figures are mean and standard deviation; [5]BMI categories: underweight < 18.50, normal range ≥ 18.55–24.99, overweight ≥ 25.00–29.99, obese (class I) ≥ 30.00–34.99, obese (class II)—severe obese ≥ 35.00–39.99 and obese (class II)—morbid obese ≥ 40.00 (according to WHO and Ministry of Health categories) [44, 45]; [6]as categorised by New Zealand government statistics groups for major ethnic groups. MELAA is an acronym for Middle Eastern/Latin American/African (http://www.stats.govt.nz/Census/2013-census/profile-and-summary-reports/infographic-culture-identity.aspx); [7]as categorised by New Zealand government statistics groups (http://www.stats.govt.nz/Census/2013-census/profile-and-summary-reports/qstats-education-training/highest-qualification.aspx); [8]as categorised by New Zealand 2013 Deprivation Index, University of Otago, Department of Public Health. Deprivation score was unknown for one woman, as her address had no meshblock listed (http://www.otago.ac.nz/wellington/departments/publichealth/research/hirp/otago020194.html); [9]a lead maternity carer (LMC) in New Zealand provides lead maternity care (is in charge). This can be either a midwife, obstetrician, or GP (https://www.midwife.org.nz/in-new-zealand/contexts-for-practice).

Table 2: Participants views and experiences of capillary blood glucose monitoring.

	Women with less tight glycaemic treatment targets $n = 20$ (% of 20)	Women with tighter glycaemic treatment targets $n = 40$ (% of 40)	Women total $n = 60$ (%)
Knew their glycaemic treatment targets	19 (98.3)	40 (100)	59 (98.3)
Viewed achieving glycaemic treatment targets as very important or important	20 (100)	39 (97.5)	59 (98.3)
Viewed documenting blood glucose results as very important or important	18 (90)	37 (92.5)	56 (93.3)
Experienced difficult fasting glycaemic treatment target (before breakfast)	12 (60)	25 (62.5)	37 (61.6)
Experienced difficult postprandial glycaemic treatment target (after dinner)	3 (15)	8 (20)	11 (18.3)

judgemental attitude by health professionals, being impatient with them, and being not believed that they had tried their hardest to stay within their recommended glycaemic treatment targets as a barrier. Inconsistent information by health professionals (10, 17%), never seeing the same health professional twice (8, 13%), and long waiting hours at the clinic (7, 12%) were also experienced as difficult (Table 4).

An increased cost for buying more vegetables, fresh fruits, and wholemeal bread was reported as a barrier by a quarter of women (15, 25%) (Table 4).

4. Discussion

In this survey, women with GDM identified enablers and barriers to achieving optimal glycaemic control. While achieving optimal glycaemic control was viewed as important, most women found it difficult to achieve their morning fasting glycaemic treatment targets, experienced hunger, and wanted the health information in their first language or visually displayed. For most women, food costs were not reported as a concern for the family budget. Being taught blood glucose testing in a group setting was considered helpful. Support from health professionals and family, friends, and work colleagues was valued. Barriers reported include long clinic waiting hours; inconsistent advice, judgemental attitudes, impatience, and not being believed by health professionals; and unhealthy food being offered by family members, friends, and work colleagues.

Health care providers recognise that teaching moments can be maximised by incorporating specific adult-learning principles and learning styles into their teaching strategies and providing written information that supports these

TABLE 3: Enablers identified by women with GDM[1].

Enablers	Women with less tight glycaemic treatment targets $n = 20$ (% of 20)	Women with tighter glycaemic treatment targets $n = 40$ (% of 40)	Women total $N = 60$ (%)
Health professional demonstrating on themselves CBGT[2]	20 (100)	40 (100)	60 (100)
Watching participants perform CBGT[2]	20 (100)	40 (100)	60 (100)
Group teaching	11 (55)	33 (82.5)	44[3] (78.5)
One to one teaching	6 (30)	6 (15)	12[3] (21.4)
Health professionals listening and explaining	6 (30)	35 (87.5)	41 (68.3)
Being ask about their CBGC[4] and reminded to do them	7 (35)	26 (65)	33 (55)
Others cooking incorporating GDM diet	11 (55)	17 (42.5)	28 (46.6)
Using Google	9 (45)	13 (32.5)	22 (36.6)
Going for walks/exercising together	6 (30)	9 (45)	15 (25)
Less costs	3 (15)	5 (12.5)	8 (13.3)

[1]Multiple answers were possible for this part of the survey; [2]capillary blood glucose testing; [3]results from 56 women; [4]capillary blood glucose concentrations.

TABLE 4: Barriers identified by women with GDM.

Barriers	Women with less tight glycaemic treatment targets $n = 20$ (% of 20)	Women with tighter glycaemic treatment targets $n = 40$ (% of 40)	Women total $n = 60$ (%)
Health information available only in English	8 (40)	25 (62.5)	33 (55)
Health information in words not visual	5 (25)	11 (27.5)	16 (26.6)
Being offered unhealthy food by family, friends, and work colleagues	5 (25)	14 (35)	23 (38.3)
Impatient, not being believed, and being judged by health professionals	7 (35)	6 (15)	13 (21.6)
Inconsistent information by health professionals	4 (20)	6 (15)	10 (16.6)
Never seeing the same health professional twice	3 (15)	5 (12.5)	8 (13.3)
Long waiting hours at clinic	4 (20)	3 (7.5)	7 (11.6)
Being hungry	14 (70)	23 (57.5)	37 (61.6)
Increased costs	7 (35)	8 (20)	15 (25)

learning styles [29]. The survey results showed that participants wished to be provided with better visual information and to have written information in their own language. Most women enjoyed group teaching sessions, although some preferred one-to-one sessions.

We found no published studies reporting on the effects of providing visual learning aids for women with gestational diabetes or the impact of having the information in their first language. One mixed-method study [30] among young people with type 1 diabetes (T1DM) in Norway found that a pictorial diary as a mobile phone app covering the topics diet, insulin dosage, physical activity, and pre- and postprandial glucose measurements all led to a change in the participants' applied knowledge about the management of their diabetes. This is an area requiring further research. For information to make sense and motivate behaviour change, it needs to be provided in a language best understood by the women with GDM [23–25, 31]. Women identified Google as a helpful tool. Health professionals need to be aware that women will access information beyond the clinic environment and the quality of this information may vary. Diabetes in Pregnancy Services should consider how they provide health information and the content of their teaching sessions. Health literacy providing clear and relevant health messages has been identified as an effective way to help people manage their own health care [31–34]. It would be challenging for Diabetes in Pregnancy Services to provide the information for women with GDM in all the languages identified through this survey. The solution may be to provide increased visual information which requires little language and/or translate the written information for the languages identified. The use of trained translators has been encouraged, as family members are often unfamiliar with the health care medical terms, may find it difficult talking about sensitive matters, and may have different degrees of English fluency [35].

Achieving adequate fasting blood glucose control prior to breakfast, also known as the dawn phenomenon [36], was identified as a challenge for most women in this survey, regardless of whether their recommended glycaemic targets were identified as less tight or tighter. In the literature, this has been identified previously for people with T1DM and T2DM [37] but we could not find any publications specifically relating to gestational diabetes. Anecdotal evidence through social media indicates that women with GDM do find this control difficult [38]. Various recommendations for achieving glycaemic control include subcutaneous insulin, walking after dinner, restricting carbohydrate intake at dinner time, late protein snack before bed time, and staying hydrated [39] but require further research for women with GDM. Two-thirds of women commented on being hungry. It is unclear from the survey if this relates to women trying to lower their morning fasting blood glucose with eating less at dinner time or eating very low carbohydrate meals. This would benefit from further exploration.

Some women identified barriers regarding health professional's attitude to not achieving adequate glycaemic control. These included judgemental attitude, not being believed when women stated that they were trying their hardest to follow all diet and pharmaceutical recommendations, and seeing a different health professional at each visit receiving inconsistent information. Findings from other qualitative studies reiterate these findings [31, 40, 41] and highlight the importance for health professional to have a woman-centred approach, not only focusing on blood glucose concentrations but investing time to listen, believing what the women say is true, and providing consistent information and continuity of care [41].

Support from family, friends, and work colleagues were appreciated by the women surveyed. These results are consistent with those of other studies [42, 43]. Barrier identification included unhealthy food being offered to them by family members, friends, and work colleagues, indicating a lack of understanding. Diabetes in Pregnancy Services may consider providing opportunity for family and friends to attend information sessions about GDM and its implication or include discussions about effective strategies for difficult situations at clinic appointments.

This study had some limitations. The participants were from two selected areas in New Zealand, and while they were a cross-sectional representation of the demographics of the New Zealand population, this did not include women living in rural or remote areas. The findings may not be generalised as different district health boards provide care for women with GDM through different models of care.

5. Conclusions

This survey identified barriers and enablers for women with GDM in achieving optimal glycaemic control from two different geographical locations in New Zealand. The results provide insights into women's views and experiences with GDM in achieving glycaemic control targets. Two-thirds of women found it difficult to achieve adequate fasting capillary blood glucose control, regardless of their recommended glycaemic targets, and identified the need for better strategies and adequate health professional and family support to manage this difficulty. Barriers for health information and literacy identified that health professionals need to consider using a women-centred and adult-learning style approach, provide visual aids, provide written information in relevant languages, and include extended family members when imparting knowledge on or teaching GDM-related skills. Long clinic waiting hours, inconsistent advice, judgemental attitudes, and not being believed by health professionals require further consideration when providing a health care service for women with GDM. Findings from this survey will be useful for developing strategies for Diabetes in Pregnancy Services to support women with GDM in achieving their glycaemic control.

Conflicts of Interest

None of the authors have any financial conflict of interests associated with this publication. Caroline A. Crowther and Julie Brown are the lead investigators for the TARGET trial in which this study is nested.

Authors' Contributions

Ruth Martis contributed to the conception and the design of the survey, recruited the women, conducted the survey, entered the data, performed the data analysis, and drafted the article and the revision of the article from coauthors' feedback. Julie Brown and Caroline A. Crowther contributed to the conception and design of the survey, provided advice on the data analysis and data interpretation, commented on all drafts of the manuscript, and approved the final version.

Acknowledgments

The authors would like to express their sincere thanks to all the women who participated. A special thank you to Jane Yates, research assistant, for the assistance with compiling the demographic information and Samuel Dobson for the Pivot Table assistance. Ruth Martis is a recipient of the University of Auckland senior health research scholarship. The TARGET trial is supported through funding from Health Research Council of New Zealand Grant 14/499. The Liggins Institute provided essential materials to enable the study to be conducted.

References

[1] S. Wild, G. Roglic, A. Green, R. Sicree, and H. King, "Global prevalence of diabetes: estimates for the year 2000 and projections for 2030," *Diabetes Care*, vol. 27, pp. 1047–1053, 2004.

[2] Ministry of Health, *Diabetes in Pregnancy: Quick Reference Guide for Health Professionals on the Screening, Diagnosis and Treatment of Gestational Diabetes in New Zealand*, Ministry of Health, Wellington, New Zealand, 2014.

[3] L. Guariguata, U. Linnenkamp, J. Beagley, D. R. Whiting, and N. H. Cho, "Global estimates of the prevalence of hyperglycaemia in pregnancy," *Diabetes Research and Clinical Practice*, vol. 103, no. 2, pp. 176–185, 2014.

[4] U. Kampmann, L. Ring Madsen, G. Oeskov Skajaa, D. Smed Iversen, N. Moeller, and P. Ovesen, "Gestational diabetes: a clinical update," *World Journal of Diabetes*, vol. 6, no. 8, pp. 1065–1072, 2015.

[5] World Health Organization (WHO), *Global Report on Diabetes. WK 810*, World Health Organization, Geneva, Switzerland, 2016.

[6] NICE, National Institute for Health and Clinical Excellence, *Diabetes in Pregnancy: Management of Diabetes and its Complications from Preconception to the Postnatal Period. NICE Guideline NG3*, National Institute for Health and Care Excellence, London, UK, 2015.

[7] HAPO Study Cooperative Research Group, B. E. Metzger, L. P. Lowe et al., "Hyperglycemia and adverse pregnancy outcomes," *New England Journal of Medicine*, vol. 358, no. 19, pp. 1991–2002, 2008.

[8] J. M. Nicklas, L. J. Miller, C. A. Zera, R. B. Davis, S. E. Levkoff, and E. W. Seely, "Factors associated with depressive symptoms in the early postpartum period among women with recent gestational diabetes mellitus," *Maternal and Child Health Journal*, vol. 17, no. 9, pp. 1665–1672, 2013.

[9] A. Lucas, R. Morley, and T. Cole, "Adverse neurodevelopmental outcome of moderate neonatal hypoglycaemia," *BMJ*, vol. 29, no. 6659, pp. 1304–1308, 1988.

[10] A. Ornoy, E. A. Reece, G. Pavlinkova, C. Kappen, and R. K. Miller, "Effect of maternal diabetes on the embryo, fetus, and children: congenital anomalies, genetic and epigenetic changes and developmental outcomes," *Birth Defects Research Part C: Embryo Today: Reviews*, vol. 105, no. 1, pp. 53–72, 2015.

[11] D. Mitanchez, C. Yzydorczyk, and U. Simeoni, "What neonatal complications should the pediatrician be aware of in case of maternal gestational diabetes?," *World Journal of Diabetes*, vol. 6, no. 5, pp. 734–743, 2015.

[12] N. Poolsup, N. Suksomboon, and M. Amin, "Effect of treatment of gestational diabetes mellitus: a systematic review and meta-analysis," *PLoS One*, vol. 9, no. 3, article e92485, 2014.

[13] M. B. Landon, C. Y. Spong, E. Thom et al., "A multicenter, randomized trial of treatment for mild gestational diabetes," *New England Journal of Medicine*, vol. 361, no. 14, pp. 1339–1348, 2009.

[14] C. A. Crowther, J. E. Hiller, J. R. Moss, A. J. McPhee, W. S. Jeffries, and J. S. Robinson, "Effect of treatment of gestational diabetes mellitus on pregnancy outcomes," *New England Journal of Medicine*, vol. 352, no. 24, pp. 2477–2486, 2005.

[15] J. Brown, N. A. Alwan, J. West et al., "Lifestyle interventions for the treatment of women with gestational diabetes," *Cochrane Database of Systematic Reviews*, vol. 5, article CD011970, 2017.

[16] Z. Nachum, N. Zafran, R. Salim et al., "Glyburide versus metformin and their combination for the treatment of gestational diabetes mellitus: a randomized controlled study," *Diabetes Care*, vol. 40, no. 2, pp. 332–337, 2017.

[17] B. Kalra, Y. Gupta, R. Singla, and S. Klara, "Use of oral anti-diabetic agents in pregnancy: a pragmatic approach," *North American Journal of Medical Sciences*, vol. 7, no. 1, pp. 6–12, 2015.

[18] R. J. Ryu, K. E. Hays, and M. F. Hebert, "Gestational diabetes mellitus management with oral hypoglycemic agents," *Seminars in Perinatology*, vol. 38, no. 8, pp. 508–515, 2014.

[19] N. Kavitha, S. De, and S. Kanagasabai, "Oral hypoglycemic agents in pregnancy: an update," *The Journal of Obstetrics and Gynecology of India*, vol. 63, no. 2, pp. 82–87, 2013.

[20] J. Parsons, K. Ismail, S. Amiel, and A. Forbes, "Perceptions among women with gestational diabetes," *Qualitative Health Research*, vol. 24, no. 4, pp. 575–585, 2014.

[21] M. K. Morrison, J. M. Lowe, and C. E. Collins, "Australian women's experiences of living with gestational diabetes," *Women and Birth*, vol. 27, no. 1, pp. 52–57, 2014.

[22] G. Trutnovsky, T. Panzitt, E. Magnet, C. Stern, U. Lang, and M. Dorfer, "Gestational diabetes: women's concerns, mood state, quality of life and treatment satisfaction," *The Journal of Maternal-Fetal & Neonatal Medicine*, vol. 25, no. 11, pp. 2464–2466, 2012.

[23] J. E. Hirst, S. T. Thach, T. D. My An, R. Forsyth, J. M. Morris, and H. E. Jeffery, "Women with gestational diabetes in Vietnam: a qualitative study to determine attitudes and health behaviours," *BMC Pregnancy and Childbirth*, vol. 12, no. 1, pp. 81–90, 2012.

[24] A. Lapolla, G. Di Cianni, A. Di Benedetto et al., "Quality of life, wishes, and needs in women with gestational diabetes: Italian DAWN pregnancy study," *International Journal of Endocrinology*, vol. 2012, Article ID 784726, 6 pages, 2012.

[25] M. Bandyopadhyay, R. Small, M. Davey, J. J. N. Oats, D. A. Forster, and A. Aylward, "Lived experience of gestational diabetes mellitus among immigrant South Asian women in Australia," *Australian and New Zealand Journal of Obstetrics and Gynaecology*, vol. 51, pp. 360–364, 2011.

[26] http://www.health.govt.nz/new-zealand-health-system/my-dhb/counties-manukau-dhb/population-counties-manukau-dhb. July 2017.

[27] http://www.health.govt.nz/new-zealand-health-system/my-dhb/canterbury-dhb/population-canterbury-dhb. July 2017.

[28] http://www.stats.govt.nz/browse_for_stats/population/census_counts/2013CensusUsuallyResidentPopulationCounts HOTP 2013Census.aspx. July 2017.

[29] S. S. Russell, "An overview of adult-learning processes," *Urologic Nursing*, vol. 26, no. 5, pp. 349–352, 370, 2006.

[30] D. H. Frøisland, E. Årsand, and F. Skårderud, "Improving diabetes care for young people with type 1 diabetes through visual learning on mobile phones: mixed-methods study," *Journal of Medical Internet Research*, vol. 14, no. 4, pp. 113–125, 2012.

[31] B. U. Devsam, F. E. Bogossian, and A. S. Peacock, "An interpretive review of women's experiences of gestational diabetes mellitus: proposing a framework to enhance midwifery assessment," *Women and Birth*, vol. 26, no. 2, pp. e69–e76, 2013.

[32] Ministry of Health, *A Framework for Health Literacy*, Ministry of Health, Wellington, New Zealand, 2015.

[33] Work base Education Trust, *Māori Health Literacy Research: Gestational Diabetes Mellitus*, Ministry of Health, Wellington, New Zealand, 2014.

[34] B. Bhavadharini, M. Deepa, S. Nallaperumal, R. M. Anjana, and V. Mohan, "Knowledge about gestational diabetes mellitus amongst pregnant women in South Tamil Nadu," *Journal of Diabetology*, vol. 8, pp. 22–26, 2017.

[35] B. Gray, "The use of interpreters, chapter 8," in *Cole's Medical Practice in New Zealand*, I. M. St. George, Ed., Medical Council of New Zealand, Wellington, New Zealand, 12th edition, 2013.

[36] M. F. Carroll and D. S. Schade, "The dawn phenomenon revisited: implications for diabetes therapy," *Endocrine Practice*, vol. 11, no. 1, pp. 55–64, 2005.

[37] F. Porcellati, P. Lucidi, G. B. Bolli, and C. G. Fanelli, "Thirty years of research on the Dawn phenomenon: lessons to optimize blood glucose control in diabetes," *Diabetes Care*, vol. 36, no. 12, pp. 3860–3862, 2013.

[38] http://www.gestationaldiabetes.co.uk/high-fasting-levels/.

[39] J. P. Sheehan, "Fasting hyperglycemia: etiology, diagnosis, and treatment," *Diabetes Technology & Therapeutics*, vol. 6, no. 4, pp. 525–533, 2004.

[40] K. Fahy, "What is woman-centred care and why does it matter?," *Women and Birth*, vol. 25, pp. 149–151, 2012.

[41] R. Janes, J. Titchener, J. Pere, and R. Pere, "Understanding barriers to glycaemic control from the patient's perspective," *Journal of Primary Health Care*, vol. 5, no. 2, pp. 114–122, 2013.

[42] T. A. Miller and M. R. DiMatteo, "Importance of family/social support and impact on adherence to diabetic therapy," *Diabetes, Metabolic Syndrome and Obesity: Targets and Therapy*, vol. 6, pp. 421–426, 2013.

[43] L. S. Mayberry and C. Y. Osborn, "Family support, medication adherence and glycemic control among adults with type 2 diabetes," *Diabetes Care*, vol. 35, pp. 1239–1245, 2012.

[44] World Health Organization (WHO), *Obesity: Preventing and Managing the Global Epidemic, Report of a WHO Consultation*, WHO Technical Report Series 894, Geneva, Switzerland, 2000.

[45] Ministry of Health, *Understanding Excess Body Weight: New Zealand Health Survey*, Ministry of Health, Wellington, New Zealand, 2015.

7

Risk of Type 2 Diabetes Mellitus following Gestational Diabetes Pregnancy in Women with Polycystic Ovary Syndrome

Joan C. Lo, Jingrong Yang, Erica P. Gunderson, Mohammad K. Hararah, Joel R. Gonzalez, and Assiamira Ferrara

Division of Research, Kaiser Permanente Northern California, Oakland, CA, USA

Correspondence should be addressed to Joan C. Lo; joan.c.lo@kp.org

Academic Editor: Daniela Foti

Background. This study examines gestational diabetes mellitus (GDM) in women with polycystic ovary syndrome (PCOS) and the risk of type 2 diabetes mellitus (DM) following GDM pregnancy. *Methods.* A cohort of 988 pregnant women with PCOS who delivered during 2002–2005 was examined to determine the prevalence and predictors of GDM, with follow-up through 2010 among those with GDM to estimate the risk of DM. *Results.* Of the 988 pregnant women with PCOS, 192 (19%) developed GDM. Multivariable predictors of GDM included older age, Asian race, prepregnancy obesity, family history of DM, preconception metformin use, and multiple gestation. Among women with PCOS and GDM pregnancy, the incidence of DM was 2.8 (95% confidence interval (CI) 1.9–4.2) per 100 person-years and substantially higher for those who received pharmacologic treatment for GDM (6.6 versus 1.5 per 100 person-years, $p < 0.01$). The multivariable adjusted risk of DM was fourfold higher in women who received pharmacologic treatment for GDM (adjusted hazard ratio 4.1, 95% CI 1.8–9.6). The five-year incidence of DM was 13.1% overall and also higher in the pharmacologic treatment subgroup (27.0% versus 7.1%, $p < 0.01$). *Conclusions.* The strongest predictors of GDM among women with PCOS included Asian race and prepregnancy obesity. Pharmacologic treatment of GDM is associated with fourfold higher risk of subsequent DM.

1. Introduction

Women with polycystic ovary syndrome (PCOS) are at increased risk for developing gestational diabetes mellitus (GDM) during pregnancy [1–6]. Both PCOS and GDM are also risk factors for type 2 diabetes mellitus [1, 2, 7–9]. Women with GDM pregnancy have a 7-fold higher risk of developing subsequent type 2 diabetes mellitus compared to women without GDM [10], with an annual incidence of 1.7–2.2% [11–13]. In women with PCOS, the risk of diabetes has been reported up to 8-fold higher compared to that in women without PCOS [7]. While fewer studies have examined diabetes risk in women with PCOS, women who experience a GDM pregnancy, impaired glucose metabolism, and glucose intolerance following GDM pregnancy has been observed [14, 15]. In this study, we examined a large, community-based population of women with PCOS and GDM pregnancy to determine the subsequent risk of diabetes and differential risk by GDM severity.

2. Materials and Methods

Kaiser Permanente Northern California (KPNC) is an integrated healthcare delivery system with over 3 million members and more than 30,000 births/year. We identified nondiabetic KPNC women with PCOS who had a delivered pregnancy during 1 January 2002 to 31 December 2005 and underwent screening for GDM during pregnancy. Women identified with GDM were followed after pregnancy delivery to 31 December 2010 for the development of type 2 diabetes mellitus, censoring at diabetes, membership disenrollment, death, or end of follow-up (whichever came first). The study was approved by the KPNC Institutional Review Board, and the requirement for informed consent was waived due to the nature of the study.

As previously described [16, 17], chart review was conducted to verify PCOS diagnosis using the 2003 ESHRE/ASRM Rotterdam criteria [9], requiring at least two of the three criteria: oligo- or amenorrhea, androgen excess,

Table 1: Baseline characteristics in pregnant women with polycystic ovary syndrome (PCOS) by gestational diabetes mellitus (GDM) status.

		988 PCOS women by GDM status			Adjusted odds of GDM	
		No GDM $N = 796$	GDM $N = 192$	p value	Adjusted* odds ratio	95% confidence interval
Age in years (mean ± standard deviation)		31.1 ± 4.5	32.9 ± 4.0	<0.01	1.11	1.06–1.15
Race/ethnicity						
White		43.5%	30.7%		Referent	
Black		4.0%	3.1%		0.95	0.36–2.49
Hispanic		26.1%	25.5%	<0.01	1.42	0.91–2.21
Asian		22.5%	38.0%		3.52	2.26–5.47
Other		3.9%	2.6%		0.89	0.31–2.51
Prepregnancy BMI						
Normal	<25.0 kg/m^2	30.7%	19.3%		Referent	
Overweight	25–29.9 kg/m^2	30.0%	25.5%	<0.01	1.42	0.86–2.33
Moderately obese	30–39.9 kg/m^2	30.2%	39.1%		2.65	1.63–4.32
Severely obese	≥40.0 kg/m^2	9.2%	16.2%		4.04	2.16–7.57
Family history of diabetes		54.7%	64.6%	0.01	1.52	1.07–2.17
Preconception metformin†		21.6%	35.9%	<0.01	1.65	1.14–2.39
Treatment with fertility drugs or IVF‡		56.7%	66.7%	0.01	1.19	0.82–1.73
Multiple gestation pregnancy		9.7%	16.7%	<0.01	1.88	1.14–3.10

*Covariates in the adjusted logistic regression model. †Administered within 3 months of conception to assist in achieving ovulatory cycles. ‡In vitro fertilization.

and polycystic ovary morphology by ultrasound. Androgen excess was defined by acne, hirsutism, and/or elevated androgen levels. Polycystic ovary morphology was verified by imaging, except for 5% of the cohort where records were unavailable to verify reproductive endocrine documentation of polycystic-appearing ovaries [16]. Patient characteristics, including preconception body mass index (BMI), metformin, fertility drugs or *in vitro fertilization* [16, 17], family history of diabetes, and pharmacologic management of GDM, were ascertained by chart review and pharmacy records.

The diagnosis of GDM was based on a 3 hr 100 g oral glucose tolerance test (OGTT) using the American Diabetes Association criteria during the study period [8]. We additionally included women with 1 hr 50 g screening glucose ≥ 180 mg/dL (10 mmol/L) who were managed as GDM patients without a 3-hr OGTT ($N = 18$). Subsequent development of type 2 diabetes was established by laboratory evidence of fasting glucose ≥ 126 mg/dL (7.0 mmol/L), HbA1C ≥ 6.5%, or treatment with a hypoglycemic agent (insulin or glyburide), except during a subsequent GDM pregnancy. Metformin treatment in the absence of laboratory criteria did not qualify for diabetes, given its known use in PCOS management. When both fasting glucose and HbA1C criteria were met, the date of diabetes was determined by fasting glucose criteria.

2.1. Statistical Methods. Differences between subgroups were compared using chi-square, Fisher exact or Student's t-tests. Multivariable logistic regression was used to examine independent predictors of GDM. For women with PCOS who experienced a GDM pregnancy, the subsequent incidence of diabetes was calculated per 100 person-years. The association of GDM pharmacotherapy and risk of subsequent diabetes mellitus was examined using Cox proportional hazard analyses, adjusted for potential confounders. Analyses were performed using SAS version 9.3 (SAS Institute, Cary, NC) or STATA version 10.2 (College Station, TX); a two-sided p value of <0.05 was chosen as the criterion for statistical significance.

3. Results

Among 1023 women with PCOS and delivered pregnancy, 988 (96.6%) underwent GDM screening. The remaining 35 women not screened for GDM included 17 who delivered extremely preterm (≤29 weeks of gestation) and 11 who were managed presumptively as GDM patients. Among the 988 women screened for GDM, 174 (17.6%) met the GDM criteria based on the 3-hour OGTT [8] and 18 with 1-hour glucose ≥ 180 mg/dL (10.0 mmol/L) following 50 g oral glucose were managed as GDM patients without a 3-hour OGTT, yielding a total of 192 (19.4%) pregnant women with PCOS and GDM. Within this subset, 57 (29.7%) received pharmacologic treatment for GDM (insulin or glyburide).

As previously described [17], the cohort was racially/ethnically diverse, with 41.0% White, 25.5% Asian, 26.0% Hispanic, 3.9% Black, and 3.6% other race. The mean age was 31.4 ± 4.4 years, and 42.4% were obese. As expected, women with PCOS who had GDM were older and more likely to be Asian compared to those without GDM (Table 1). They were also more likely to be obese, have a family history of diabetes, receive preconception metformin, undergo fertility treatment, and experience multiple gestation. In multivariable logistic regression analyses adjusted for these clinical factors, predictors of GDM included older age, Asian race, family history of diabetes, moderate and

Table 2: Baseline characteristics and incident diabetes mellitus (DM) in women with polycystic ovary syndrome (PCOS) and gestational diabetes mellitus (GDM) pregnancy.

	186* PCOS women with GDM by subsequent DM status			Adjusted relative rate of DM following GDM pregnancy	
	No diabetes $N = 161$	Diabetes $N = 25$	p value	Adjusted hazard ratio	95% confidence interval
Age, years (mean ± standard deviation)	32.9 ± 4.1	33.3 ± 3.4	0.57	1.01	0.91–1.12
Race/ethnicity					
White	31.1%	32.0%		Referent	
Black	3.1%	0.0%		—[$]	
Hispanic	23.0%	40.0%	0.44	1.38[$]	0.51–3.74
Asian	39.8%	28.0%		1.96	0.55–6.94
Other	3.1%	0.0%		—[$]	
Prepregnancy BMI (kg/m^2)	31.6 ± 7.6	37.5 ± 7.1	<0.01	1.09	1.03–1.15
Family history of diabetes	62.7%	80.0%	0.12	1.59	0.56–4.46
Preconception metformin[†]	34.2%	48.0%	0.18	0.91	0.39–2.11
Pharmacologic treatment for GDM	23.6%	60.0%	<0.01	4.10	1.75–9.57

*One woman with no follow-up after delivery and 5 women with incident DM during the first year after delivery were not included. †Administered within 3 months of conception to assist in achieving ovulation. $Women of other ($N = 5$) or Black ($N = 5$) race were included with the 47 women of Hispanic ethnicity for these analyses.

severe prepregnancy obesity, preconception metformin use, and multiple gestation, with severe obesity and Asian race as the strongest risk factors (Table 1). Although treatment with fertility drugs or in vitro fertilization for conception may be markers for PCOS severity (and hence metabolic perturbation), fertility treatment was no longer associated with risk of GDM in adjusted analyses.

Among the 192 women with PCOS and GDM pregnancy, 191 (99.5%) remained health plan members following delivery. There were five incident cases of type 2 diabetes within the first year, followed by 25 cases during follow-up. Because these five cases may represent preexisting undiagnosed diabetes, the remaining analyses focus on the 25 incident cases beyond the first year among 186 PCOS GDM women (total follow-up 951.9 person-years). Those who developed diabetes had significantly higher BMI and were much more likely to have received pharmacologic therapy for GDM, whereas differences in preconception metformin use and family history of diabetes were not significant (Table 2).

Figure 1 shows the incidence of diabetes per year of follow-up for the first five years after pregnancy delivery. The overall incidence of diabetes was 2.8 (CI 1.9–4.2) per 100 person-years during follow-up through 2010. The overall incidence was more than 4-fold higher if pharmacologic GDM treatment was required (6.6 versus 1.5 per 100 person-years, $p < 0.01$) compared to no pharmacologic treatment for GDM. Among the 122 women with PCOS and GDM who had complete 5-year follow-up postdelivery, the cumulative 5-year risk of diabetes was 13.1% overall and 27.0% versus 7.1% ($p < 0.01$) for those with and without pharmacologic GDM treatment, respectively. Adjusted for age, race/ethnicity, prepregnancy BMI, family history of diabetes, and preconception metformin use, pharmacologic treatment for GDM was associated with a 4-fold higher rate of incident diabetes (hazard ratio 4.1, CI 1.8–9.6; Table 2).

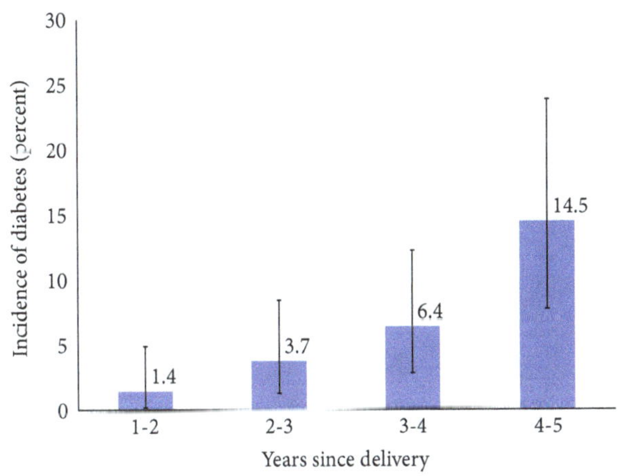

Figure 1: Incidence of diabetes mellitus by year of follow-up after pregnancy delivery among women with PCOS and gestational diabetes mellitus.

4. Discussion

Among nearly 1000 women with Rotterdam diagnosis-confirmed PCOS, we found a high prevalence of GDM at 19%, 2-3 times higher than the KPNC background rate of 6%–8% [18]. Our prevalence of GDM among women with PCOS is higher than previously estimated at 14% when PCOS was identified solely by coded diagnosis [3], without chart review for greater cohort specificity. We found that women with PCOS who were of Asian race had significantly higher risk of GDM, consistent with previous observations for the general population [18]. For women with PCOS who experienced a GDM pregnancy, the subsequent incidence of diabetes was 2.8 per 100 person-years overall and fourfold higher if pharmacologic treatment for GDM was required. In other GDM cohorts not selected for

PCOS, insulin therapy has been associated with 3-5-fold higher risk of postdelivery diabetes compared to no insulin therapy [19–21].

It is estimated that 10%–50% of women with GDM develop diabetes during the 5-year interval following delivery [12, 22]. A prospective study that excluded preexisting diabetes based on prepregnancy glycemia measurements reported a diabetes incidence rate of 1.8 per 100 person-years among GDM women assessed on average within ten years after their last pregnancy [11]. Diabetes incidence rates of 1.7–2.2 per 100 person-years have also been reported in other GDM populations not selected for PCOS status [12, 13]. Our data suggest the risk of diabetes among PCOS women with prior GDM is much higher. While racial/ethnic differences in diabetes risk were not observed in our study, the numbers within each non-White subgroup were limited. Others have found differential diabetes risk conferred by GDM pregnancy for White compared to Asian women [23] and higher risk among African American women [24], not considering PCOS status. While Asian race is a predictor of GDM in women with PCOS [5], among the broader population of women with GDM irrespective of PCOS status, Asian race is also a predictor of subsequent type 2 diabetes [12].

Our study has some limitations. Although postpartum diabetes surveillance is likely greater for PCOS women, the variable rate of diabetes screening in routine clinical care during the period of our study (including the use of fasting glucose and/or hemoglobin A1C rather than that of an oral glucose tolerance test) may contribute to potential underestimation of diabetes incidence. Furthermore, women diagnosed with diabetes in their first postpartum year were not included. We also did not examine relevant postpartum factors such as weight trajectory (or postpartum weight retention), physical activity, lactation, or subsequent reproductive care (including metformin) that may have influenced diabetes risk. Nonetheless, this is one of the first studies from a large US healthcare delivery system examining GDM and subsequent diabetes risk in women with chart-confirmed PCOS, where receipt of pharmacologic GDM therapy was associated with a 4-fold higher risk of subsequent diabetes. Collectively, these findings emphasize the importance of systematic diabetes screening in this high-risk population [1] and further studies examining racial/ethnic differences in the outcome, the role of androgen excess, weight status, and modifiable risk factors.

Conflicts of Interest

Joan C. Lo has received research funding from Amgen and Sanofi, and Assiamira Ferrara has received research funding from Takeda, unrelated to this study. The remaining authors have nothing to disclose.

Acknowledgments

The authors thank Drs. Seth Feigenbaum, Grace Lee, and Susan Peng for the physician chart review. This study was funded by the National Institute of Child Health and Human Development, National Institute of Health (R01HD052966).

References

[1] R. S. Legro, S. A. Arslanian, D. A. Ehrmann et al., "Diagnosis and treatment of polycystic ovary syndrome: an endocrine society clinical practice guideline," *The Journal of Clinical Endocrinology and Metabolism*, vol. 98, no. 12, pp. 4565–4592, 2013.

[2] B. C. Fauser, B. C. Tarlatzis, R. W. Rebar et al., "Consensus on women's health aspects of polycystic ovary syndrome (PCOS): the Amsterdam ESHRE/ASRM-Sponsored 3rd PCOS Consensus Workshop Group," *Fertility and Sterility*, vol. 97, no. 1, pp. 28–38.e25, 2012, e25.

[3] J. C. Lo, S. L. Feigenbaum, G. J. Escobar, J. Yang, Y. M. Crites, and A. Ferrara, "Increased prevalence of gestational diabetes mellitus among women with diagnosed polycystic ovary syndrome: a population-based study," *Diabetes Care*, vol. 29, no. 8, pp. 1915–1917, 2006.

[4] M. Ashrafi, F. Sheikhan, A. Arabipoor, R. Hosseini, F. Nourbakhsh, and Z. Zolfaghari, "Gestational diabetes mellitus risk factors in women with polycystic ovary syndrome (PCOS)," *European Journal of Obstetrics, Gynecology, and Reproductive Biology*, vol. 181, pp. 195–199, 2014.

[5] M. L. Pan, L. R. Chen, H. M. Tsao, and K. H. Chen, "Relationship between polycystic ovarian syndrome and subsequent gestational diabetes mellitus: a nationwide population-based study," *PLoS One*, vol. 10, no. 10, article e0140544, 2015.

[6] Y. J. Zhang, H. Jin, Z. L. Qin et al., "Predictors of gestational diabetes mellitus in Chinese women with polycystic ovary syndrome: a cross-sectional study," *Gynecologic and Obstetric Investigation*, vol. 81, no. 3, pp. 220–224, 2016.

[7] A. E. Joham, S. Ranasinha, S. Zoungas, L. Moran, and H. J. Teede, "Gestational diabetes and type 2 diabetes in reproductive-aged women with polycystic ovary syndrome," *The Journal of Clinical Endocrinology and Metabolism*, vol. 99, no. 3, pp. E447–E452, 2014.

[8] American Diabetes Association, "Gestational diabetes mellitus," *Diabetes Care*, vol. 27, Supplement 1, pp. S88–S90, 2004.

[9] The Rotterdam ESHRE/ASRM-Sponsored PCOS Consensus Workshop Group, "Revised 2003 consensus on diagnostic criteria and long-term health risks related to polycystic ovary syndrome," *Fertility and Sterility*, vol. 81, no. 1, pp. 19–25, 2004.

[10] L. Bellamy, J. P. Casas, A. D. Hingorani, and D. Williams, "Type 2 diabetes mellitus after gestational diabetes: a systematic review and meta-analysis," *Lancet*, vol. 373, no. 9677, pp. 1773–1779, 2009.

[11] E. P. Gunderson, C. E. Lewis, A. L. Tsai et al., "A 20-year prospective study of childbearing and incidence of diabetes in young women, controlling for glycemia before conception: the Coronary Artery Risk Development in Young Adults (CARDIA) Study," *Diabetes*, vol. 56, no. 12, pp. 2990–2996, 2007.

[12] A. J. Lee, R. J. Hiscock, P. Wein, S. P. Walker, and M. Permezel, "Gestational diabetes mellitus: clinical predictors and long-term risk of developing type 2 diabetes: a retrospective cohort study using survival analysis," *Diabetes Care*, vol. 30, no. 4, pp. 878–883, 2007.

[13] A. H. Xiang, B. H. Li, M. H. Black et al., "Racial and ethnic disparities in diabetes risk after gestational diabetes mellitus," *Diabetologia*, vol. 54, no. 12, pp. 3016–3021, 2011.

[14] S. Palomba, A. Falbo, T. Russo et al., "The risk of a persistent glucose metabolism impairment after gestational diabetes mellitus is increased in patients with polycystic ovary syndrome," *Diabetes Care*, vol. 35, no. 4, pp. 861–867, 2012.

[15] C. Capula, E. Chiefari, A. Vero, D. P. Foti, A. Brunetti, and R. Vero, "Prevalence and predictors of postpartum glucose intolerance in Italian women with gestational diabetes mellitus," *Diabetes Research and Clinical Practice*, vol. 105, no. 2, pp. 223–230, 2014.

[16] S. L. Feigenbaum, Y. Crites, M. K. Hararah, M. P. Yamamoto, J. Yang, and J. C. Lo, "Prevalence of cervical insufficiency in polycystic ovarian syndrome," *Human Reproduction*, vol. 27, no. 9, pp. 2837–2842, 2012.

[17] M. Yamamoto, S. L. Feigenbaum, Y. Crites et al., "Risk of preterm delivery in non-diabetic women with polycystic ovarian syndrome," *Journal of Perinatology*, vol. 32, no. 10, pp. 770–776, 2012.

[18] A. Ferrara, H. S. Kahn, C. P. Quesenberry, C. Riley, and M. M. Hedderson, "An increase in the incidence of gestational diabetes mellitus: Northern California, 1991-2000," *Obstetrics & Gynecology*, vol. 103, no. 3, pp. 526–533, 2004.

[19] K. Baptiste-Roberts, B. B. Barone, T. L. Gary et al., "Risk factors for type 2 diabetes among women with gestational diabetes: a systematic review," *The American Journal of Medicine*, vol. 122, no. 3, pp. 207–214.e4, 2009, e204.

[20] N. W. Cheung and D. Helmink, "Gestational diabetes: the significance of persistent fasting hyperglycemia for the subsequent development of diabetes mellitus," *Journal of Diabetes and its Complications*, vol. 20, no. 1, pp. 21–25, 2006.

[21] K. Lobner, A. Knopff, A. Baumgarten et al., "Predictors of postpartum diabetes in women with gestational diabetes mellitus," *Diabetes*, vol. 55, no. 3, pp. 792–797, 2006.

[22] C. Kim, K. M. Newton, and R. H. Knopp, "Gestational diabetes and the incidence of type 2 diabetes: a systematic review," *Diabetes Care*, vol. 25, no. 10, pp. 1862–1868, 2002.

[23] G. Mukerji, M. Chiu, and B. R. Shah, "Impact of gestational diabetes on the risk of diabetes following pregnancy among Chinese and South Asian women," *Diabetologia*, vol. 55, no. 8, pp. 2148–2153, 2012.

[24] Y. Wang, L. Chen, R. Horswell et al., "Racial differences in the association between gestational diabetes mellitus and risk of type 2 diabetes," *Journal of Women's Health*, vol. 21, no. 6, pp. 628–633, 2012.

8

Height and Risk of Gestational Diabetes Mellitus: Results from the Healthy Baby Cohort Study

Hui Li,[1] Lulu Song,[1] Lijun Shen,[1] Bingqing Liu,[1] Xiaoxuan Zheng,[1] Lina Zhang,[1] Youjie Wang ,[1] Zhongqiang Cao ,[2] and Shunqing Xu[3]

[1]*Department of Maternal and Child Health, School of Public Health, Tongji Medical College, Huazhong University of Science and Technology, Wuhan, Hubei 430030, China*
[2]*Wuhan Children's Hospital (Wuhan Maternal and Child Healthcare Hospital), Tongji Medical College, Huazhong University of Science and Technology, Wuhan, Hubei 430030, China*
[3]*Key Laboratory of Environment and Health, Ministry of Education & Ministry of Environmental Protection, and State Key Laboratory of Environmental Health, School of Public Health, Tongji Medical College, Huazhong University of Science and Technology, Wuhan, Hubei 430030, China*

Correspondence should be addressed to Youjie Wang; wangyoujie@mails.tjmu.edu.cn and Zhongqiang Cao; bestfriends985@163.com

Academic Editor: Daniela Foti

Background. The aim of this study was to examine the association between height and plasma glucose level, as well as risk of GDM among Chinese women. *Methods.* A total of 6941 pregnant Chinese women were recruited from the Healthy Baby Cohort study in Hubei Province, China, in 2012–2014. Measured height was categorized into four groups according to the quartile distribution (≤158.0 cm, 158.1–161.0 cm, 161.1–164.0 cm, and >164.0 cm). GDM was defined based on the International Association of the Diabetes in Pregnancy Study Group criteria. Linear regression was used to estimate the association between height and plasma glucose levels. Logistic regression was used to calculate odds ratios (ORs) and 95% confidence intervals (CIs) for the association between height and GDM. *Results.* The prevalence of GDM was 14.7% in our study. Height was inversely associated with the 1 h and 2h plasma glucose levels (all P value for trend < 0.05), but not with fasting plasma glucose levels. A significant negative trend was found between height and risk of GDM (P value for trend < 0.05), and each centimeter increase in height was associated with 2% (OR: 0.98; 95% CI: 0.96, 0.99) lower risk of GDM. Women in the highest quartile of height (>164.0 cm) had 23% (OR: 0.77; 95% CI: 0.64, 0.94) lower risk of developing GDM than those in the shortest quartile of height (≤158.0 cm), after adjusting for potential confounders. *Conclusions.* Our findings suggested that height was negatively associated with risk of GDM among Chinese women. The difference in plasma glucose levels is present in the 1 h and 2 h plasma glucose, but not with fasting plasma glucose.

1. Introduction

Gestational diabetes mellitus (GDM) is characterized by glucose intolerance with onset or first recognition during pregnancy [1]. The prevalence of GDM ranged from 9.3% to 25.5% among 15 collaborating centers using the International Association of the Diabetes and Pregnancy Study Group (IADPSG) criteria [2]. GDM is not only related to adverse pregnancy outcomes [3] but it is also associated with adverse long-term health effects on both mothers and their offspring [4, 5]. Identification of women at risk of GDM may allow early health monitoring and intervention.

Adult height is determined by the combination of genetic and environmental factors [6]. Studies have suggested that height was negatively associated with glucose tolerance in adults [7, 8]. Furthermore, a meta-analysis has demonstrated that shorter height was associated with the development of type 2 diabetes [9]. Given that GDM and type 2 diabetes share several similar pathogenic processes [10, 11], it is plausible that shorter height may also increase the risk of GDM.

Previous studies have shown an inverse relationship between height and risk of GDM in several countries [7, 12–15], but not all [16, 17]. However, due to the variations in height among different ethnic and socioeconomic groups [14], their results might not generalize to Chinese women. In addition, the different diagnostic criteria for GDM may affect the results. To our knowledge, the association between height and risk of GDM using the International Association of the Diabetes in Pregnancy Study Group (IADPSG) criteria has not been previously investigated in the Chinese population.

Therefore, we examined the association between height and plasma glucose level, as well as risk of GDM among pregnant Chinese women based on data from the Healthy Baby Cohort (HBC) study.

2. Methods

2.1. Study Participants. The HBC study was conducted at the Women and Children Medical and Healthcare Center of Wuhan City in the Hubei Province, China. This ongoing prospective cohort study is designed to assess the environmental and genetic factors that affect child health and development. Briefly, a total of 11,311 pregnant women who gave birth at this hospital were recruited between September 2012 and October 2014. Each participant was required to provide blood and urine samples and complete a standard questionnaire by a face-to-face interview at the time of institutional delivery. In the present study, we excluded participants with a history of diabetes ($n = 6$), those with missing information on height or other important covariates ($n = 70$), or those with missing values for fasting, 1 h, and 2 h plasma glucose ($n = 4294$). The final analytic sample included 6941 women. Except for alcohol consumption before pregnancy, the main characteristics of the women with OGTT results (6941) and the women without OGTT results (4294) on height (161.26 ± 4.52 cm versus 161.06 ± 4.54 cm), age at delivery (28.48 ± 3.46 years versus 27.77 ± 4.01 years), prepregnancy BMI (20.69 ± 2.75 kg/m^2 versus 20.27 ± 2.59 kg/m^2), education level (college or above rate: 73.6% versus 76.5%), employment status (employed rate: 84.4% versus 74.7%), exposure to passive smoking during pregnancy (88.3% versus 86.2%), smoking before pregnancy (0.5% versus 1.1%), and taking physical activity (yes: 87.7% versus 89.4%) were statistically different.

The study was approved by the Medical Ethics Committee of the School of Public Health, Tongji Medical College, Huazhong University of Science and Technology. All participants provided written informed consent at recruitment.

2.2. Assessment of Height. The height was measured without shoes, using a stadiometer, and recorded to the nearest 0.1 centimeter (cm) during the first antenatal care visit in the hospital. We categorized height into four groups according to the quartile distribution (≤158.0 cm, 158.1–161.0 cm, 161.1–164.0 cm, and >164.0 cm).

2.3. Diagnosis of GDM. In this study, all pregnant women underwent a 75 g 2 h oral glucose tolerance test (OGTT) in the morning after overnight fasting of at least 8 hours at 24–28 gestational weeks. Fasting, 1 h, and 2 h plasma glucose levels were measured at the Women and Children Medical and Healthcare Center of Wuhan City using the Roche Modular P800 Automatic Biochemistry Analyzer. According o the IADPSG criteria [18], women were diagnosed with GDM if they met any of the following cutoff points: fasting plasma glucose ≥ 5.1 mmol/l, 1 h plasma glucose ≥ 10.0 mmol/l, or 2 h plasma glucose ≥ 8.5 mmol/l.

2.4. Assessment of Covariates. Data on demographic characteristics (maternal age, educational level, and employment status) and lifestyle factors (alcohol consumption before pregnancy, smoking before pregnancy, passive smoking during pregnancy, and physical activity during pregnancy) were collected by questionnaires. Passive smoking was defined as exposure second-hand smoking more than once per week and for >15 min per time. Information on parity was obtained from medical records. Prepregnancy weight was self-reported at the first antenatal care visit (usually at the first trimester). Prepregnancy body mass index (BMI) was calculated as self-reported prepregnancy weight in kilograms divided by the measured height in square meters.

2.5. Statistical Analysis. Continuous variables were described as mean ± standard deviation (SD), and categorical variables were presented as a number and percentage. To compare the differences between the GDM group and non-GDM group, Student's t-test was used for continuous variables, and chi-square test was used for categorical variables.

Differences in mean fasting, 1 h, and 2 h plasma glucose levels among height quartiles were compared by analysis of covariance. Dunnett's test was used for post hoc analysis. Linear regression models were used to estimate the association of fasting, 1 h, and 2 h plasma glucose levels with height. Logistic regression models were used to estimate odds ratios (ORs) and 95% confidence intervals (CIs) for the association between height and risk of GDM. Models were fit using height as a categorical variable, based on the quartile distribution of height, and the lowest quartile was used as the reference group. Covariates was selected based on established or potential associations with GDM [4, 5], including maternal age (continuous), prepregnancy BMI (continuous), educational level (high school or below, college or above), employment status (employed or unemployed), parity (primiparous or multiparous), alcohol consumption before pregnancy (yes or no), smoking before pregnancy (yes or no), passive smoking during pregnancy (yes or no), and physical activity frequency during pregnancy (never/rarely, 1-2 days/week, 3-4 days/week, and 5-6 days/week or daily). In order to test for linear trend between height and plasma glucose levels or risk of GDM, we estimated the statistical significance by assigning the median values of each quartile of maternal height and fitting this as a continuous variable in a separate regression model.

To assess a potential effect modification, we performed subgroup analyses to examine the association between height and risk of GDM stratified by maternal age (<28 or ≥28 years, the median value of age at delivery), prepregnancy BMI (<24

Table 1: Characteristics of the study participants according to occurrence of gestational diabetes mellitus.

	GDM	Non-GDM	P value
Number of participants	1017	5924	—
Age at delivery (years)	29.56 ± 3.88	28.30 ± 3.35	<0.001[a]
Height (cm)	160.80 ± 4.63	161.34 ± 4.50	<0.001[a]
Prepregnancy BMI (kg/m^2)	21.52 ± 3.08	20.55 ± 2.66	<0.001[a]
Educational level			<0.001[b]
High school or below	319 (31.4)	1513 (25.5)	
College or above	698 (68.6)	4411 (74.5)	
Employment status			0.006[b]
Employed	829 (81.5)	5030 (84.9)	
Unemployed	188 (18.5)	894 (15.1)	
Parity			<0.001[b]
Primiparous	854 (84.0)	5365 (90.6)	
Multiparous	163 (16.0)	559 (9.4)	
Alcohol consumption before pregnancy			0.872[b]
Yes	21 (2.1)	127 (2.1)	
No	996 (97.9)	5797 (97.9)	
Smoking before pregnancy			0.263[b]
Yes	8 (0.8)	30 (0.5)	
No	1009 (99.2)	5894 (99.5)	
Passive smoking during pregnancy			0.461[b]
Yes	112 (11.0)	700 (11.8)	
No	905 (89.0)	5224 (88.2)	
Physical activity during pregnancy			0.510[b]
Never or rarely	105 (10.3)	631 (10.7)	
1-2 days/week	82 (8.1)	556 (9.4)	
3-4 days/week	83 (8.2)	426 (7.2)	
5-6 days/week	13 (1.3)	90 (1.5)	
Daily	734 (72.2)	4221 (71.3)	

Data are mean ± SD or numbers (percentages). BMI: body mass index; GDM: gestational diabetes mellitus. [a]Derived from Student's t-test. [b]Derived from chi-square test.

or ≥ 24 kg/m^2, the cutoff value of overweight for Chinese adults [19]), educational level (high school or below, college or above), and parity (primiparous or multiparous). Tests for interaction across subgroup were conducted using the Wald test.

All analyses were performed using SAS 9.4 software (SAS Institute Inc., Cary, NC, USA). A two-tailed P value < 0.05 was considered statistically significant.

3. Results

Among the 6941 women, the mean age at delivery was 28.5 (SD: 3.5) years, the mean height was 161.3 (SD: 4.5) cm, and 89.6% were primiparous. In total, 1017 (14.7%) women were diagnosed with GDM based on the IADPSG criteria used in the present study. Differences in distribution of the characteristics between GDM group and non-GDM group are presented in Table 1. Women with GDM were older and shorter, had lower educational level and higher prepregnancy BMI, and were more likely multiparous (all P values < 0.05).

Table 2 shows the mean fasting, 1 h, and 2 h plasma glucose levels according to height quartiles. Mean 1 h and 2 h plasma glucose levels decreased linearly with increasing height (all P values for trend < 0.001) without adjustment for confounders. After adjustment for potential confounders, the height was still inversely associated with the 1 h and 2 h plasma glucose levels (all P values for trend < 0.001). Post hoc analyses suggested that women with taller height had lower 1 h and 2 h plasma glucose levels than those with shorter height (158.1–161.0 cm versus ≤158.0 cm, $P < 0.05$; 161.1–164.0 cm versus ≤158.0 cm, $P < 0.05$; >164.0 cm versus ≤158.0 cm, $P < 0.05$).

Table 3 presents the relationship between height and fasting, 1 h, and 2 h plasma glucose levels. Linear associations of height with 1 h and 2 h plasma glucose levels were identified (all P values < 0.001). After controlling for potential confounders, every centimeter increase in height was

Table 2: Mean plasma glucose levels according to height quartiles.

Plasma glucose (mmol/l)	Height quartiles (cm) ≤158.0 n (1936)	158.1–161.0 n (1789)	161.1–164.0 n (1567)	>164.0 n (1649)	P for trend[b]
Unadjusted					
Fasting	4.44 ± 0.50	4.45 ± 0.53	4.44 ± 0.50	4.47 ± 0.50	0.253
1 h	7.36 ± 1.63	7.29 ± 1.67	7.22 ± 1.63[a]	7.12 ± 1.59[a]	<0.001
2 h	6.63 ± 1.36	6.51 ± 1.30[a]	6.40 ± 1.28[a]	6.34 ± 1.21[a]	<0.001
Adjusted for age, prepregnancy BMI, educational level, occupational status, parity, alcohol consumption before pregnancy, smoking before pregnancy, passive smoking during pregnancy, and physical activity during pregnancy					
Fasting	4.44 ± 0.48	4.45 ± 0.51	4.44 ± 0.51	4.47 ± 0.49	0.131
1 h	7.34 ± 1.58	7.29 ± 1.57	7.23 ± 1.58[a]	7.14 ± 1.58[a]	<0.001
2 h	6.61 ± 1.28	6.51 ± 1.27[a]	6.41 ± 1.27[a]	6.35 ± 1.26[a]	<0.001

Data are mean ± SD. [a]$P < 0.05$ for the comparison with the shortest quartile of height by using analysis of covariance and Dunnett's test for post hoc analysis. [b]P values for trend were performed by assigning the median values of each quartile of height and fitting this as a continuous variable in a separate regression model.

Table 3: Regression coefficients (95% CIs) of plasma glucose levels for every centimeter increase in height.

Plasma glucose (mmol/l)	Unadjusted regression coefficient[a] (95% CI)	P value	Adjusted regression coefficient[b] (95% CI)	P value
Fasting	0.0018 (−0.0009, 0.0045)	0.184	0.0023 (−0.0003, 0.0049)	0.087
1 h	−0.0197 (−0.0282, −0.0112)	<0.001	−0.0157 (−0.0240, −0.0075)	<0.001
2 h	−0.0256 (−0.0324, −0.0189)	<0.001	−0.0231 (−0.0297, −0.0165)	<0.001

CI: confidence intervals. [a]Not adjusted for any confounders. [b]Adjusted for maternal age, prepregnancy BMI, educational level, employment status, parity, alcohol consumption before pregnancy, smoking before pregnancy, passive smoking during pregnancy, and physical activity during pregnancy.

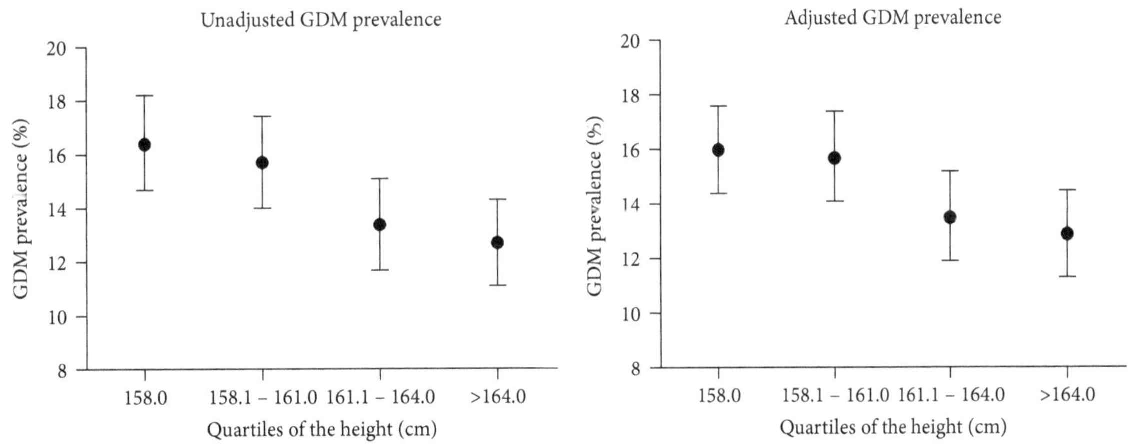

(a) Unadjusted GDM prevalence

(b) Adjusted GDM prevalence

Figure 1: Unadjusted and adjusted gestational diabetes mellitus (GDM) prevalence according to height quartiles. (a) Association between height and unadjusted prevalence of GDM; (b) association between height and prevalence of GDM after adjusting for maternal age, prepregnancy BMI, educational level, employment status, parity, alcohol consumption before pregnancy, smoking before pregnancy, passive smoking during pregnancy, and physical activity during pregnancy. The vertical bars are 95% confidence intervals.

associated with a linear change in 1 h plasma glucose levels with −0.0157 mmol/l (95% CI: −0.0240, −0.0075) and in 2 h plasma glucose levels with −0.0231 mmol/l (95% CI: −0.0297, −0.0165). No significant association was observed between height and fasting plasma glucose levels before and after adjusting for potential confounding variables.

The unadjusted and adjusted prevalence of GDM according to height quartiles are shown in Figure 1. There was a descending linear relationship between height and prevalence of GDM before and after adjustment for potential confounders (P value for trend < 0.05).

Table 4 shows the unadjusted and adjusted ORs and 95% CIs for GDM according to height quartiles. A significant negative trend was found between height and risk of GDM (P value for trend < 0.05), and each centimeter increase in height was associated with 2% (OR: 0.98; 95% CI: 0.96,

Table 4: ORs (95% CIs) for the association between height and gestational diabetes mellitus.

Height quartiles (cm)	Number of participants	Number of GDM cases	Unadjusted OR[a] (95% CI)	Adjusted OR[b] (95% CI)
≤158.0	1936	317	1.00 (reference)	1.00 (reference)
158.1–161.0	1789	281	0.95 (0.80, 1.13)	0.98 (0.82, 1.17)
161.1–164.0	1567	210	0.79 (0.65, 0.96)	0.82 (0.67, 0.99)
>164.0	1649	209	0.74 (0.61, 0.90)	0.77 (0.64, 0.94)
Per 1 cm increase in height	—	—	0.97 (0.96, 0.99)	0.98 (0.96, 0.99)
P values for trend[c]	—	—	<0.001	0.002

OR: odds ratio; CI: confidence intervals; GDM: gestational diabetes mellitus. [a]Not adjusted for any confounders. [b]Adjusted for maternal age, prepregnancy BMI, educational level, occupational status, parity, alcohol consumption before pregnancy, smoking before pregnancy, passive smoking during pregnancy, and physical activity during pregnancy. [c]*P* values for trend were performed by assigning the median values of each quartile of maternal height and fitted this as a continuous variable in a separate regression model.

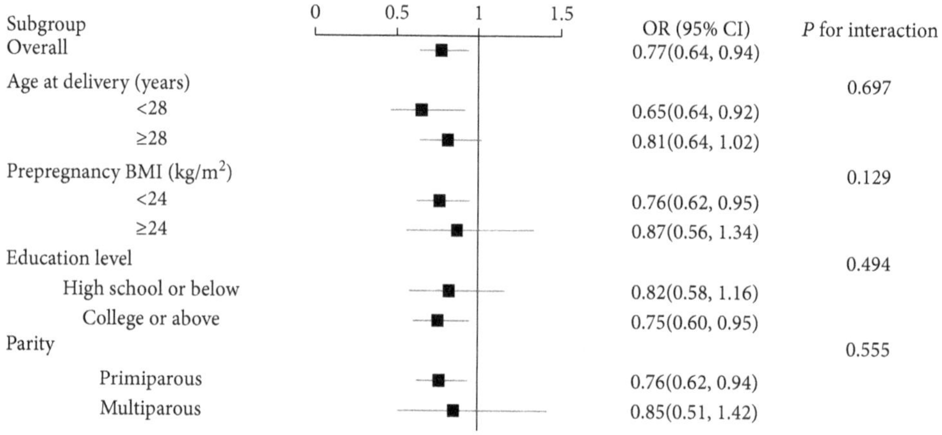

Figure 2: Subgroup analysis of associations between the highest quartile of height and gestational diabetes mellitus (GDM). Odds ratios for GDM are comparison of the highest quartile of height with the shortest quartile of height. Analyses were adjusted for maternal age, prepregnancy BMI, educational level, employment status, parity, alcohol consumption before pregnancy, smoking before pregnancy, passive smoking during pregnancy, and physical activity during pregnancy. Horizontal lines are 95% confidence intervals.

0.99) lower risk of GDM. After adjustment for potential confounders, women in the highest quartile of height (>164.0 cm) had lower risk of GDM with an adjusted OR of 0.77 (95% CI: 0.64, 0.94), compared with those in the shortest quartile height (≤158.0 cm).

3.1. Subgroup Analyses. The inverse relationship between height and risk of GDM was generally similar across the subgroup stratified by maternal age, prepregnancy BMI, educational level, and parity (all *P* values for interaction > 0.05) (Figure 2).

4. Discussion

In this study, we investigated the association between height and risk of GDM among Chinese women. We observed height was negatively associated with risk of GDM after adjustment for potential confounders. In addition, we found that height was inversely associated with the 1 h and 2 h plasma glucose levels, but not with fasting plasma glucose levels.

Several studies have investigated the association between height and GDM, and the findings were inconsistent. The Omega Cohort Study including 1644 American women suggested an inverse relationship between self-reported height and risk of GDM based on the National Diabetes Data Group (NDDG) diagnostic criteria independent of age, race/ethnicity, education, and prepregnancy BMI [12]. Similarly, the relationship between height and risk of GDM using the NDDG criteria was observed in a study of 2772 Greek women and a study of 9005 Korean women [7, 13]. A study recruited 126,861 American women and shown that the risk of GDM decreased linearly with increasing height using the American Diabetes Association Criteria [14]. However, in their study, height data were measured or self-reported. Branchtein et al. investigated 4973 Brazilian women and found a negative association between height and GDM using the 1988 World Health Organization (WHO) criteria [15]. In contrast, a study of 1635 women from Hungary reported no significant association between height and risk of GDM according to the 1998 WHO criteria [16]. The DALI study including 971 women found that decreased height was associated with significantly decreased risk of GDM using the IADPSG criteria [17]. These discrepancies across these studies may be due to the differences in height among ethnic groups, diagnostic criteria for GDM, race/ethnicity, and sample size.

The mechanisms underlying the relationship between height and risk of GDM are not clear. GDM is characterized by pancreatic β-cell dysfunction and insulin resistance [10]. Shorter adult stature predicts impaired β-cell function and insulin resistance [7, 20], which was associated with an increased risk of GDM. In addition, intrauterine nutrition and childhood nutrition are important determinants of adult height [6, 21]. Inadequate intrauterine and childhood nutrition might increase risk of diabetes during adulthood [22–24]. Our study had no information on intrauterine and childhood nutrition, which prevented us from exploring whether height or nutrition has an effect on GDM. Further studies are needed to investigate the association between height and risk of GDM independent of intrauterine and childhood nutrition.

Low socioeconomic status during childhood was reported to be related with shorter adult height [25]. Studies have suggested that individuals who grew up in low socioeconomic status were more likely to develop diabetes in later life [26, 27]. Given that educational level is considered as a reliable marker of socioeconomic status during childhood [28], we adjusted educational level in our study and found that the significant association between height and risk of GDM still remained. In addition, we performed a subgroup analysis according to educational level and found that the inverse association between height and risk of GDM was consistent across the subgroup stratified by educational level. Therefore, our results suggested that the association between height and risk of GDM could not be fully explained by socioeconomic status during childhood.

Interestingly, we observed that height was inversely correlated with 1 h and 2 h plasma glucose levels, but not with fasting plasma glucose levels. Our findings were in agreement with a study from Brazil, reporting a negative association of height with 1 h and 2 h plasma glucose levels but not with fasting glucose levels without adjusting any [15]. Similarly, two studies conducted in Australia and Poland suggested that shorter women have higher 2 h plasma glucose levels than taller women, but not fasting plasma glucose levels [29, 30].

We found height was negatively associated with 1 h and 2 h plasma glucose, but not with fasting plasma glucose. A possible reason for this may be the different metabolisms of a standard dose of glucose during OGTT among taller and shorter women. Women with shorter stature have a lower mass of metabolically active tissues in response to a 75 g OGTT compared with women with taller stature [31].

Our study had several strengths, including a large sample size and a wide range of potential confounders. In addition, the diagnosis of GDM in our study was based on the measure of OGTT, performed with unified instruments at one hospital, which minimized the misclassification of GDM and non-GDM cases.

However, some limitations should be considered. First, some characteristics of the women with OGTT results and without OGTT results were statistically different, which might introduce selection bias, potentially reducing the generalization of this analysis. However, the differences were relatively small. Due to the large sample of the women with OGTT results (6941) and the women without OGTT results (4294), a slight difference would lead to a P value < 0.05. Moreover, the participants did not know the research purpose at the stage of data collecting; it was unlikely that women with shorter height tended to take or not take the OGTT test in this study. Second, although a variety of known risk factors of GDM were taken into account in the analyses of our study, it is not possible to rule out the residual confounding attributable to unmeasured factors, such as early-life nutrition factors, history of GDM, family history of diabetes, and maternal dietary intakes during pregnancy. Third, height and GDM might be jointly determined by genetic factors, but we are unable to examine their association.

5. Conclusion

Our result suggested that height was negatively associated with risk of GDM in pregnant Chinese women, independent of potential confounders. The difference in plasma glucose levels is present in the 1 h and 2 h plasma glucose, but not with fasting plasma glucose.

Conflicts of Interest

None of the authors had any personal or financial conflicts of interest.

Acknowledgments

The authors gratefully thank all the participants from the Healthy Baby Cohort and the staffs of the Women and Children Medical and Healthcare Center of Wuhan. This study was supported by the National Natural Science Foundation of China (91643207, 81273083) and Hubei Province Health & Family Planning Scientific Research Project (WJ2017Z001).

References

[1] American Diabetes Association, "Diagnosis and classification of diabetes mellitus," *Diabetes Care*, vol. 37, Supplement 1, pp. S81–S90, 2014.

[2] D. A. Sacks, D. R. Hadden, M. Maresh et al., "Frequency of gestational diabetes mellitus at collaborating centers based on IADPSG consensus panel–recommended criteria: the Hyperglycemia and Adverse Pregnancy Outcome (HAPO) study," *Diabetes Care*, vol. 35, no. 3, pp. 526–528, 2012.

[3] M. I. Schmidt, B. B. Duncan, A. J. Reichelt et al., "Gestational diabetes mellitus diagnosed with a 2-h 75-g oral glucose tolerance test and adverse pregnancy outcomes," *Diabetes Care*, vol. 24, no. 7, pp. 1151–1155, 2001.

[4] E. A. Reece, G. Leguizamón, and A. Wiznitzer, "Gestational diabetes: the need for a common ground," *Lancet*, vol. 373, no. 9677, pp. 1789–1797, 2009.

[5] T. A. Buchanan, A. H. Xiang, and K. A. Page, "Gestational diabetes mellitus: risks and management during and after pregnancy," *Nature Reviews Endocrinology*, vol. 8, no. 11, pp. 639–649, 2012.

[6] K. Silventoinen, "Determinants of variation in adult body height," *Journal of Biosocial Science*, vol. 35, no. 2, pp. 263–285, 2003.

[7] E. Anastasiou, M. Alevizaki, S. J. Grigorakis, G. Philippou, M. Kyprianou, and A. Souvatzoglou, "Decreased stature in gestational diabetes mellitus," *Diabetologia*, vol. 41, no. 9, pp. 997–1001, 1998.

[8] D. C. Brown, C. D. Byrne, P. M. S. Clark et al., "Height and glucose tolerance in adult subjects," *Diabetologia*, vol. 34, no. 7, pp. 531–533, 1991.

[9] M. Janghorbani, F. Momeni, and M. Dehghani, "Hip circumference, height and risk of type 2 diabetes: systematic review and meta-analysis," *Obesity Reviews*, vol. 13, no. 12, pp. 1172–1181, 2012.

[10] C. D. Malchoff, "Diagnosis and classification of diabetes mellitus," *Diabetes Care*, vol. 35, Supplement 1, pp. S64–S71, 2012.

[11] S. E. Kahn, "The relative contributions of insulin resistance and beta-cell dysfunction to the pathophysiology of type 2 diabetes," *Diabetologia*, vol. 46, no. 1, pp. 3–19, 2003.

[12] C. B. Rudra, T. K. Sorensen, W. M. Leisenring, E. Dashow, and M. A. Williams, "Weight characteristics and height in relation to risk of gestational diabetes mellitus," *American Journal of Epidemiology*, vol. 165, no. 3, pp. 302–308, 2007.

[13] H. C. Jang, H. K. Min, H. K. Lee, N. H. Cho, and B. E. Metzger, "Short stature in Korean women: a contribution to the multifactorial predisposition to gestational diabetes mellitus," *Diabetologia*, vol. 41, no. 7, pp. 778–783, 1998.

[14] J. Brite, E. J. Shiroma, K. Bowers et al., "Height and the risk of gestational diabetes: variations by race/ethnicity," *Diabetic Medicine*, vol. 31, no. 3, pp. 332–340, 2014.

[15] L. Branchtein, M. I. Schmidt, M. C. G. Matos et al., "Short stature and gestational diabetes in Brazil," *Diabetologia*, vol. 43, no. 7, pp. 848–851, 2000.

[16] Á. G. Tabák, Z. Kerényi, E. Nagy, Z. Bosnyák, E. Madarasz, and G. Tamás, "Height and gestational diabetes mellitus," *Diabetic Medicine*, vol. 19, no. 4, pp. 344-345, 2002.

[17] L. Mendoza, J. Harreiter, D. Simmons et al., "Risk factors for hyperglycemia in pregnancy in the DALI study differ by period of pregnancy and OGTT time point," *European Journal of Endocrinology*, vol. 179, no. 1, pp. 39–49, 2018.

[18] International Association of Diabetes and Pregnancy Study Groups Consensus Panel, B. E. Metzger, S. G. Gabbe et al., "International association of diabetes and pregnancy study groups recommendations on the diagnosis and classification of hyperglycemia in pregnancy," *Diabetes Care*, vol. 33, no. 3, pp. 676–682, 2010.

[19] C. Chen and F. Lu, "The guidelines for prevention and control of overweight and obesity in Chinese adults," *Biomedical and Environmental Sciences*, vol. 17, pp. 1–36, 2003.

[20] J. Vangipurapu, A. Stancakova, R. Jauhiainen, J. Kuusisto, and M. Laakso, "Short adult stature predicts impaired beta-cell function, insulin resistance, Glycemia, and type 2 diabetes in Finnish men," *The Journal of Clinical Endocrinology and Metabolism*, pp. jc.2016–jc.2933, 2016.

[21] J. M. Perkins, S. V. Subramanian, G. Davey Smith, and E. Ozaltin, "Adult height, nutrition, and population health," *Nutrition Reviews*, vol. 74, no. 3, pp. 149–165, 2016.

[22] E. H. Yeung, F. B. Hu, C. G. Solomon et al., "Life-course weight characteristics and the risk of gestational diabetes," *Diabetologia*, vol. 53, no. 4, pp. 668–678, 2010.

[23] D. J. P. Barker, K. M. Godfrey, P. D. Gluckman, J. E. Harding, J. A. Owens, and J. S. Robinson, "Fetal nutrition and cardiovascular disease in adult life," *Lancet*, vol. 341, no. 8850, pp. 938–941, 1993.

[24] S. Bartz and M. Freemark, "Pathogenesis and prevention of type 2 diabetes: parental determinants, breastfeeding, and early childhood nutrition," *Current Diabetes Reports*, vol. 12, no. 1, pp. 82–87, 2012.

[25] A. J. Barros, C. G. Victora, B. L. Horta, H. D. Goncalves, R. C. Lima, and J. Lynch, "Effects of socioeconomic change from birth to early adulthood on height and overweight," *International Journal of Epidemiology*, vol. 35, no. 5, pp. 1233–1238, 2006.

[26] V. Tsenkova, T. Pudrovska, and A. Karlamangla, "Childhood socioeconomic disadvantage and prediabetes and diabetes in later life: a study of biopsychosocial pathways," *Psychosomatic Medicine*, vol. 76, no. 8, pp. 622–628, 2014.

[27] S. Stringhini, G. D. Batty, P. Bovet et al., "Association of lifecourse socioeconomic status with chronic inflammation and type 2 diabetes risk: the Whitehall II prospective cohort study," *PLoS Medicine*, vol. 10, no. 7, article e1001479, 2013.

[28] D. Blane and I. White, *Education, Social Circumstances and Mortality. Health and Social Organization: Towards a Health Policy for the Twenty-First Century.*, pp. 171–187, Routledge, London, 1996.

[29] R. G. Moses and M. T. Mackay, "Gestational diabetes: is there a relationship between leg length and glucose tolerance?," *Diabetes Care*, vol. 27, no. 5, pp. 1033–1035, 2004.

[30] J. Ogonowski and T. Miazgowski, "Are short women at risk for gestational diabetes mellitus?," *European Journal of Endocrinology*, vol. 162, no. 3, pp. 491–497, 2010.

[31] W. Rathmann, K. Strassburger, G. Giani, A. Doring, and C. Meisinger, "Differences in height explain gender differences in the response to the oral glucose tolerance test," *Diabetic Medicine*, vol. 25, no. 11, pp. 1374–13755, 2008.

Temporal Trends in Gestational Diabetes Prevalence, Treatment, and Outcomes at Aarhus University Hospital, Skejby, between 2004 and 2016

Per Glud Ovesen,[1] Jens Fuglsang,[1] Mette Bisgaard Andersen,[1] Charlotte Wolff,[1] Olav Bjørn Petersen,[1] and H. David McIntyre[2,3]

[1]*Department of Obstetrics and Gynecology, Aarhus University Hospital, Aarhus, Denmark*
[2]*Faculty of Medicine, University of Queensland, Brisbane, QLD, Australia*
[3]*Danish Diabetes Academy, Odense University Hospital, Odense, Denmark*

Correspondence should be addressed to Per Glud Ovesen; per.ovesen@dadlnet.dk

Academic Editor: Eusebio Chiefari

Background. The prevalence of gestational diabetes (GDM) is increasing worldwide. The most important risk of GDM in pregnancy is excessive fetal growth, increasing the risk of complications during delivery as well as long-term complications like obesity and diabetes in both the mother and the offspring. *Method.* All women with GDM who delivered a singleton between 2004 and 2016 were included. The treatment of GDM patients sought to achieve normal blood glucose levels, primarily by diet and exercise. If the glycemic targets were not reached, insulin therapy was initiated. Birth weight and birth weight Z-score was calculated corrected for gender and gestational age at delivery. *Results.* The study included 1910 women. The number of GDM women increased significantly each year over the course of the study, as did the proportion requiring insulin therapy. Birth weight and birth weight Z-score fell significantly over the years largely due to a decrease in large for gestational age frequency from 29% to around 19%. *Conclusion.* During the last 13 years, the number of women diagnosed with GDM has increased. Furthermore, the proportion of GDM women receiving insulin treatment has increased. The birth weight in diet-treated women has been virtually normal for the last 5 years of the reported period.

1. Introduction

The prevalence of gestational diabetes (GDM) has been increasing in many parts of the world, with much of this increase attributed to increasing maternal overweight and obesity during pregnancy and to older age at child bearing [1–3].

The most important risk of GDM in pregnancy is excessive fetal growth. Glucose passes through the placenta to the fetus and consequently the fetus develops hyperinsulinemia. Insulin stimulates fetal growth and the extra glucose is stored as body fat causing macrosomia and increasing the risk of birth trauma, shoulder dystocia, and delivery by caesarean section. Long-term complications include the risk of diabetes in the mother and obesity and diabetes in the offspring. Many reports from the last two decades have outlined such risks, thereby emphasizing the need for attention and intervention to address such complications. In this report, we describe the temporal trends for women with GDM in a Danish university hospital setting.

Differing criteria for GDM diagnosis [4, 5] make global comparisons difficult, but in Aarhus, Denmark, the same criterion for GDM diagnosis (2-hour venous plasma glucose after a 75 g glucose load $\geq$ 9.0 mmol/L) has been used since 2004 [6]. This retrospective cohort study from the Aarhus University Hospital at Skejby aims to document the temporal trends in GDM prevalence, describe patterns of GDM treatment, and outline the pregnancy outcomes for women with GDM and their babies from 2004 to 2016.

Aarhus University Hospital, Skejby, is the principal secondary and tertiary hospital for the mid region of Jutland. Women diagnosed with GDM requiring insulin therapy are routinely referred from regional hospitals for care at Aarhus

Table 1: Nutrition therapy for women with gestational diabetes (The 3 Q's).

Nutrition therapy for women with gestational diabetes (The 3 Q's)	
Quality	Protein 10–20%, lipids maximum 25–40%, carbohydrate 45–60%
Quantity	Individualized, but a minimum of 175 g carbohydrate per day
FreQuency	Three small-to-moderate-size meals and two to four snacks

University Hospital, Skejby (the area covers some 1.3 mio. persons). Pregnant women from the local uptake area (approximately 325, 000 persons) are referred on diagnosis of GDM. From the regional hospitals, women are referred only when insulin treatment is required or other complications develop, usually around gestational week 30 but with large individual variation. The hospital has between 4500 and 5000 deliveries per year; numbers are increasing slightly over time.

2. Materials and Methods

The cohort included all women with GDM who delivered a singleton at Aarhus University Hospital, Skejby between 2004 and 2016.The basis of GDM treatment is glycemic control. At the 1st visit, GDM patients received a glucose monitor and were instructed in its use. Patients were taught to check their glucose level before and 1½ hour after breakfast and dinner. The glycemic targets were <6.0 mmol/L before meals and <8.0 mmol/L 1½ h postprandial. All women received dietary advice from a dietician at the time of diagnosis. Specific nutrition/food recommendations were individualized but based on "the 3 Q's": Quality, Quantity and freQuency and self-monitoring of blood glucose. Recommended dietary macronutrient composition consisted of 45–60% carbohydrates, 10–20% protein, and a maximum of 40% lipids (Table 1). Quantities were individualized based on clinical parameters including pregestational body mass index, hunger, plasma glucose levels, weight gain, and ketone levels. A minimum of 175 g carbohydrate/day was recommended. Weight loss was not recommended; however, for obese women, modest energy restriction by 30% of estimated energy needs was advised to improve glycemic control without ketonuria and reduce maternal weight gain. Regarding the frequency of meals, carbohydrate was distributed throughout the day in three small-to-moderate-size meals and in between two to four snacks. Because of the increased morning insulin resistance, carbohydrate is often less well tolerated at breakfast than other meals. An evening snack may be needed to prevent accelerated ketosis overnight (Table 2). The intention of advising three small-to-moderate-size meals and two to four snacks was to decrease the risk of high postprandial glucose levels with less glucose excursions and thereby reducing fetal hyperglycemia and thus the risk of macrosomia. All patients were advised to undertake daily moderate physical exercise for 30 minutes.

If the glycemic targets were not reached, insulin therapy was initiated using premixed insulin aspart 30%/insulin NPH 70% (Novomix30) before breakfast and dinner. Insulin doses were adjusted according to blood sugar levels, measurements of HbA1c, and ultrasonographic estimates of fetal growth. When insulin therapy is added to nutrition therapy, a goal is to maintain carbohydrate consistency at meals and snacks to facilitate insulin adjustments.

Table 2: Example of carbohydrate distribution on a diet of 1800 kcal/day.

	Carbohydrates (g)	% carbohydrates calories
Breakfast	30	15
Morning snack	20	10
Lunch	50	25
Afternoon snack	35	15
Dinner	50	25
Bedtime snack	20	10

Patients attended the outpatients' clinic every 2 to 5 weeks. Telephone consultations could replace physical visits, if appropriate. Usually, patients had frequent telephone consultations the first weeks after commencing insulin therapy.

This retrospective cohort study was approved by the Danish Health Authorities (jr. 3-3013-360/1) and the Danish Data Protection Agency (jr. 1-16-02-271-13). Data were extracted from computerized hospital databases, complemented by direct data abstraction from clinical records as required. To facilitate presentation of the data, births were grouped by year of delivery into birth periods as follows: period 1: 2004–2008; period 2: 2009–2012; period 3: 2013–2016.

The majority of descriptive and outcome variables are presented in their original form. Birth weight standard deviation (SD or "Z") score was calculated as: (Z-score = individual birth weight − mean birth weight/SD birth weight), corrected for gender and gestational age at delivery [7]. Large for gestational age (LGA) and small for gestational age (SGA) were defined as a birth weight Z-score ≥ 1.3 or ≤ − 1.3, respectively. The remainder of the neonates were considered appropriate for gestational age (AGA). Preterm birth was defined as delivery before 37 completed gestational weeks [8].

Data distributions were verified by visual analysis of histograms and Q-Q plots. Sample size for all analyses was sufficient to allow for parametric statistical analysis [9]. Statistical analysis was performed using chi-squared tests for categorical variables (reported as n (%)) and analysis of variance for continuous variables (reported as mean (SD)). Statistical significance was accepted at the 5% level on two-tailed testing.

3. Results

The study included 1910 women. Numbers of births in each period were as follows: period 1: 2004–2008 (n = 497); period

TABLE 3: Maternal characteristics.

Variable	Period 1: 2004–2008		Period 2: 2009–2012		Period 3: 2013–2016	
	GDM	All	GDM	All	GDM	All
Total births = 1910	497	21,513	624	17,911	789	18,174
GDM (%)	2.3%		3.5%		4.3%	
Maternal age (years)	32.3	30.0	32.2	30.2	31.7	30.1
Maternal BMI (kg/m^2)	29.2	23.8	28.1*	23.7	28.0**	23.4
Insulin treated n (%)	94 (18.9)		127 (20.2)		218 (26.8)*	
Danish born Caucasian (%)	86.5	93.2	85.6	93.6	85.9	94.0

Characteristics of women included in the cohort. Data are presented as mean (SD) or n (%).$^*p < 0.05$ versus period 1; $^{**}p < 0.01$ versus period 1.

TABLE 4: Pregnancy outcomes—mother and infant.

Variable	Period 1: 2004–2008 $n = 497$	Period 2: 2009–2012 $n = 624$	Period 3: 2013–2016 $n = 789$
Gestation at delivery (days)	272 (13)	272 (13)	274 (11)
Delivery mode			
Simple vaginal n (%)	306 (61.6)	432 (68.4)	551 (69.8)
Vacuum extraction n (%)	0 (0)	2 (0.3)	18 (2.3)*
Elective C-section n (%)	109 (21.9)	98 (15.7)*	105 (13.3)*
Emergency C-section n (%)	68 (13.7)	85 (13.6)	112 (14.2)
Not recorded n (%)	14 (2.8)	9 (1.4)	3 (0.4)
Birth weight (grams)	3605 (582)	3465 (589)**	3524 (554)*
Birth weight Z-score	0.64 (1.40)	0.30 (1.35)***	0.26 (1.27)***
SGA/AGA/LGA (%)	8/63/29	8/73/19***	9/73/18***
Length (cm)	51.9 (2.7)	51.3 (2.8)**	51.5 (2.7)
Abdominal circumference (cm)	33.5 (2.2)	33.2 (2.8)	33.3 (2.3)
Head circumference (cm)	35.1 (1.7)	34.9 (1.9)	34.9 (1.7)
Placental weight (g)	718 (174)	673 (187)***	687(203)**
Apgar (5minutes)	9.9 (0.6)	9.9 (0.7)	9.8 (0.8)

Maternal and infant outcomes. Data are reported as mean (SD) for continuous variables and n (%) for categorical variables. Statistical comparisons performed using one-way ANVOA followed by unpaired t-tests with Bonferroni correction for continuous variables and Chi squared tests for categorical variables. $^*p < 0.05$ versus period 1; $^{**}p < 0.01$ versus period 1; $^{***}p < 0.001$ versus period 1.

2: 2009–2012 ($n = 624$); period 3: 2013–2016 ($n = 789$). Missing data were more common in period 1 but comprised a maximum of 2% of cases across all variables reported. No data imputation was undertaken. Maternal baseline characteristics are reported in Table 3, and maternal and infant pregnancy outcomes are noted in Table 4.

The number of GDM women treated each year increased significantly over the course of the study, as did the proportion requiring insulin therapy. Interestingly, this cannot be related to increasing maternal overweight/obesity as the mean maternal BMI in GDM women actually fell slightly but significantly over the three periods.

Concerning pregnancy outcomes, the timing of delivery (mean 38.9 weeks) remained constant over time, but the elective caesarean section fell and the simple vaginal delivery rate increased in the periods after 2008. Emergency caesarean section rates remained unchanged at 14% of all deliveries.

Birth weight and birth weight Z-score fell significantly in periods 2 and 3 compared to period 1, with no major changes in head or abdominal circumference. As can be seen in the breakdown of birth weight into SGA/AGA/LGA in Table 3, this was due largely to a decrease in LGA frequency from 29% to around 19%, with a concurrent increase in AGA, but no increase in SGA babies. Similar temporal trends were evident for both diet- and insulin-treated women. Insulin-treated women (mean (SD) BW Z-score: 1.0 (1.5)) had significantly larger babies than those treated with diet alone (BW Z-score 0.2 (1.2); $p < 0.001$) (Figure 1).

To confirm the birth period-related changes noted above, analyses were also performed using year of birth as a

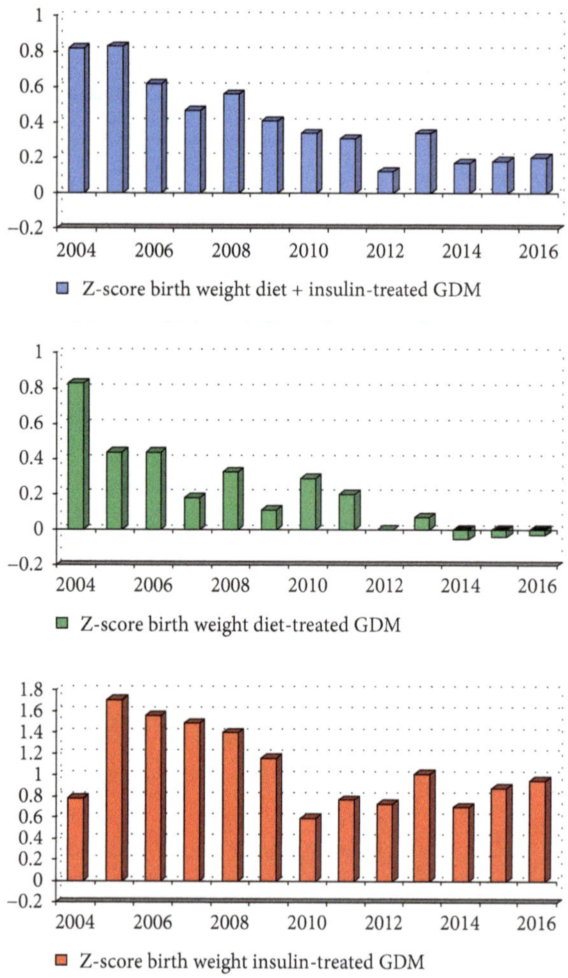

Figure 1: Z-score for birth weight.

grouping variable (rather than birth period). These showed the same temporal trends as noted above (data not shown).

4. Discussion

The present data demonstrate that during the last 13 years, the number of women diagnosed with GDM has increased. Furthermore, not only the number but also the proportion of GDM women receiving insulin treatment has increased. Finally, our results demonstrate a decline in the average birth weight in both diet treated and insulin treated GDM women.

4.1. GDM Prevalence. The increasing number of women diagnosed with GDM is not unexpected. This phenomenon is known on a large scale not only in industrialized countries but also on a worldwide scale [10, 11]. The reason could be sought in increasing obesity and age among women at child bearing. In our cohort, however, we observed a minor decrease in average BMI among pregnant women with GDM, thus other factors may contribute to our findings. Through the close national obstetrical network [12], knowledge on GDM, its diagnosis, and its consequences for women and their newborns, has been disseminated throughout not only the obstetrical care at the hospitals but even into the nationwide antenatal health care program. Hence, a national awareness concerning GDM exists amongst all caregivers the pregnant women meet in the antenatal program. This vigilance probably does add to the identification and screening of women at risk for GDM. Many women were also referred from neighbouring hospitals for insulin therapy. This number may be expected to increase when overall numbers increase.

4.2. Insulin Treatment of GDM. The absolute number and the proportion of women receiving insulin therapy has also increased during the period studied. Increasing absolute numbers would be a natural consequence of the overall increase in women diagnosed with GDM. As the percentages of women receiving insulin also have increased, other explanations must also exist. The average BMI has fallen, primarily due to an increased number of women in the normal BMI category and a decrease in women in the overweight category, rather than to changes in the numbers of women in the extremes of the BMI range (data not shown). Diagnostic criteria for the diagnosis of GDM have not changed in the periods reported.

We hypothesize that increased GDM awareness may have led treating doctors to initiate or adjust insulin therapy not only on the basis of pre and postprandial glucose levels but also due to regular ultrasonographic evaluation of fetal growth/abdominal circumference. It is a well-known clinical experience that some mothers do experience excess fetal growth despite normal or near-normal levels of glucose and HbA1c.

Finally, patients referred from neighbouring hospitals to our tertiary center are those who exhibit the most severe variants of GDM. Centralized treatment of women requiring insulin therapy, introduction of formalized agreements between secondary and tertiary hospitals, and revision of guidelines regarding GDM treatment are all actions that encourage the secondary hospitals to pay more attention to GDM care. Unfortunately, our data do not allow us to identify those patients referred specifically for insulin treatment from neighbouring hospitals. Also, our data do not allow us to discern HbA1c, daily blood sugar levels, or the total daily insulin requirements among pregnant women with GDM. Many pregnant women with GDM maintain a normal HbA1c level for long periods, and the utility of HbA1c as a marker of GDM control is not well established. Future studies should explore if more pregnant women with GDM are put on a low-insulin dose treatment during GDM pregnancy. Finally, one could surmise that as the same team members in our team for pregnant women with diabetes, including the dietician, have been working together for more than 15 years, clinical experience has been accumulated and probably has an impact on daily clinical work.

4.3. Birth Weights. Among GDM mothers, the average BW Z-score declined over time. We observed that the number of LGA infants declined with an increase in AGA infants. Thus, the average birth weight tended to normalize without an increase in SGA newborns. We conclude that the effect of interventions has been to normalize birth weights among those GDM women who would otherwise have given birth to the largest babies. This is a preferable outcome.

As can be seen from Figure 1, the birth weight in diet-treated women has been virtually normal for the last 5 years of the reported period. Although the birth weight is decreasing towards normal, some challenges remain in the insulin-treated group. In gestational diabetes, *early* and *sufficient* intervention with insulin is the key to achieve a good neonatal/obstetrical outcome when diet therapy fails to provide adequate glycemic control. Nevertheless, the time frame for treatment is very limited. Many women are reluctant to start insulin therapy, hoping that more intensive dietary management will achieve acceptable glycemic control. Although we do not have data on the gestational week of initiation of insulin therapy, we believe that this postponement of insulin treatment renders the time left to achieve normal birth weight limited. Another obstacle may be slow titration of insulin therapy. This is often commenced cautiously due to concerns about the risk of hypoglycemia, with a consequent delay in achieving optimal glycemic control.

4.4. Strength and Weaknesses. For the present data, it is a strength that all data on the DM diagnosis has been reviewed during the pregnancy by one of the two main consultants treating pregnant women with GDM. Birth weights have been captured contemporarily.

Some limitations regarding the diagnosis of GDM have been discussed above as has the pattern in referrals from other hospitals. Furthermore, our source data contain limited information about ethnicity. For example adopted individuals are not readily identified.

4.5. External Validity. The present study is a one-center study and thus, in principle, is valid for Aarhus University Hospital, Skejby, only.

As stated above, though, a national societal vigilance on the detection and treatment of GDM is prevailing. National guidelines on the antenatal care and treatment of pregnancies complicated by GDM exist, and the interhospital cooperation between caregivers to GDM pregnant women is high. Thus, the clinical approach is very similar on a nationwide base for the treatment of pregnant women with GDM [13].

5. Conclusion

We here present data that show a decline in birth weights towards the normal range in GDM women. Noteworthy is the shift from LGA newborns to AGA newborns without increasing the number of SGA newborns.

At the same time, an increasing number of women are diagnosed with GDM, and an increased proportion of patients with GDM receive insulin therapy.

We speculate that a general societal awareness of GDM has contributed to a better identification of women at risk. Future studies should aim at investigating the patterns among women receiving insulin therapy; especially insulin dosage regimens in relation to birth weights of the neonates deserve to be scrutinized.

Conflicts of Interest

None of the authors had any personal or financial conflict of interest.

Acknowledgments

Per Glud Ovesen was financially supported by the Novo Nordisk Foundation. H. David McIntyre was financially supported by the Danish Diabetes Academy.

References

[1] U. Kampmann, L. R. Madsen, G. O. Skajaa, D. S. Iversen, N. Moeller, and P. Ovesen, "Gestational diabetes: a clinical update," *World Journal of Diabetes*, vol. 6, no. 8, pp. 1065–1072, 2015.

[2] K. Benhalima, C. Mathieu, A. Van Assche et al., "Survey by the European Board and College of Obstetrics and Gynaecology on screening for gestational diabetes in Europe," *European Journal of Obstetrics & Gynecology, and Reproductive Biology*, vol. 201, pp. 197–202, 2016.

[3] B. S. Buckley, J. Harreiter, P. Damm et al., "Gestational diabetes mellitus in Europe: prevalence, current screening practice and barriers to screening. A review," *Diabetic Medicine*, vol. 29, no. 7, pp. 844–854, 2012.

[4] International Association of Diabetes and Pregnancy Study Groups Consensus Panel, B. E. Metzger, S. G. Gabbe et al., "International association of diabetes and pregnancy study groups recommendations on the diagnosis and classification of hyperglycemia in pregnancy," *Diabetes Care*, vol. 33, no. 3, pp. 676–682, 2010.

[5] "Committee opinion no. 504: screening and diagnosis of gestational diabetes mellitus," *Obstetrics & Gynecology*, vol. 118, no. 3, pp. 751–753, 2011.

[6] D. M. Jensen, P. Damm, B. Sorensen et al., "Clinical impact of mild carbohydrate intolerance in pregnancy: a study of 2904 nondiabetic Danish women with risk factors for gestational diabetes mellitus," *American Journal of Obstetrics and Gynecology*, vol. 185, no. 2, pp. 413–419, 2001.

[7] K. Marsal, P. H. Persson, T. Larsen, H. Lilja, A. Selbing, and B. Sultan, "Intrauterine growth curves based on ultrasonically estimated foetal weights," *Acta Paediatrica*, vol. 85, no. 7, pp. 843–848, 1996.

[8] International Association of Diabetes in Pregnancy Study Group (IADPSG) Working Group on Outcome Definitions, D. S. Feig, R. Corcoy et al., "Diabetes in pregnancy outcomes: a systematic review and proposed codification of definitions," *Diabetes/Metabolism Research and Reviews*, vol. 31, no. 7, pp. 680–690, 2015.

[9] S. G. Kwak and J. H. Kim, "Central limit theorem: the cornerstone of modern statistics," *Korean Journal of Anesthesiology*, vol. 70, no. 2, pp. 144–156, 2017.

[10] J. A. Lavery, A. M. Friedman, K. M. Keyes, J. D. Wright, and C. V. Ananth, "Gestational diabetes in the United States: temporal changes in prevalence rates between 1979 and 2010," *BJOG*, vol. 124, no. 5, pp. 804–813, 2017.

[11] Y. Zhu and C. Zhang, "Prevalence of gestational diabetes and risk of progression to type 2 diabetes: a global perspective," *Current Diabetes Reports*, vol. 16, no. 1, p. 7, 2016.

[12] Dansk Selskab for Obstetrik og Gynækologi (DSOG), *Sandbjerg guideline: Behandling af gestationel diabetes mellitus*, 2007, http://gynobsguideline.dk/sandbjerg/Behandling%20af%20gestationel%20diabetes%20mellitus.pdf.

[13] C. Jeppesen, H. T. Maindal, J. K. Kristensen, P. G. Ovesen, and D. R. Witte, "National study of the prevalence of gestational diabetes mellitus among Danish women from 2004 to 2012," *Scandinavian Journal of Public Health*, vol. 45, no. 8, pp. 811–817, 2017.

10

Higher Concentrations of BCAAs and 3-HIB are Associated with Insulin Resistance in the Transition from Gestational Diabetes to Type 2 Diabetes

Ulrika Andersson-Hall,[1] Carolina Gustavsson,[1] Anders Pedersen,[2] Daniel Malmodin,[2] Louise Joelsson,[1] and Agneta Holmäng[1]

[1]*Institute of Neuroscience and Physiology, Sahlgrenska Academy, University of Gothenburg, Gothenburg, Sweden*
[2]*Swedish NMR Centre, University of Gothenburg, Gothenburg, Sweden*

Correspondence should be addressed to Ulrika Andersson-Hall; ulrika.andersson.hall@gu.se

Academic Editor: Yoshifumi Saisho

Aim. Determine the metabolic profile and identify risk factors of women transitioning from gestational diabetes mellitus (GDM) to type 2 diabetes mellitus (T2DM). *Methods.* 237 women diagnosed with GDM underwent an oral glucose tolerance test (OGTT), anthropometrics assessment, and completed lifestyle questionnaires six years after pregnancy. Blood was analysed for clinical variables (e.g., insulin, glucose, HbA1c, adiponectin, leptin, and lipid levels) and NMR metabolomics. Based on the OGTT, women were divided into three groups: normal glucose tolerance (NGT), impaired glucose tolerance (IGT), and T2DM. *Results.* Six years after GDM, 19% of subjects had T2DM and 19% IGT. After BMI adjustment, the IGT group had lower HDL, higher leptin, and higher free fatty acid (FFA) levels, and the T2DM group higher triglyceride, FFA, and C-reactive protein levels than the NGT group. IGT and T2DM groups reported lower physical activity. NMR measurements revealed that levels of branched-chain amino acids (BCAAs) and the valine metabolite 3-hydroxyisobyturate were higher in T2DM and IGT groups and correlated with measures of insulin resistance and lipid metabolism. *Conclusion.* In addition to well-known clinical risk factors, BCAAs and 3-hydroxyisobyturate are potential markers to be evaluated as predictors of metabolic risk after pregnancy complicated by GDM.

1. Introduction

Gestational diabetes mellitus (GDM), defined as glucose intolerance with onset or first recognition during pregnancy [1], occurs in up to 14% of pregnancies every year [2]. Although in most women glucose tolerance returns to normal after delivery, the frequency of GDM correlates with the prevalence of type 2 diabetes mellitus (T2DM), and women with GDM have increased risk for T2DM later in life. The 10-year risk is ~40%, and the incidence is highest in the first 5 years after pregnancy [3]. In both GDM and T2DM, chronic insulin resistance and pancreatic β-cell dysfunction play crucial pathogenic roles. Pregnancy, an inherently insulin-resistant state, may reveal a preexisting deficiency in insulin secretion and insulin sensitivity and relative β-cell failure. Thus, the stress of pregnancy may reveal a predisposition to T2DM and provide early signs useful for preventing chronic diseases.

Comprehensive metabolic profiling (metabolomics) has provided unique insights into the mechanisms of insulin resistance. For example, branched-chain amino acids (BCAAs) and the aromatic amino acids (AAAs) are strongly associated with metabolic disease [4]. The BCAA-related metabolite cluster is tightly associated with the incidence of T2DM in cross-sectional and case-control studies and across multiple ethnic groups and geographies. Altered flux through the BCAA catabolic pathway, rather than BCAA concentrations per se, appears to be especially important. Considerable evidence implicates free fatty acids (FFAs) and other lipids that contribute to metabolic disease and insulin resistance.

These results raise the possibility that lipids and BCAAs and interactions between BCAAs, FFAs, and glucose oxidative pathways have combined effects [5]. Metabolomics has potential prognostic power and may provide insights into the mechanisms of insulin resistance and T2DM.

Recently, we characterized the metabolic transition profile from pregnancy to postpartum by mass spectrometry-based metabolomics in women with GDM [6]. These women had significantly higher postpartum levels of BCAAs (especially valine) than women with healthy pregnancies, and their circulating lipids did not return to normal levels after pregnancy. BCAAs were not elevated during pregnancy and therefore increased postpartum.

3-Hydroxy-isobutyrate (3-HIB), a catabolic intermediate of the BCAA valine, may be released from muscle cells and regulates transendothelial transport and muscle cell uptake of FFAs [7, 8]. Thus, 3-HIB may be a signalling metabolite that connects the regulation of FFA flux to BCAA catabolism. This novel hypothesis might explain how increased BCAA levels cause insulin resistance and diabetes.

In this study, we compared the metabolic profiles of women who had impaired glucose tolerance (IGT) or T2DM or were normoglycaemic 6 years after GDM. We hypothesized that alterations in BCAA metabolism interact with lipid metabolism and glucose oxidative pathways to induce insulin resistance and diabetes.

2. Methods

2.1. Subjects. The study was approved by the ethics committee at the University of Gothenburg (402-08/750-15). Informed consent was obtained from all participants. Data were collected retrospectively from women in the Gothenburg area who were diagnosed with GDM from 2005 to 2009 ($N = 542$). Upon contact, women were invited to participate in the study. 378 women were briefly interviewed by telephone and asked to come to a follow-up visit. 237 women completed this visit at 5.6 ± 0.5 years after pregnancy (Figure 1). Follow-up participants were less frequently of non-Nordic ethnicity ($P < 0.001$) and had lower pregestational body mass index (BMI) and a lower fasting glucose value at GDM diagnosis ($P < 0.01$) than women who could not be reached or chose not to participate. If a woman had GDM during two pregnancies during the study interval, only data from the first pregnancy and follow-up were analysed (Figure 1).

2.2. Protocol. At follow-up, fasting blood samples were collected for all women, and those who had not previously been diagnosed with diabetes or who did not have a diagnostic fasting plasma glucose value underwent a 2 h 75 g OGTT. Venous blood for analysis of plasma glucose and serum insulin was collected at 0, 30, 60, 90, and 120 minutes. Capillary glucose was measured at 0 and 120 minutes as a backup in case venous sampling was unsuccessful. Fasting serum and plasma blood samples were used for further analysis.

Anthropometric measurements (weight, height, waist, and hip circumference) and resting blood pressure were determined, and participants were asked to complete questionnaires during the visit. A self-administered dietary questionnaire was used to assess energy intake (EI) during the 3 previous months [9]. The questionnaire has a semi-quantitative food frequency design and was validated in Swedish men and women against a 4-day food record and 24 h energy expenditure and nitrogen excretion [9]. Basal metabolic rate (BMR) was calculated with Henry's equation [10]; subjects with an EI/BMR ratio < 0.95 or > 3.0 were excluded. Physical activity was assessed by asking participants to rate the activity level between 0 and 4 at work and 1 and 4 at leisure with clear description of each level. To create an overview of activity level, reported activities at leisure and work were added to give a maximum of 8. Only fully and correctly completed questionnaires were used for analysis. In a subgroup of women ($n = 87$), fat mass, fat-free mass and body fat % was measured with air displacement plethysmography (BOD POD, software version 5.4.0, COSMED) at a second visit. Data from the GDM pregnancy were collected from medical records. BMI at the start of pregnancy was calculated from the weight recorded at the first antenatal visit performed during gestational weeks 6–12 and BMI change as the difference between BMI at follow-up and BMI at the start of pregnancy.

2.3. Glucose Tolerance Groups. Based on fasting and 2 h glucose values from the OGTT at the 6-year follow-up, three groups were created: normal glucose tolerance (NGT), IGT (including impaired fasting glucose or impaired glucose tolerance), and T2DM (including subjects with previously diagnosed T2DM). Classification was based on venous glucose levels according to the 1999 WHO guidelines [11]. In those subjects where venous glucose levels were not obtained, capillary glucose measurements were used to calculate corresponding venous values as described [12]. These values are only used for diagnosis and are not included in the analysis. Individuals with type 1 DM (T1DM) at follow-up, confirmed with antibody tests (GADA and IA-2A), were excluded from the main analysis but were included in a subgroup analysis of ketone metabolism.

2.4. Biochemical Measurements. HbA1c was analysed immediately with a point-of-care analyser (Afinion AS100; Axis-Shield, Oslo, Norway). Glucose, insulin, cholesterol (total, low-density lipoprotein (LDL), high-density lipoprotein (HDL)), triglycerides, leptin, adiponectin, C-reactive protein, and FFAs were analysed at the accredited Clinical Chemistry Laboratory, Sahlgrenska University Hospital (International Standard ISO 15189:2007). ELISA was used to measure adiponectin (Human Adiponectin ELISA kit, Millipore, Billerica, MA; interassay coefficient of variation, 7.0% at 10.5 mg/L) and leptin (Human Leptin Quantikine, R&D Systems; interassay coefficient of variation, 8.0% at 9 μg/L). All other assays were routinely done with a cobas modular system (Roche Diagnostics). Homeostatic model assessment of insulin resistance (HOMA-IR) was calculated as (fasting glucose $\times$ fasting insulin)/22.5 [13]. Adipose tissue insulin resistance (ADIPO-IR) was calculated as fasting FFA $\times$ fasting insulin [14]. Due to occasional technical problems either with blood sampling or blood analysis, full sets

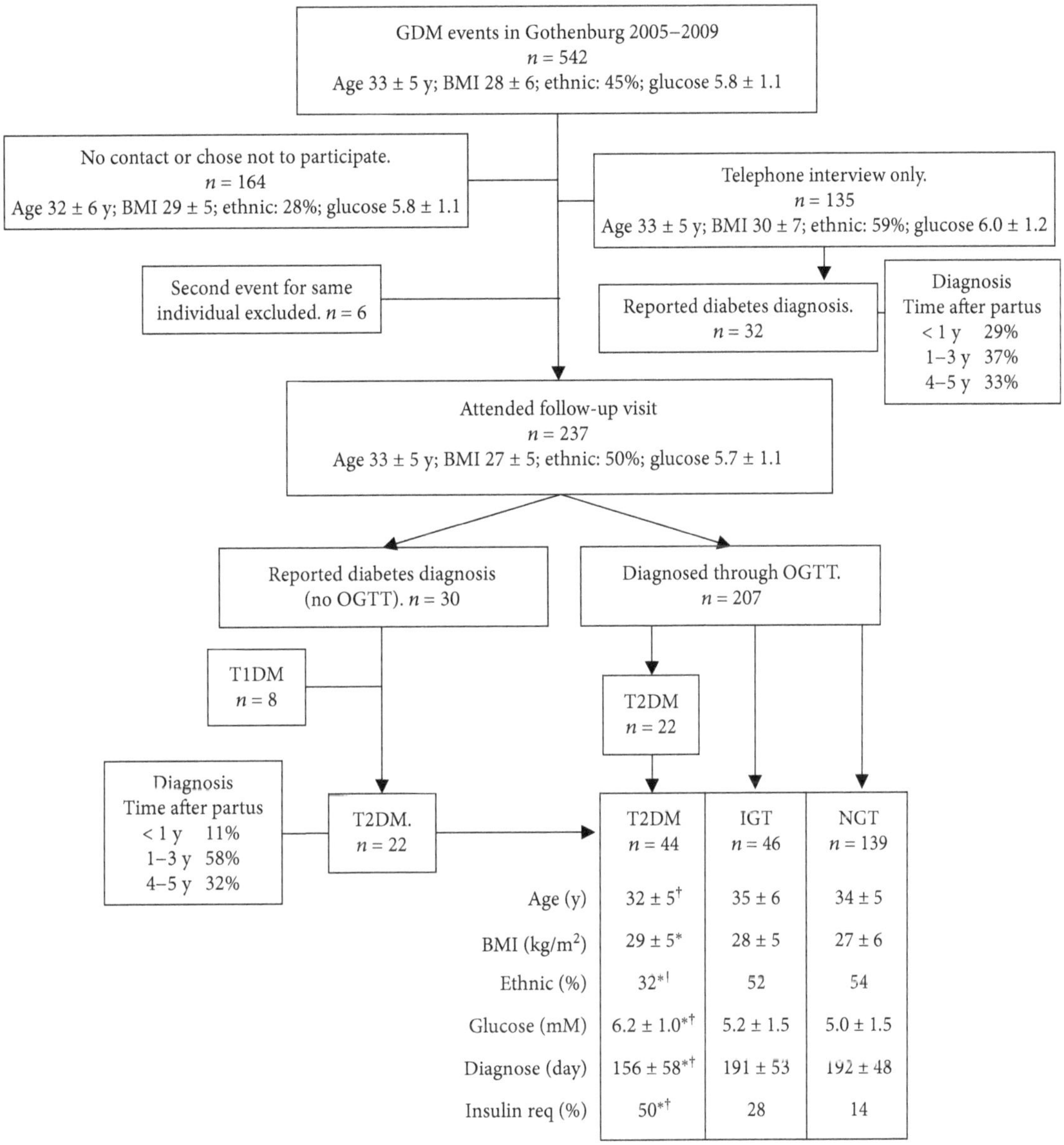

FIGURE 1: Flow chart of study population and pregnancy data. Age, age at partus; BMI, BMI at start of pregnancy (kg/m^2); ethnic, % Nordic ethnicity; glucose, fasting p-glucose (mM) at time of GDM diagnosis; diagnose, gestational age at time of GDM diagnosis; and insulin req, required insulin treatment during GDM pregnancy. $^*P < 0.05$ versus NGT. $^\dagger P < 0.05$ versus IGT. Values are mean ± SD.

for analysis were not available for all parameters at all time points. See Table 1 for *n* numbers.

2.5. NMR Spectroscopy. 224 fasting serum samples were available for NMR analysis after all other blood analysis was performed. NMR data were acquired on a Bruker 800 MHz spectrometer equipped with a 3 mm TCI CryoProbe and a cooled SampleJet sample changer using the "zgespe" pulse sequence encoding a one-dimensional ^{1}H experiment with suppression of water and J-modulation by excitation sculpting and perfect echo, respectively, and T2 filtering with a CPMG pulse train. For each sample, 128 scans were collected into 65k points with an acquisition time of 2.04 seconds, relaxation delay of 3 seconds, sweep width of 20 ppm, and a total CPMG pulse train of 193 ms (total experimental time, 12 minutes 4 seconds). The temperature was kept at 6°C in the sample changer and at 25°C during acquisition. Spectral data were processed with TopSpin 3.5pl6 (Bruker BioSpin), zero filling once, and 0.3 Hz line broadening before Fourier transform. Representative samples for the different groups were subjected to two-dimensional NMR data acquisition using ^{1}H-^{1}H TOCSY ("mlevgpphw5"), ^{1}H,^{13}C-HSQC ("hsqcetgpsisp2.2"), and two-dimensional Jres ("jresgpprqf") experiments. Two-dimensional results for 3-HIB are shown in Supplementary Materials (available here). Experimental details are available on request. Processed one-dimensional data were imported into MATLAB 2016a (MathWorks) and aligned with icoshift [15], and peaks were integrated with an in-house MATLAB routine. NMR integrals were expressed as a percentage of NGT. Two-dimensional data, the human metabolome database [16] and Chenomx 8.3 (Chenomx Inc.) were used to annotate metabolite peaks.

Table 1: Anthropometry, blood pressure (BP), clinical blood measurements, and self-reported lifestyle data at follow-up 6 years after GDM pregnancy.

Variable	NGT			IGT			T2DM			*P*			*P* (BMI adjusted)		
	n	Mean	SD	*n*	Mean	SD	*n*	Mean	SD	IGT versus NGT	T2D versus NGT	T2D versus IGT	IGT versus NGT	T2D versus NGT	T2D versus IGT
Anthropometry and blood pressure															
BMI (kg/m^2)	139	26.1	4.8	46	29.4	4.5	44	29.1	5.8	<0.001	0.002				
BMI change (kg/m^2)	139	−0.4	3.0	46	1.8	3.1	44	−0.4	3.5	<0.001		0.003	0.001		
Waist (cm)	137	87.5	10.8	45	94.2	16.2	44	94.6	14.5	0.007	0.004				
Hip (cm)	137	102.3	9.7	45	108.4	9.1	44	107.1	11.8	0.002	0.02				
Waist : hip ratio	137	0.9	0.1	45	0.9	0.1	44	0.9	0.1						
Body fat (%)	59	32.9	7.9	16	40.5	6.6	12	38.5	13.2	0.007					
Fat mass (kg)	59	23.4	9.5	16	32.3	10.7	12	31.8	15.8	0.01	0.04				
Fat-free mass (kg)	59	45.6	5.4	16	46.0	6.7	12	45.9	6.0						
BP systolic (mmHg)	138	113.9	12.8	46	122.9	14.0	44	119.2	14.2	<0.001			0.02		
BP diastolic (mmHg)	138	74.9	9.6	46	78.6	9.8	44	78.1	10.6						
Clinical blood measurements															
b-HbA1c (mmol/mol)	139	37.1	3.7	45	38.4	3.8	44	52.6	18.8		<0.001	<0.001		<0.001	<0.001
p-glucose fasting (mM)	138	5.4	0.4	43	6.1	0.4	44	8.2	3.5	0.02	<0.001	<0.001	0.02	<0.001	<0.001
p-glucose 2 h (mM)	128	5.5	1.1	42	7.8	1.6	12	11.8	3.9	<0.001	<0.001	<0.001	<0.001	<0.001	<0.001
s-insulin fasting (mU/L)	134	8.0	4.2	43	14.4	9.5	44	12.8	7.4	<0.001	<0.001		<0.001	0.003	
s-insulin 2 h (mU/L)	121	44.7	37.7	40	87.1	57.1	12	85.3	58.4	<0.001	0.008		<0.001	0.01	
HOMA-IR	133	1.9	1.0	43	3.8	2.7	43	4.9	3.4	<0.001	<0.001	0.04	<0.001	<0.001	0.004
s-total cholesterol (mM)	137	4.7	0.8	45	4.7	0.8	43	4.7	0.7						
s-HDL (mM)	138	1.5	0.3	45	1.3	0.3	44	1.4	0.4	0.001	0.04		0.04		
s-LDL (mM)	138	2.9	0.8	45	3.1	0.7	44	3.0	0.6						
s-triglycerides (mM)	137	0.9	0.5	45	1.2	0.5	44	1.4	1.4		<0.001			0.002	
s-leptin (mg/L)	134	18.2	11.8	42	29.3	12.9	44	24.4	22.4	<0.001	0.04		0.03		
s-adiponectin (ug/L)	137	17.8	14.5	41	18.1	15.9	44	14.2	12.9						
Leptin : adiponectin 10^{-3}	137	1.86	1.95	41	2.83	2.52	44	3.51	3.67		0.001			0.02	
s-C-reactive protein (mg/L)	137	2.1	3.6	43	3.1	3.1	44	5.5	8.2		<0.001			0.008	0.007
p-free fatty acids (mM)	138	0.43	0.18	41	0.56	0.20	44	0.59	0.22	0.001	<0.001		0.001	<0.001	
ADIPO-IR (mM·pM)	134	24.1	17.6	40	53.6	38.2	44	55.7	40.5	<0.001	<0.001		<0.001	<0.001	
Questionnaires															
Physical activity	120	4.0	1.1	38	3.3	1.0	34	3.4	1.3	0.008	0.02		0.009	0.02	
Energy intake (kcal)	88	2390	561	31	2366	735	17	2258	610						
Protein intake (g/kg)	88	1.4	0.4	31	1.2	0.4	17	1.4	0.5						
Fat intake (g/kg)	88	1.6	0.5	31	1.3	0.4	17	1.5	0.5						
Carbohydrate intake (g/kg)	88	3.7	1.2	31	3.2	1.3	17	3.4	1.3						

The women were divided into glucose tolerance groups based on follow-up OGTT. Statistical analyses were done with ANOVA (*P*) and ANCOVA (BMI-adjusted *P*). BMI change refers to change from start of pregnancy to follow-up. Macronutrient intake expressed as g/kg body weight. b, whole blood; p, plasma; s, serum.

TABLE 2: NMR metabolites at follow-up 6 years after GDM pregnancy.

%	NGT		IGT		T2DM		*P*			*P* (BMI adjusted)		
	Mean	SD	Mean	SD	Mean	SD	IGT versus NGT	T2D versus NGT	T2D versus IGT	IGT versus NGT	T2D versus NGT	T2D versus IGT
Phenylalanine	100.0	45.4	121.8	43.8	117.1	49.1	0.02					
Tyrosine	100.0	25.1	109.6	26.9	111.6	26.7		0.03				
Glucose	100.0	20.7	112.1	18.1	159.5	79.6		<0.001	<0.001		<0.001	<0.001
Mannose	100.0	25.9	113.4	26.2	144.3	59.5		<0.001	<0.001		<0.001	<0.001
Glycerol	100.0	43.1	127.5	48.6	140.7	71.1	0.006	<0.001		0.007	<0.001	
Glycine	100.0	27.0	88.1	19.1	89.6	25.6	0.02	0.05		0.04		
Citrate	100.0	31.0	111.5	23.9	117.3	25.7		0.002			0.002	
Pyruvate	100.0	80.6	141.3	78.2	119.4	73.7	0.008			0.01		
Acetoacetate	100.0	105.8	115.7	103.9	253.1	348.8		<0.001	0.001		<0.001	0.001
3-HIB	100.0	54.7	128.2	52.7	131.5	75.5	0.02	0.006		0.005	0.002	
Valine	100.0	19.2	108.2	15.1	109.5	21.6	0.04	0.01			0.05	
Isoleucine	100.0	22.1	109.0	19.0	115.7	28.5		<0.001			0.001	
Leucine	100.0	18.2	111.2	13.6	113.4	22.7	0.002	<0.001		0.01	0.001	

Metabolites significantly different between groups are shown. Data is expressed as % of NGT. Statistics are performed using ANOVA (P) and ANCOVA (BMI-adjusted P). $n = 137$ for NGT, $n = 43$ for IGT, and $n = 44$ for T2DM.

2.6. Statistical Analysis. Pregnancy data were analysed with one-way ANOVA and post hoc Tukey analysis or chi-square test (binary variables). Follow-up measurements were analysed with ANOVA and ANCOVA (BMI as covariate). To predict the likelihood of T2DM from pregnancy data, variables were analysed by binary regression (outcome T2DM, yes/no). For association of follow-up variables with insulin resistance, a stepwise forward linear regression model was built with HOMA-IR as the dependant variable. All variables in Table 1 that are not direct measures of glucose metabolism (glucose, insulin, and HbA1c) plus metabolites from Table 2 involved in fat and amino acid metabolism were entered as predictors. Ketone bodies did not correlate with HOMA-IR and were excluded. Bivariate and partial correlations (BMI as control variable) were further performed. $P < 0.05$ was considered significant. All values are mean ± SD unless otherwise stated.

3. Results

3.1. Risk Factors for T2DM 6 Years after GDM. After the follow-up OGTT, 58% had NGT ($n = 139$), 19% IGT ($n = 46$), 19% T2DM ($n = 44$), and 3% T1DM ($n = 8$). In the T2DM group, BMI at start of pregnancy was higher than in the NGT group (Figure 1), GDM was diagnosed earlier, fasting glucose was higher at GDM diagnosis, and higher percentages required insulin during pregnancy or were non-Nordic.

By logistic regression, the strongest prediction model for development of T2DM included fasting glucose at GDM diagnosis ($P = 0.001$, Exp(B) = 1.92), gestational age at diagnosis ($P = 0.004$, Exp(B) = 0.99), and insulin treatment ($P = 0.03$ Exp(B) = 2.5). These factors predicted 81% of T2DM cases 6 years later.

3.2. Clinical Characteristics and Physical Activity. Anthropometric and clinical data at the 6-year follow-up are shown in Table 1. Women with IGT or T2DM had higher BMI than normoglycaemic women, but only in the IGT group did BMI increase from prepregnancy to follow-up ($P < 0.001$). Anthropometric measurements were all higher in the IGT and T2DM groups than in the NGT group.

As expected, glucose, insulin, and HOMA-IR were higher in the IGT and T2DM groups even after BMI adjustment. HbA1c was significantly increased in T2DM only. HDL was lower and leptin was higher in the IGT and T2DM groups than in the NGT group, but only the differences between IGT and NGT were significant after BMI adjustment. FFA and ADIPO-IR, reflecting inability of insulin to suppress peripheral lipolysis, were higher in the IGT and T2DM groups, and the difference was highly significant even after BMI adjustment; there were no differences in total cholesterol or LDL. The leptin : adiponectin ratio and C-reactive protein (CRP) were both higher in T2DM, independent of BMI. Physical activity was higher in the NGT group than in the other groups, even after BMI adjustment, and correlated with several metabolic parameters (BMI, waist circumference, hip circumference, HbA1c, fasting insulin, 2-hour OGTT glucose, HOMA-IR, HDL, leptin, ADIPO-IR, and CRP). After adjustment for BMI, significant correlations remained for hip circumference ($r = -0.22$, $P = 0.003$), HOMA-IR ($r = -0.23$, $P = 0.002$), ADIPO-IR ($r = -0.20$, $P = 0.007$), and CRP ($r = -0.20$, $P = 0.005$). Self-reported dietary intake did not differ in the groups.

3.3. Metabolomics. NMR metabolomics of serum samples from the 6-year follow-up showed significant differences between groups (Table 2). Metabolites that differed significantly after BMI adjustment are shown in Figure 2. All three BCAAs were significantly increased in the T2DM group after

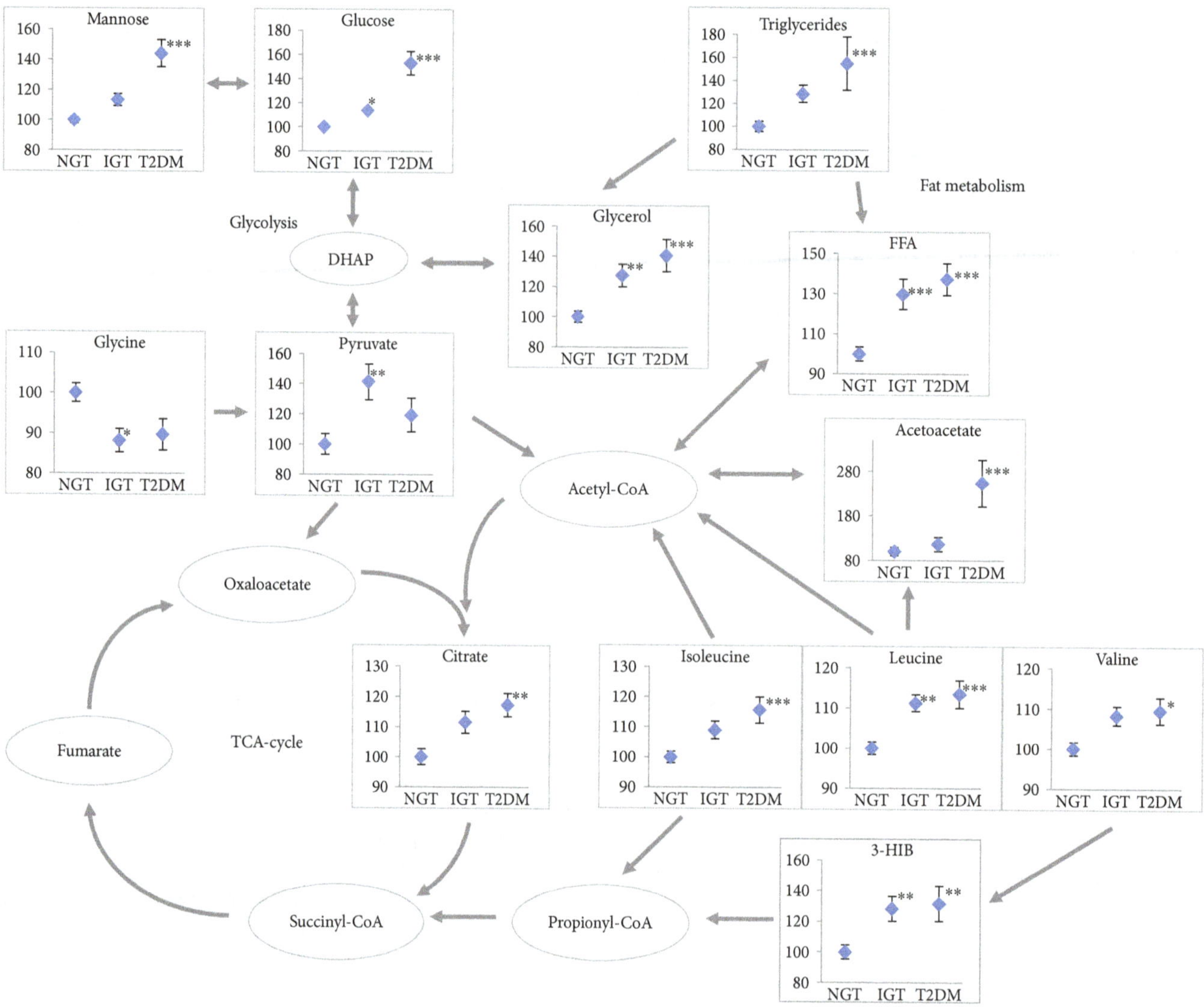

FIGURE 2: Map of metabolites that differed significantly between groups after BMI adjustment 6 years after a GDM pregnancy. Values are percent of NGT (mean ± SEM). $n = 137$ for NGT, $n = 43$ for IGT, and $n = 44$ for T2DM. $^{*}P < 0.05$, $^{**}P < 0.01$, and $^{***}P < 0.001$ versus NGT by ANCOVA with BMI as covariate.

BMI adjustment, and there was a tendency to increase for all BCAAs in the IGT group, but only the increase in leucine was significant. 3-HIB increased by ~30% in both the IGT and T2DM groups. AAA concentrations were significantly elevated in IGT (Tyr) and in T2DM (Phe) by ANOVA but not after BMI adjustment.

Figure 3 shows correlations of BCAAs and 3-HIB with glucose and lipid metabolism measurements that remained significant after BMI was introduced as a covariate. 3-HIB correlated with all glucose and insulin measurements, whereas BCAAs mainly correlated with fasting values (Figure 3(a)). For lipid metabolites and adipokines, 3-HIB correlated only with triglycerides and its breakdown/precursor metabolites glycerol and FFA. All BCAAs correlated positively with triglycerides, glycerol, and the leptin : adiponectin ratio and inversely with HDL. Of the BCAAs and 3-HIB, only leucine correlated with body fat percentage ($P < 0.01$, $R = 0.3$, $n = 89$).

For AAAs, Tyr correlated with fasting insulin ($P < 0.001$, $R = 0.31$) and the leptin : adiponectin ratio ($P < 0.001$, $R = 0.28$), whereas Phe did not correlate with any glucose metabolism or lipid parameters after BMI adjustment.

Other group differences included for T2DM increased mannose, acetoacetate, glycerol, and citrate and for IGT increased pyruvate and glycerol and decreased glycine.

3.4. Regression Model to Predict HOMA-IR. To predict HOMA-IR variance, follow-up variables that correlated with HOMA-IR but are not direct measurements of glucose metabolism were analysed in a regression model. These included BMI, BMI change, age, blood pressure, waist and hip circumference, waist : hip ratio, triglycerides, cholesterol, HDL, LDL, CRP, leptin, adiponectin, leptin : adiponectin ratio, FFA, phenylalanine, tyrosine, glycine, valine, leucine, isoleucine, 3-HIB, and physical activity. After stepwise analysis, the model contained eight variables that gave an

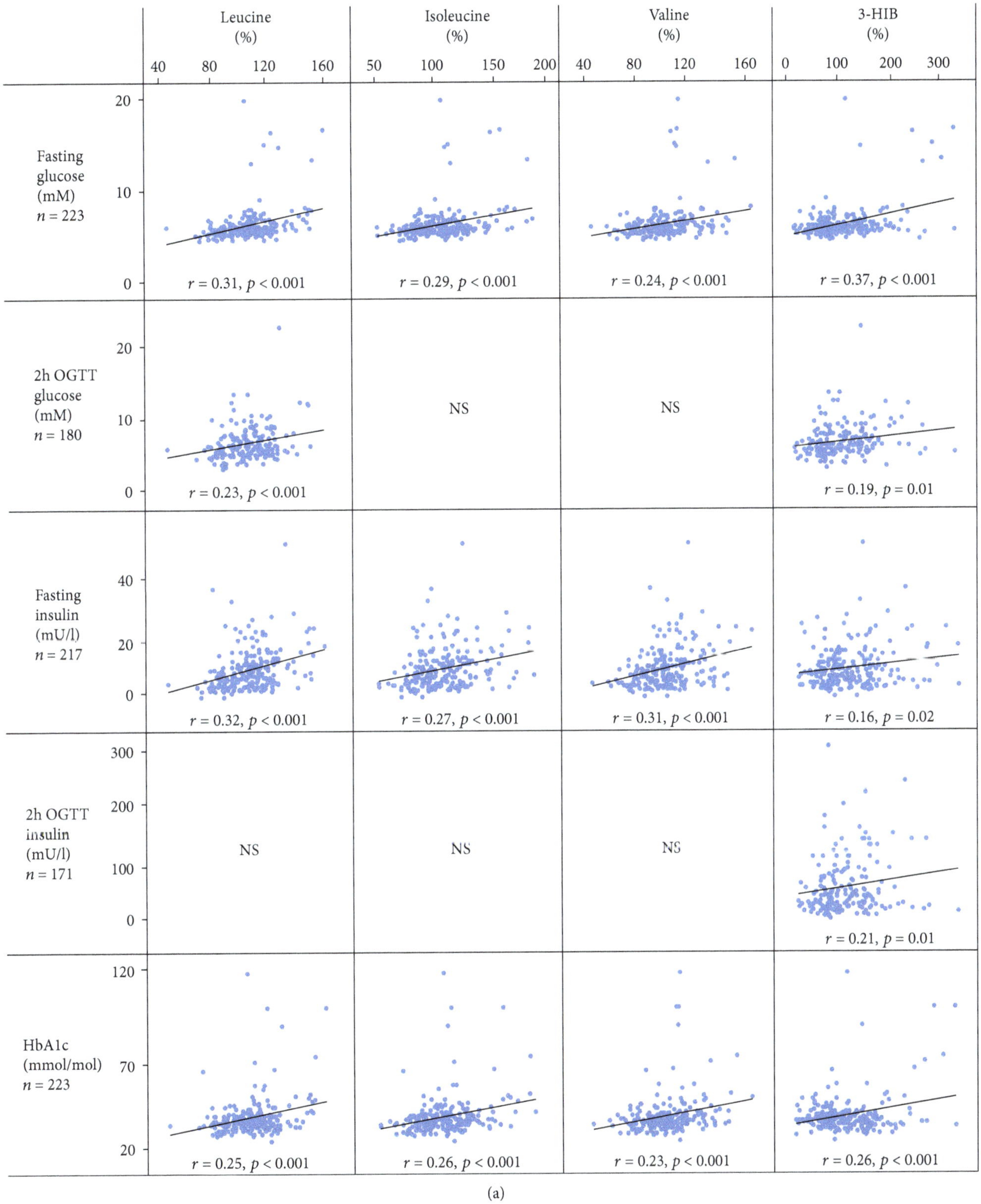

(a)

Figure 3: Continued.

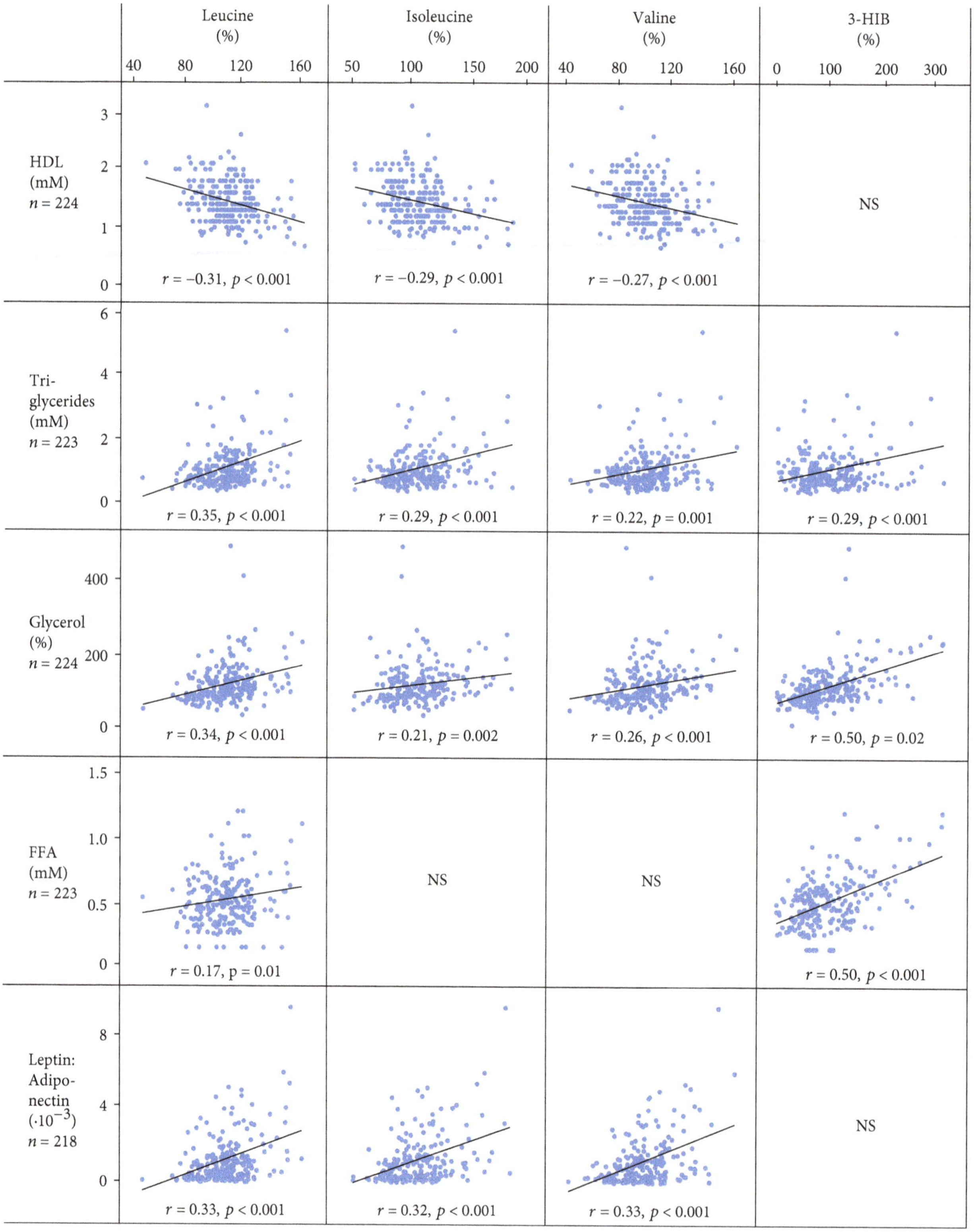

(b)

FIGURE 3: Correlations between glucose (a) and lipid (b) metabolism measurements and BCAAs, 3-HIB, and AAAs 6 years after GDM pregnancy. All three groups (NGT, IGT, and T2DM) were included. Only correlations that were significant after BMI adjustment are shown ($P < 0.05$).

adjusted $R^2 = 0.62$ (Table 3). The three variables with the highest contribution to explain HOMA-IR variance were triglycerides ($\beta = 0.35$, $P < 0.001$), waist circumference ($\beta = 0.31$, $P < 0.001$), and 3-HIB ($\beta = 0.19$, $P < 0.001$). Other contributing variables were age, serum CRP, diastolic blood pressure, physical activity, and BMI change.

TABLE 3: Stepwise linear regression model with HOMA-IR as dependent variable and follow-up variables as independent variables.

Variables included in model	β	P
s-triglycerides (mM)	0.35	<0.001
Waist (cm)	0.31	<0.001
3-HIB (%)	0.19	<0.001
Age (y)	−0.18	<0.001
s-C-reactive protein (mg/L)	0.15	0.008
Diastolic BP (mmHg)	0.13	0.01
Physical activity	−0.12	0.01
BMI change (kg/m^2)	0.11	0.02

Out of 22 variables, 8 remained in the final model to predict HOMA-IR variance; $R = 0.80$, $R^2 = 0.64$, and adjusted $R^2 = 0.62$.

3.5. T1DM and Ketone Metabolism. Eight women were diagnosed with T1DM 6 years after GDM. This group had higher levels of acetoacetate and acetate than the NGT group (Figure 4) and the highest level of 3-HIB; no differences in BCAAs were found (data not shown). For the whole population, 3-HIB correlated with acetoacetate ($P < 0.001$, $R = 0.386$, $n = 232$).

4. Discussion

This study shows that the metabolic profile in women with IGT or T2DM differs substantially from that of women with NGT 6 years after GDM. At follow-up, 22% of the women had developed diabetes (19% T2DM and 3% T1DM) and 19% had IGT. Women with IGT and diabetes had an increased clinical risk profile (higher fasting glucose and insulin treatment during pregnancy) and developed diabetes at an earlier gestational age than those who remained normoglycaemic after pregnancy. These clinical risk factors, which have been shown in other follow-up studies [17], predicted 81% of T2DM cases 6 years after GDM pregnancy.

The IGT and T2DM groups had significant differences in amino acids. AAAs and BCAAs were increased and glycine was decreased. The increases for T2DM in leucine, isoleucine, valine, and 3-HIB were significant after BMI adjustment, but those in tyrosine and phenylalanine were not. The BMI-independent differences in precursors and intermediates such as mannose, glucose, glycine, pyruvate, and citrate point to a possible dysregulation of glycolysis and the TCA-cycle. Changes in triglycerides, glycerol, and FFA suggest dysfunctional fat metabolism. In regression models, the risk factors mainly associated with HOMA-IR are in order of importance triglycerides, waist circumference, 3-HIB, age, CRP, diastolic blood pressure, physical activity, and change in BMI from pregnancy to follow-up.

Disturbed AA metabolism has long been considered a feature of obesity and associated metabolic disease; obese people have higher blood levels of the BCAAs (leucine, isoleucine, and valine) and AAA (phenylalanine and tyrosine) but lower levels of glycine than lean people [18]. We obtained similar results but after BMI adjustment, some of these significances disappeared, linking the metabolism of BCAAs, triglycerides/fatty acids cycle, and glycolysis more strongly to the reduced insulin sensitivity and increased risk of IGT and T2DM per se. Only leucine correlated with body fat percentage. Levels of leucine, isoleucine, and valine are increased as early as 7 years before T2DM development [19]. In one study, BCAAs were elevated 6–9 weeks postpartum in GDM women who were at highest risk for T2DM [20]. Evidently, this metabolic profile precedes the onset of disease rather than being a consequence of T2DM.

BCAAs differ from other AAs in that they are initially catabolized primarily in skeletal muscle not in liver [21]. Indeed, ~50% of skeletal muscle AA uptake consists of BCAAs, since leucine, isoleucine, and valine avoid the hepatic metabolism of substrates immediately after absorption from the intestine [22]. Complete catabolism of BCAAs requires several enzymatic steps. As with most AAs, the final step results in acetyl-CoA, propionyl-CoA, and succinyl-CoA formed from catabolism of isoleucine, leucine, valine, methionine, citrate, and fatty acids—all of which were significantly higher in T2DM than NGT subjects in our study. While some reactions are reversible, leucine, isoleucine, and valine cannot be resynthesized. The catabolic pathways of these BCAAs share two catabolic enzymes in the first step; thereafter, the pathways diverge. The ketogenic leucine product, isovaleryl-CoA, is finally catabolized to acetyl-CoA and acetoacetate. Both valine and isoleucine are considered glucogenic, being metabolized to propionyl-CoA and acetyl-CoA, respectively.

One important step in valine metabolism is generation of 3-HIB, which can be released from tissues. Elevated plasma concentrations of 3-HIB in 3-day fasted subjects and in T1DM patients fasted overnight reflect augmented valine degradation from net body protein breakdown [23]. Since 3-HIB can serve as a gluconeogenic substrate [24], elevated plasma 3-HIB may have a physiologic function in fasting. The increased postabsorptive plasma 3-HIB levels in our subjects with diabetes may reflect increased protein breakdown as a consequence of relative insulin deficiency due to insufficient insulin secretion in relation to insulin resistance, which would also explain increased ketone body production [25]. The tight connection to fasting is also shown by the strong correlation between 3-HIB and both fasting glucose and insulin. Acetoacetate and 3-HIB were correlated and were elevated in both T1DM and T2DM women, whereas only 3-HIB was elevated in the IGT group. The high 3-HIB levels in the circulation and in skeletal muscle in diabetic subjects may lead to excess FFA uptake into muscle [7] and to incomplete lipid degradation [26], resulting in impaired fat oxidation and accumulation of lipotoxic intermediates, which adds to the metabolic inflexibility, impaired insulin signalling, and insulin resistance [7]. Consistent with these findings, 3-HIB had a strong linear correlation with triglycerides, glycerol, FFA, and ADIPO-IR. Interestingly, 3-HIB and body fat were not correlated. The tight relationship of BCAAs to metabolism in skeletal muscle, the most important tissue for insulin resistance, might also explain the strong correlations between 3-HIB and 2 h OGTT glucose and insulin, HOMA-IR, and HbA1c that we found.

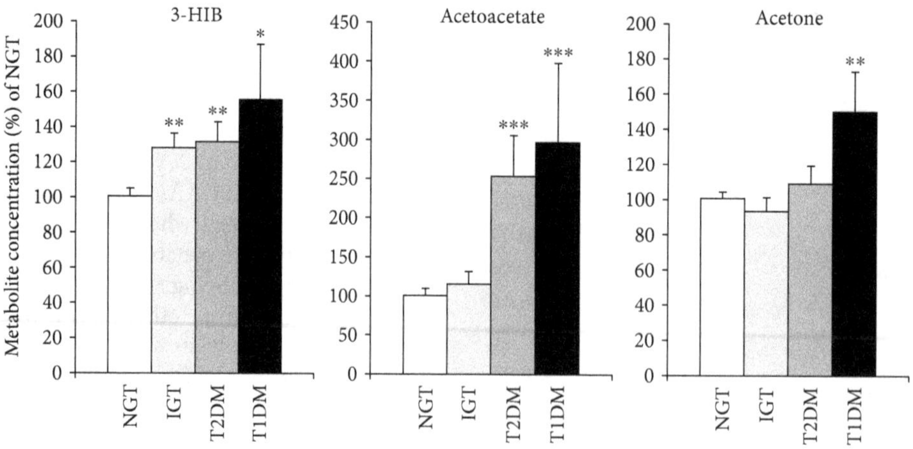

FIGURE 4: 3-HIB and ketone concentrations in T1DM ($n = 8$), T2DM ($n = 44$), and IGT ($n = 43$) versus NGT ($n = 137$). $^{*}P < 0.05$, $^{**}P < 0.01$, and $^{***}P < 0.001$ versus NGT by ANCOVA with BMI as covariate.

Increased BCAA and 3-HIB levels can either be explained by increased protein breakdown and/or decreased catabolism of BCAAs and 3-HIB. In a recent study, several genes involved in BCAA catabolism were downregulated in muscle from insulin-resistant subjects [26]; the highest correlation was seen with *MUT* and *ALDH6A1*, both involved in valine catabolism downstream of 3-HIB. Consistent with this finding, we found a 10–15% increase in BCAAs but a 30% increase in HIB, suggesting 3-HIB accumulation due to impaired catabolism. Experimentally induced defects in MUT reduced cellular respiration and lipid oxidation, eventually leading to lipid accumulation in muscle and insulin resistance [26]. These results together with our findings point to BCAAs, particularly 3-HIB, as a sensitive and early marker for impaired glucose and lipid metabolism.

American Diabetes Association guidelines for postpartum glucose testing were revised in 2017 to include a 75 g OGTT at 4–12 weeks postpartum and thereafter every 1–3 years for women with a prior GDM diagnosis, and more frequent testing if screening results fall within the prediabetes ranges [27]. Low rates of postpartum glucose testing after GDM have been reported for several cohorts of women, despite national guidelines requiring glucose monitoring, and transition to primary care; fewer than half of women with GDM receive postpartum glucose testing [28]. In our study, all women visited the maternal clinic 6–8 weeks postpartum for a 3-day self-monitored glucose profile and a nonfasting glucose sample. They were then given a medical referral and advised to contact primary care for annual follow-up starting 1 year postpartum. Nevertheless, only 42% of our women visited a primary care physician for aftercare during the study period, confirming the reported low rates of follow-up with glucose testing and primary care visits after delivery [28]. Possible reasons for the low follow-up rate include logistical difficulties in administering an OGTT, a time-consuming and inconvenient procedure, fear of receiving a diagnosis of diabetes, and failure to attend the postpartum follow-up examination [20].

Pharmaceutical intervention and lifestyle modifications are as effective in delaying or preventing the onset of T2DM after a GDM pregnancy as they are in other cases of reduced glucose tolerance [29, 30]. In our study, a high level of self-reported physical activity was significantly more common in the NGT group, even after BMI adjustment, and correlated negatively with waist circumference, HOMA-IR, fasting insulin and glucose, and HbA1c, suggesting a strong preventive or delaying effect of IGT. Thus, to identify women at high risk for diabetes after GDM is critical for individual risk stratification and early prevention after delivery (e.g., with increased physical activity).

With the availability and advancement of methods such as NMR and mass spectrometry, several other nonglucose metabolites associated with insulin resistance have been identified, such as 2-hydroxybutyrate (interestingly also linked to amino acid metabolism and the TCA cycle in similarity with 3-HIB), lipid signalling molecules, and fatty acids [31, 32]. The identification of BCAAs, 3-HIB, and these other metabolites in insulin resistance might provide further information in mechanistic studies of metabolic disease, as well as provide different combinations of markers for early prediction of disease and for evaluation of therapeutic interventions.

A limitation of the study is a potential recruitment bias out of the total Gothenburg GDM population, possibly due to language difficulties in the non-Nordic ethnic population. However, this factor is not likely to affect comparisons between glucose tolerance groups or correlations of metabolic parameters.

5. Conclusion

Metabolic risk scores that can identify women at the highest risk for transitioning from GDM to IGT and T2DM are needed. A cost-effective and easy-to-use strategy must be adopted by healthcare givers to reach these women and offer individualized prevention programs. A single blood sample taken annually to analyse one or a few metabolites, in addition to well-known clinical risk factors, would be beneficial but is currently unavailable. Thus, 3-HIB is an interesting metabolite warranting further evaluation as one of a suite of markers for insulin resistance beyond the risk associated with obesity and might improve the prediction of future metabolic risk.

Abbreviations

3-HIB:	3-Hydroxyisobutyrate
AA:	Amino acid
AAA:	Aromatic amino acid
ADIPO-IR:	Adipose tissue insulin resistance
BCAA:	Branched-chain amino acid
BMR:	Basic metabolic rate
EI:	Energy intake
FFA:	Free fatty acids
GDM:	Gestational diabetes mellitus
IGT:	Impaired glucose tolerance
NGT:	Normal glucose tolerance
OGTT:	Oral glucose tolerance test
T2DM:	Type 2 diabetes mellitus.

Conflicts of Interest

The authors declare no conflict of interest.

Authors' Contributions

Agneta Holmäng designed the study; Ulrika Andersson-Hall, Carolina Gustavsson, and Louise Joelsson collected experimental samples and data; Anders Pedersen and Daniel Malmodin performed NMR analysis; and Ulrika Andersson-Hall and Agneta Holmäng interpreted the data and wrote the manuscript.

Acknowledgments

The authors thank Linda Rilby, RNM at Department of Obstetrics, Sahlgrenska University Hospital, for expert technical assistance. This work was supported by grants from the Swedish Research Council (12206), the Swedish Diabetes Association Research Foundation, and the Swedish Federal Government LUA/ALF agreement.

References

[1] B. E. Metzger, D. R. Coustan, and Organizing Committee, "Summary and recommendations of the fourth international workshop-conference on gestational diabetes mellitus," *Diabetes Care*, vol. 21, Supplement 2, pp. B161–B167, 1998.

[2] C. Kim, K. M. Newton, and R. H. Knopp, "Gestational diabetes and the incidence of type 2 diabetes: a systematic review," *Diabetes Care*, vol. 25, no. 10, pp. 1862–1868, 2002.

[3] J. Lauenborg, T. Hansen, D. M. Jensen et al., "Increasing incidence of diabetes after gestational diabetes: a long-term follow-up in a Danish population," *Diabetes Care*, vol. 27, no. 5, pp. 1194–1199, 2004.

[4] J. R. Bain, R. D. Stevens, B. R. Wenner, O. Ilkayeva, D. M. Muoio, and C. B. Newgard, "Metabolomics applied to diabetes research: moving from information to knowledge," *Diabetes*, vol. 58, no. 11, pp. 2429–2443, 2009.

[5] D. M. Muoio and C. B. Newgard, "Molecular and metabolic mechanisms of insulin resistance and β-cell failure in type 2 diabetes," *Nature Reviews Molecular Cell Biology*, vol. 9, no. 3, pp. 193–205, 2008.

[6] E. Chorell, U. A. Hall, C. Gustavsson et al., "Pregnancy to postpartum transition of serum metabolites in women with gestational diabetes," *Metabolism*, vol. 72, pp. 27–36, 2017.

[7] C. Jang, S. F. Oh, S. Wada et al., "A branched-chain amino acid metabolite drives vascular fatty acid transport and causes insulin resistance," *Nature Medicine*, vol. 22, no. 4, pp. 421–426, 2016.

[8] L.-A. L. S. Harris, G. I. Smith, B. W. Patterson et al., "Alterations in 3-hydroxyisobutyrate and FGF21 metabolism are associated with protein ingestion–induced insulin resistance," *Diabetes*, vol. 66, no. 7, pp. 1871–1878, 2017.

[9] A. Lindroos, L. Lissner, and L. Sjostrom, "Validity and reproducibility of a self-administered dietary questionnaire in obese and non-obese subjects," *European Journal of Clinical Nutrition*, vol. 47, no. 7, pp. 461–481, 1993.

[10] C. J. Henry, "Basal metabolic rate studies in humans: measurement and development of new equations," *Public Health Nutrition*, vol. 8, no. 7A, pp. 1133–1152, 2005.

[11] World Hearth Organization, *Definition and Diagnosis of Diabetes Mellitus and Intermediate Hyperglycemia: Report of a WHO/IDF Consultation*, World Hearth Organization, 2006.

[12] C. Ignell and K. Berntorp, "Evaluation of the relationship between capillary and venous plasma glucose concentrations obtained by the HemoCue Glucose 201+ system during an oral glucose tolerance test," *Scandinavian Journal of Clinical and Laboratory Investigation*, vol. 71, no. 8, pp. 670–675, 2011.

[13] T. M. Wallace, J. C. Levy, and D. R. Matthews, "Use and abuse of HOMA modeling," *Diabetes Care*, vol. 27, no. 6, pp. 1487–1495, 2004.

[14] A. Gastaldelli, M. Gaggini, and R. A. DeFronzo, "Role of adipose tissue insulin resistance in the natural history of type 2 diabetes: results from the San Antonio metabolism study," *Diabetes*, vol. 66, no. 4, pp. 815–822, 2017.

[15] F. Savorani, G. Tomasi, and S. B. Engelsen, "*i*coshift: a versatile tool for the rapid alignment of 1D NMR spectra," *Journal of Magnetic Resonance*, vol. 202, no. 2, pp. 190–202, 2010.

[16] D. S. Wishart, T. Jewison, A. C. Guo et al., "HMDB 3.0—the human metabolome database in 2013," *Nucleic Acids Research*, vol. 41, no. D1, pp. D801-D807, 2013.

[17] M. Ekelund, N. Shaat, P. Almgren, L. Groop, and K. Berntorp, "Prediction of postpartum diabetes in women with gestational diabetes mellitus," *Diabetologia*, vol. 53, no. 3, pp. 452–457, 2010.

[18] P. Felig, E. Marliss, and G. F. Cahill Jr., "Plasma amino acid levels and insulin secretion in obesity," *The New England Journal of Medicine*, vol. 281, no. 15, pp. 811–816, 1969.

[19] T. J. Wang, M. G. Larson, R. S. Vasan et al., "Metabolite profiles and the risk of developing diabetes," *Nature Medicine*, vol. 17, no. 4, pp. 448–453, 2011.

[20] A. Allalou, A. Nalla, K. J. Prentice et al., "A predictive metabolic signature for the transition from gestational diabetes mellitus to type 2 diabetes," *Diabetes*, vol. 65, no. 9, pp. 2529–2539, 2016.

[21] E. L. Dillon, "Nutritionally essential amino acids and metabolic signaling in aging," *Amino Acids*, vol. 45, no. 3, pp. 431–441, 2013.

[22] A. Goichon, P. Chan, S. Lecleire et al., "An enteral leucine supply modulates human duodenal mucosal proteome and decreases the expression of enzymes involved in fatty acid beta-oxidation," *Journal of Proteomics*, vol. 78, pp. 535–544, 2013.

[23] A. Avogaro and D. M. Bier, "Contribution of 3-hydroxyisobutyrate to the measurement of 3-hydroxybutyrate in human plasma: comparison of enzymatic and gas-liquid chromatography-mass spectrometry assays in normal and in diabetic subjects," *Journal of Lipid Research*, vol. 30, no. 11, pp. 1811–1817, 1989.

[24] J. Letto, M. E. Brosnan, and J. T. Brosnan, "Valine metabolism gluconeogenesis from 3-hydroxyisobutyrate," *Biochemical Journal*, vol. 240, no. 3, pp. 909–912, 1986.

[25] J. J. Robert, B. Beaufrere, J. Koziet et al., "Whole body de novo amino acid synthesis in type I (insulin-dependent) diabetes studied with stable isotope-labeled leucine, alanine, and glycine," *Diabetes*, vol. 34, no. 1, pp. 67–73, 1985.

[26] C. Lerin, A. B. Goldfine, T. Boes et al., "Defects in muscle branched-chain amino acid oxidation contribute to impaired lipid metabolism," *Molecular Metabolism*, vol. 5, no. 10, pp. 926–936, 2016.

[27] American Diabetes Association, "*Standards of medical care in diabetes—2017*: summary of revisions," *Diabetes Care*, vol. 40, Supplement 1, pp. S4–S5, 2017.

[28] J. A. Bernstein, L. McCloskey, C. M. Gebel, R. E. Iverson, and A. Lee-Parritz, "Lost opportunities to prevent early onset type 2 diabetes mellitus after a pregnancy complicated by gestational diabetes," *BMJ Open Diabetes Research & Care*, vol. 4, no. 1, article e000250, 2016.

[29] Q. Gong, E. W. Gregg, J. Wang et al., "Long-term effects of a randomised trial of a 6-year lifestyle intervention in impaired glucose tolerance on diabetes-related microvascular complications: the China Da Qing Diabetes Prevention Outcome Study," *Diabetologia*, vol. 54, no. 2, pp. 300–307, 2011.

[30] W. C. Knowler, E. Barrett-Connor, S. E. Fowler et al., "Reduction in the incidence of type 2 diabetes with lifestyle intervention or metformin," *The New England Journal of Medicine*, vol. 346, no. 6, pp. 393–403, 2002.

[31] E. Ferrannini, A. Natali, S. Camastra et al., "Early metabolic markers of the development of dysglycemia and type 2 diabetes and their physiological significance," *Diabetes*, vol. 62, no. 5, pp. 1730–1737, 2013.

[32] D. Tripathy, J. E. Cobb, W. Gall et al., "A novel insulin resistance index to monitor changes in insulin sensitivity and glucose tolerance: the ACT NOW study," *The Journal of Clinical Endocrinology & Metabolism*, vol. 100, no. 5, pp. 1855–1862, 2015.

11

Mean Platelet Volume and Gestational Diabetes Mellitus

Zhongwei Zhou, Hongmei Chen, Mingzhong Sun, and Huixiang Ju

Department of Clinical Laboratory, Affiliated Yancheng Hospital, School of Medicine, Southeast University, Yancheng, Jiangsu 224001, China

Correspondence should be addressed to Huixiang Ju; jhxycsy@163.com

Academic Editor: Suat Simsek

Aim. To evaluate the association between mean platelet volume (MPV) and gestational diabetes mellitus (GDM). *Methods.* A systematic literature search was performed in PubMed, EMBASE, Web of Science, and The Cochrane Library up to 4 September 2017. Pooled standardized mean differences (SMD) and 95% confidence interval (CI) were calculated using a random-effect model. *Results.* Nineteen studies comprising 1361 GDM patients and 1911 normal pregnant women were included. MPV was increased in GDM patients when compared with healthy pregnant women (SMD: 0.79; 95% CI: 0.43–1.16; $P < 0.001$). Subgroup analyses revealed that such trend was consistent in the third-trimester (SMD: 1.35; 95% CI: 0.72–1.98), Turkish (SMD: 0.81; 95% CI: 0.43–1.19), and Italian (SMD: 2.78; 95% CI: 2.22–3.34) patients with GDM and the patients diagnosed based on Carpenter and Coustan criteria (SMD: 1.04; 95% CI: 0.42–1.65). Significantly higher MPV also were observed within cross-sectional studies (SMD: 0.99; 95% CI: 0.49–1.49). Remarkable between-study heterogeneity and potential publication bias were observed in this meta-analysis; however, sensitivity analysis indicated that the results were not unduly influenced by any single study. *Conclusions.* GDM patients are accompanied by increased MPV, strengthening the clinical evidence that MPV may be a predictive marker for GDM.

1. Introduction

Gestational diabetes mellitus (GDM), one of the most prevalent pregnancy complications, is defined as varying degrees of impaired glucose intolerance that is initially recognized in pregnancy [1]. According to different definition and criteria, GDM affects 4–18% pregnant women [2]. Although glucose intolerance may return to normal after pregnancy in most women with GDM, a certain proportion of pregnant women will develop into or are at greatest risk for progression to type 2 diabetes mellitus (T2DM) [3, 4]. And like T2DM, GDM patients generally have different levels of insulin resistance and chronic low-grade inflammation, which trigger vascular injury and dysfunction and subsequent platelet activation [5, 6]. Therefore, the level of platelet activation may be associated with severity of GDM.

Mean platelet volume (MPV), an easily and inexpensive parameter derived from routine blood counts, is usually used to evaluate platelet morphology and can be used as an indicator of platelet activity [7]. Elevated MPV has been demonstrated to be related to cardiovascular diseases and its risk factors such as T2DM, hypertension, and nonalcoholic fatty liver disease (NAFLD) [8–11]. Recently, a substantial number of studies measured MPV levels in women with GDM to evaluate whether it can be used as an indicator to monitor and assess the development of GDM. However, studies of the association between MPV and GDM yielded inconsistent findings. Some studies observed that GDM patients had significantly increased MPV compared with healthy pregnant women [12, 13], whereas other studies reported no association between MPV and GDM [14, 15]. Furthermore, some groups found decreased MPV values in patients with GDM [16, 17]. In light of these inconsistent findings, we undertook a meta-analysis to provide a more comprehensive conclusion of the association between MPV and GDM.

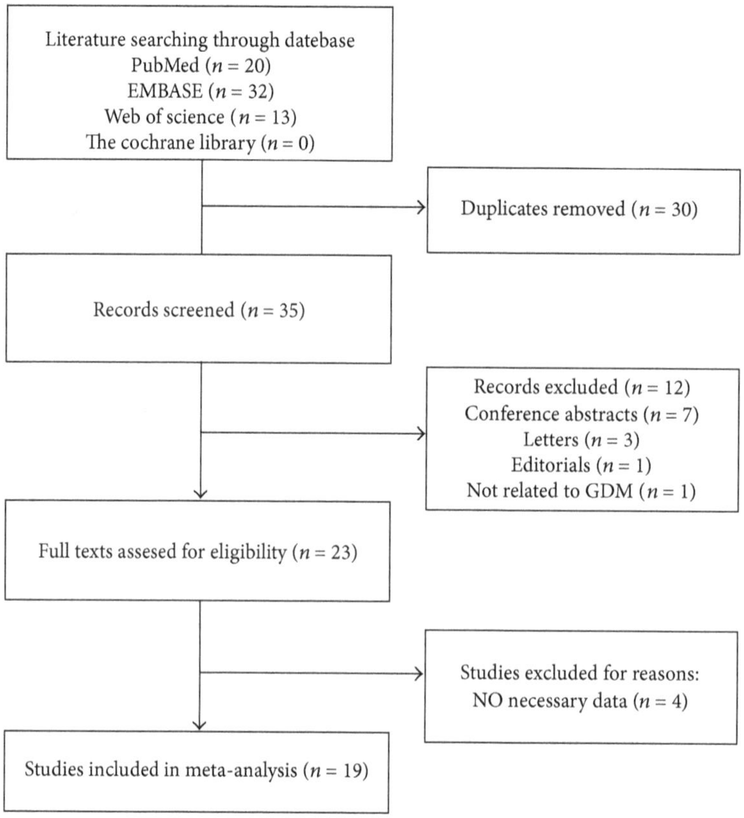

FIGURE 1: Flow chart of the study selection process.

2. Methods

2.1. Search Strategy. A systematic search on literature was performed on electronic databases including PubMed, EMBASE, Web of Science, and The Cochrane Library up until 4 September 2017. The search terms included ("gestational diabetes mellitus" OR gestational diabetes OR "GDM") AND ("mean platelet volume" OR MPV). In addition, the bibliographies from these relevant articles were also manually searched for additional eligible studies.

2.2. Study Selection. Studies were considered eligible if they met the following criteria: (1) studies compared the MPV between GDM patients and healthy pregnant women with normal glucose tolerance (NGT), (2) case and control subjects all did not have a previous history of diabetes or present pregnant complications, or (3) studies were published in English or Chinese. Studies were excluded if they were reviews, editorials, letters to the editor, case reports, conference abstracts, or studies on animals or cell lines.

2.3. Data Extraction and Quality Assessment. Two investigators (Zhongwei Zhou and Hongmei Chen) independently reviewed all identified studies and extracted the data using a predefined form and confirmed by a third reviewer (Huixiang Ju). Disagreement was resolved by discussion among all researchers. The following information was abstracted from each eligible study: the first author's name, year of publication, study location, study design, trimester of MPV measurement, average age and body mass index (BMI) of GDM patients, diagnosis criteria of GDM, sample size of the case and control group, and mean and standard deviation (SD) of MPV. If studies did not offer mean and SD of MPV, the corresponding authors were contacted. When the request was not responded, transformations were made by standard formulas.

The quality of the study was evaluated using a modified criteria based on the Newcastle-Ottawa Quality Assessment Scale (NOS) for observational studies suggested by van Dijk et al. [18], which was modified to accommodate the topic of this review. A study that met 7 or more points would be considered as a high-quality study.

2.4. Statistical Analysis. Standardized mean differences (SMD) and 95% confidence interval (CI) in MPV between GDM patients and controls were calculated and estimated for each study. A random-effect model was chosen for pooling of data. This is because if there is a significant heterogeneity between studies, the random-effect model would be more conservative than the fixed-effect model [19]. Heterogeneity across included studies was assessed using the I^2 index, and an I^2 index of 25%, 50%, and 75% would indicate small, moderate, and high heterogeneity, respectively [20]. To explore the potential source of heterogeneity, subgroup analysis was carried out by the trimester of MPV measurement, study location, and study design.

Sensitivity analysis was performed to evaluate the influence of each study on the pooled measures by omitting one

Table 1: Main characteristics of the studies included in this meta-analysis.

References	Study location	Study design	Case group		Control group		MPV measurement trimester	Average age of GDM patients (years)	Average BMI of GDM patients (kg/m^2)	GDM criteria	Quality score
			Sample size	MPV levels	Sample size	MPV levels					
Kebapcilar et al., 2016 [12]	Turkey	Case-control	101	9.16 ± 1.04	138	7.42 ± 0.80	Second	26.1	26.9	C&C	8
Sahbaz et al., 2016 [13]	Turkey	Case-control	59	8.93 ± 0.98	60	8.39 ± 1.11	Third	31.4	26.3	C&C	3
Yıldız et al., 2016 [14]	Turkey	Cross-sectional	53	9.98 ± 1.22	35	10.05 ± 1.15	NA	31.5	27.9	C&C	7
Zhu et al., 2015 [15]	China	Case-control	36	10.76 ± 2.02	36	11.07 ± 0.90	Second	31.2	NA	ADA	8
Gorar et al., 2017 [16]	Turkey	Cross-sectional	110	10.4 ± 0.74	159	10.6 ± 0.74	Second	33.0	NA	C&C	4
Yang et al., 2015 [17]	China	Cross-sectional	302	9.0 ± 1.47	310	9.3 ± 1.41	NA	30.6	21.2	ADA	7
Baldane et al., 2015 [21]	Turkey	Cross-sectional	114	10.2 ± 1.05	76	9.9 ± 1.27	Second	29.4	NA	C&C	5
Gur et al., 2015 [22]	Turkey	Cross-sectional	16	10.9 ± 1.0	167	9.6 ± 1.0	Second	29.0	27.1	NDDG	8
Erdogan et al., 2014 [23]	Turkey	Case-control	68	10.5 ± 2.94	61	11.2 ± 1.14	Second	31.8	NA	NDDG	5
Iyidir et al., 2014 [24]	Turkey	Case-control	30	8.8 ± 1.0	38	8.1 ± 0.70	Third	33.7	NA	C&C	8
Maconi et al., 2012 [25]	Italy	Cross-sectional	25	11.9 ± 1.90	100	8.3 ± 1.10	Third	31.4	NA	NA	2
Sak et al., 2012 [26]	Turkey	Case-control	42	8.9 ± 1.90	35	7.8 ± 2.0	Third	31.2	28.6	ADA	6
Erikci et al., 2008 [27]	Turkey	Cross-sectional	34	9.3 ± 1.45	45	8.1 ± 0.66	Third	29.5	NA	ADA	4
Bozkurt et al., 2006 [28]	Turkey	Cross-sectional	100	9.4 ± 1.6	100	8.3 ± 1.1	Third	31	NA	C&C	5
Yin et al., 2005 [29]	China	Cross-sectional	21	9.5 ± 1.6	20	8.7 ± 1.6	Third	27.1	NA	NA	5
Çeltik et al., 2016 [30]	Turkey	Case-control	105	8.66 ± 1.15	40	8.27 ± 0.92	Second	33.4	27.7	ADA	7
Çeltik et al., 2016 [30]	Turkey	Case-control	105	9.59 ± 1.34	40	8.95 ± 1.98	Third	33.4	27.7	ADA	
Soydinc et al., 2013 [31]	Turkey	Cross-sectional	42	9.28 ± 0.35	33	7.71 ± 0.19	Third	32.5	28.5	C&C	8
Erdem et al., 2013 [32]	Turkey	Cross-sectional	58	9.43 ± 1.09	219	8.53 ± 0.99	Second	30.1	NA	C&C	6
Köflüfl et al., 2010 [33]	Turkey	Cross-sectional	45	8.67 ± 1.43	239	8.19 ± 0.85	Second	31.2	NA	NDDG	5

MPV: mean platelet volume; GDM: gestational diabetes mellitus; BMI: body mass index; C&C: Carpenter and Coustan; NDDG: National Diabetes Data Group; ADA: American Diabetes Association; NA: not available.

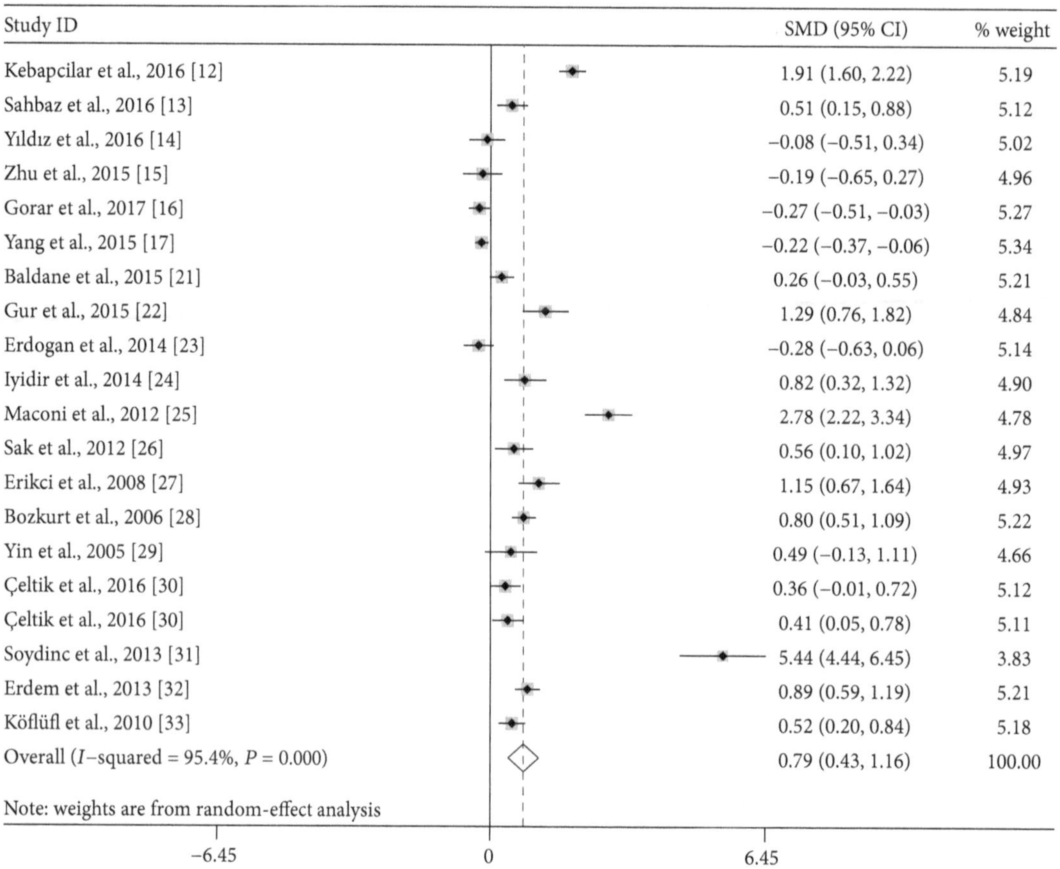

Figure 2: Overall meta-analysis of mean platelet volume in gestational diabetes mellitus patients compared with healthy pregnant women. SMD: standardized mean differences; CI: confidence interval.

single study in each turn and recalculating the pooled SMD for the remainders. Publication bias was evaluated by inspection of funnel plots and Egger's test.

All analyses were performed using Stata 14.0 (StataCorp LP, College Station, TX, USA), and $P < 0.05$ was considered to be statistically significant.

3. Results

3.1. Study Selection and Study Characteristics. The electronic database search of PubMed, EMBASE, Web of Science, and The Cochrane Library yielded a total of 65 records. After removing duplicates and reading the titles and abstracts, 23 appropriate articles were identified for full-text scrutiny. The 4 articles were further excluded for lack of necessary data. Finally, 19 studies (20 results) met the criteria to be included in the present meta-analysis [12–17, 21–33], and a flowchart showed the selection process (Figure 1).

The 19 included studies were published from 2005 to 2017 covering 1361 GDM patients and 1911 normal pregnant women. The main characteristics of these studies included in the present meta-analysis are presented in Table 1. Among these, twelve cross-sectional and seven case-control studies (8 results) were included. Fifteen studies were carried out in Turkey, three in China, and one in Italy. Several different criteria were used to define GDM, and among them, Carpenter and Coustan (C&C) criteria were used in nine studies, National Diabetes Data Group (NDDG) in three studies, and American Diabetes Association (ADA) in five studies. Nine studies measured MPV values during the second trimester and the same number during the third trimester. The results of quality evaluation showed that the mean score across included studies was 5.8. Eight studies were scored greater than or equal to 7 out of 9 which were considered as high-quality studies. However, two studies, Maconi et al. [25] and Sahbaz et al. [13], were graded 2 and 3, respectively.

3.2. Main Association of MPV with GDM. We performed a random-effect meta-analysis on the extracted 19 studies. The results showed that MPV values were significantly increased in GDM patients when compared with healthy pregnant women (Figure 2, SMD: 0.79; 95% CI: 0.43, 1.16; $P < 0.001$). Sensitivity analysis showed that no individual study significantly influenced the difference on MPV values between GDM patients and healthy pregnant women. However, significant and high-level heterogeneity among studies was found in this meta-analysis ($I^2 = 95.4$, $P < 0.001$).

3.3. Subgroup Analyses. Subgroup analyses were performed based on the trimester of MPV measurement, study location, the defined criteria of GDM, and study design. As shown in Figure 3, stratified analyses indicated that the third-trimester patients had significantly higher MPV than did

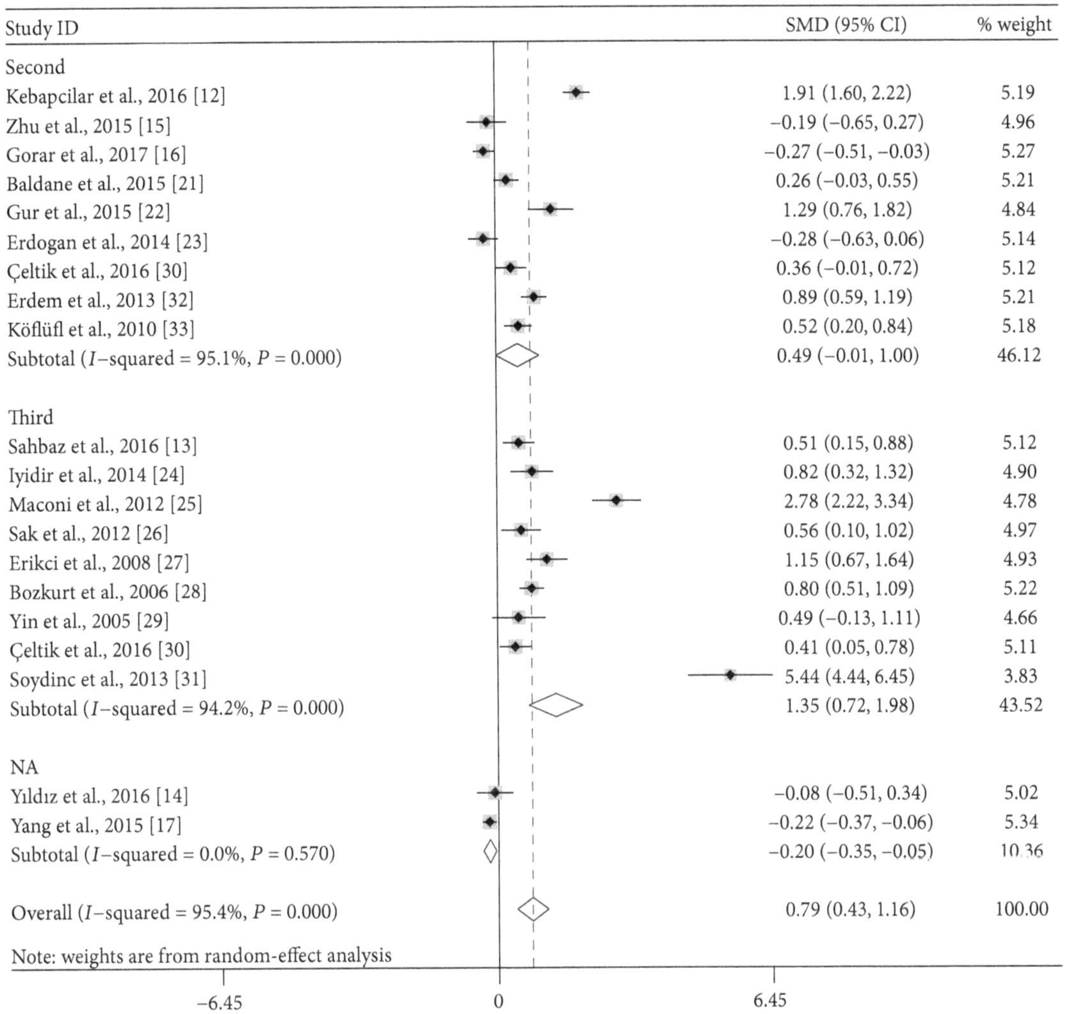

FIGURE 3: Subgroup analysis of mean platelet volume (MPV) in gestational diabetes mellitus patients compared with healthy pregnant women when stratified by the trimester of MPV measurement. SMD: standardized mean differences; CI: confidence interval; NA: not available.

healthy pregnant women (SMD: 1.35; 95% CI: 0.72–1.98), while the difference did not reach statistical significance during the second trimester (SMD: 0.49; 95% CI: −0.01–1.00). When the studies were classified to three subgroups according to study location, both Turkish (SMD: 0.81; 95% CI: 0.43–1.19) and Italian (SMD: 2.78; 95% CI: 2.22–3.34) patients had significantly higher MPV compared with the control, but the difference was not observed between Chinese women with and without GDM (SMD: −0.07; 95% CI: −0.41-0.28) (Figure 4). When stratifying by the defined criteria of GDM, patients defined by C&C criteria had significantly higher MPV compared with the control (SMD: 1.04; 95% CI: 0.42–1.65), but those defined by other criteria had not (Figure 5). The significant difference was also observed in the subgroup of cross-sectional studies (SMD: 0.99; 95% CI: 0.49–1.49), but not within the subgroup of case-control studies (SMD: 0.52; 95% CI: −0.02–1.05) (Figure 6).

3.4. Publication Bias. Visual inspection of funnel plots showed asymmetry in this meta-analysis (Figure 7). Egger's test further showed that there was potential publication bias in this meta-analysis ($P = 0.004$).

4. Discussion

This meta-analysis demonstrated that MPV was significantly increased in GDM patients compared with healthy pregnant women overall. Although potential publication bias might exist in the included studies, sensitivity analysis indicated that the results were not unduly influenced by any single study. These findings suggest that women with GDM may be accompanied by increased MPV levels. To the best of our knowledge, this is the first meta-analysis on this subject, which provides clinical evidence that MPV may be a predictive marker for GDM.

In the meta-analysis, subgroup analysis was used to analyze the potential factors contributing to heterogeneity and obtain further information from different subpopulations. When stratifying by the trimester of MPV measurement, we observed significantly increased MPV in GDM patients in the third trimester. Significantly higher MPV was also

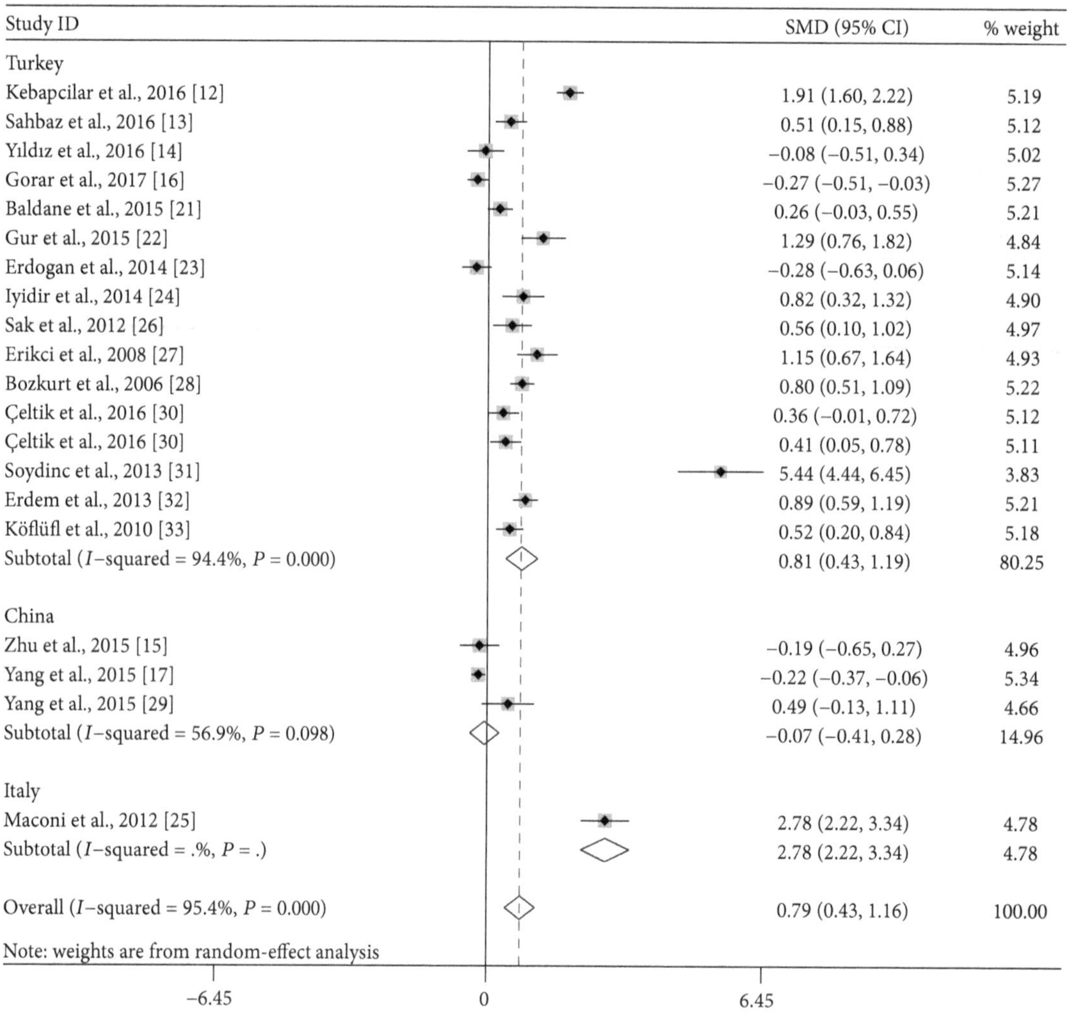

FIGURE 4: Subgroup analysis of mean platelet volume (MPV) in gestational diabetes mellitus patients compared with healthy pregnant women when stratified by study location. SMD: standardized mean differences; CI: confidence interval.

observed in Turkish and Italian women with GDM and the subgroups of cross-sectional studies and C&C criteria defined for GDM patients. These results suggest that there may be varying levels of MPV in different stages of pregnancy and GDM patients with different ethnic backgrounds, and study design and the diagnostic criteria of GDM might also influence the results of MPV. Although subgroup analyses were carried out to explore some potential sources, we still found high levels of heterogeneity in all the subgroups but studies with the Chinese patient group in which heterogeneity was moderately reduced. As data on some potential confounders such as BMI, insulin resistance index, and lifestyle are limited in the eligible studies included in the meta-analysis, which prevented us from further analyzing whether these factors were confounders affecting the outcome of this meta-analysis. Therefore, the results of this meta-analysis should be cautiously interpreted.

The pathophysiologic mechanism for increased MPV observed in GDM is not yet fully elucidated. However, several plausible explanations may account for their relationship. It has been suggested that insulin resistance is a major determinant of platelet activation which can be measured by MPV [6, 34]. Normal pregnancy is characterized by physiological insulin resistance that begins in the second trimester and peaks in the third trimester, which causes increased insulin secretion [35]. GDM is the result of increased insulin production which cannot compensate for the increased insulin resistance [36]. In this study, we found that although GDM patients had higher MPV levels than those in the control in the second trimester, the difference did not reach statistical significance, while such difference was dramatically significant during the third trimester. The diverse results of MPV levels just matched the level of insulin resistance in different trimesters. In support of this theory, two studies [12, 21] included in the present meta-analysis demonstrated that there was a significant positive correlation between MPV and homoeostasis model assessment of insulin resistance (HOMA-IR). Another plausible mechanism is the intimate connection between platelet activation and inflammation. Platelet-derived inflammatory mediators, such as soluble CD40 ligand and CD36, were considered to have significant effects on the release of cytokines and chemokines and the enhancement of the inflammatory process when the platelet is activated [37]. On the other hand, there is evidence

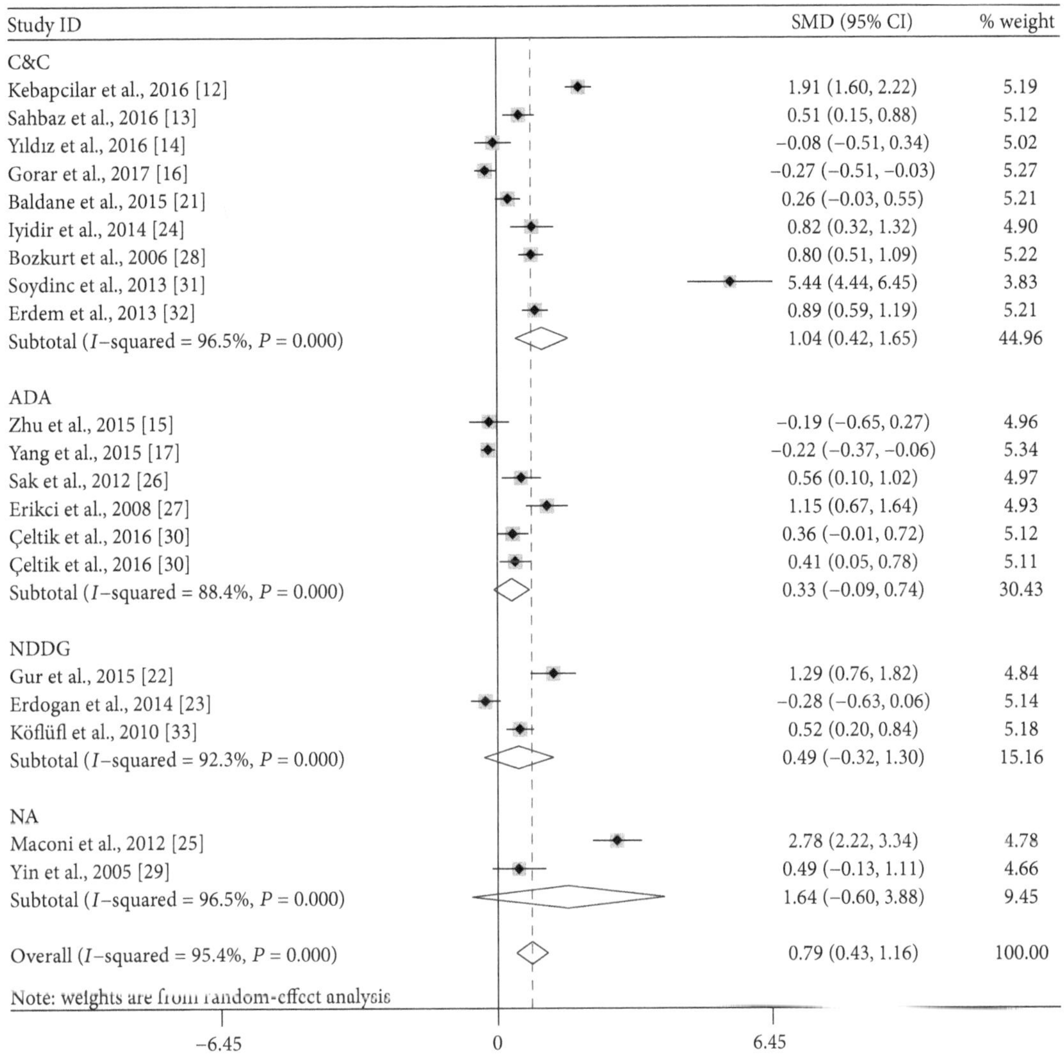

Figure 5: Subgroup analysis of mean platelet volume (MPV) in gestational diabetes mellitus patients compared with healthy pregnant women when stratified by the defined criteria of GDM. SMD: standardized mean differences; CI: confidence interval; NA: not available.

that leukocytes can release the platelet-activating factor to induce platelet activation [38]. And it has been shown that GDM is a chronic inflammatory condition, with increased proinflammatory cytokines like TNF-α, IL-6, CRP, IL-1β, and IL-18 [5, 39]. In a prospective study, increased early pregnancy leukocyte count was shown to be independently associated with the risk of GDM [40]. In this sense, MPV may serve as an indicator of chronic inflammatory status of GDM.

There are several limitations in this meta-analysis. First, all the included studies were observational; therefore, a causal link between MPV and GDM cannot be established. Second, as most of the studies included in this meta-analysis were carried out in Turkey (15 out of 19), the pooled outcome of the meta-analysis might not be representative of the total global population. Third, the asymmetric funnel plot suggested that the potential publication bias may be present among studies, so the significant differences of MPV between GDM patients and healthy pregnant women may be overestimated. However, sensitivity analysis indicated that no individual study significantly influenced the difference on MPV levels between patients and controls. In addition, it should be acknowledged that the asymmetric funnel plot is not always created by publication bias but can also be caused by low-quality studies and significant heterogeneity among studies [41, 42]. Most recently, Zwetsloot et al. [43] revealed that the funnel plot of the SMD plotted is susceptible to distortion, resulting in overestimation in publication bias assessments. Finally, due to a lack of appropriate quality-assessment tool for observational studies, our assessment of study quality was based on the modified NOS, which may lead to arbitrary results [44]. But the quality score was not used in the meta-analyses, such as subgroup analyses, as we thought that it may be better suited to assessing different aspects of methodology of a study in an independent manner.

5. Conclusion

In conclusion, this meta-analysis demonstrated that GDM patients are accompanied by increased MPV, which suggests

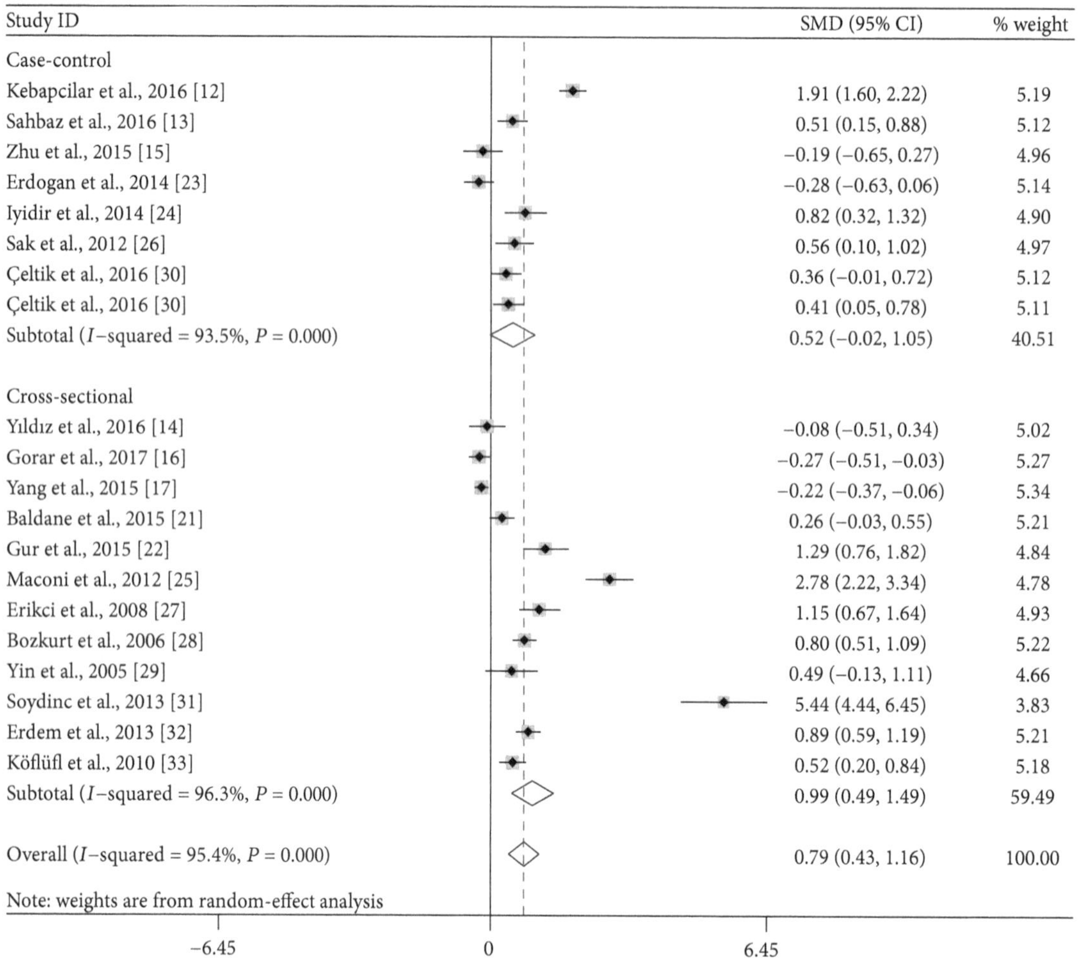

FIGURE 6: Subgroup analysis of mean platelet volume (MPV) in gestational diabetes mellitus patients compared with healthy pregnant women when stratified by study design. SMD: standardized mean differences; CI: confidence interval.

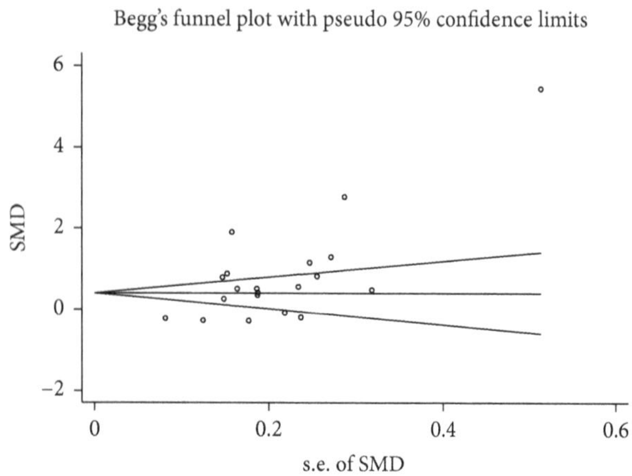

FIGURE 7: Begg's funnel plot of included studies for potential publication bias between gestational diabetes mellitus patients and healthy pregnant women. SMD: standardized mean differences; s.e.: standard error.

MPV may be used as an indicator to monitor and evaluate the development of GDM. However, the results should be cautiously interpreted because of the potential publication bias and substantial between-study heterogeneity, and further prospective, multicenter cohort studies are required to confirm these findings.

Conflicts of Interest

The authors declare no conflict of interest.

Authors' Contributions

Zhongwei Zhou and Hongmei Chen contributed equally to this work.

References

[1] D. Simmons, "Prevention of gestational diabetes mellitus: where are we now?," *Diabetes, Obesity and Metabolism*, vol. 17, no. 9, pp. 824–834, 2015.

[2] T. Cundy, E. Ackermann, and E. A. Ryan, "Gestational diabetes: new criteria may triple the prevalence but effect on outcomes is unclear," *BMJ*, vol. 348, article g1567, 2014.

[3] Y. Zhu and C. Zhang, "Prevalence of gestational diabetes and risk of progression to type 2 diabetes: a global perspective," *Current Diabetes Reports*, vol. 16, no. 1, p. 7, 2016.

[4] B. Akinci, A. Celtik, S. Yener, and S. Yesil, "Prediction of developing metabolic syndrome after gestational diabetes mellitus," *Fertility and Sterility*, vol. 93, no. 4, pp. 1248–1254, 2010.

[5] T. L. Hernandez, R. E. Van Pelt, M. A. Anderson et al., "Women with gestational diabetes mellitus randomized to a higher-complex carbohydrate/low-fat diet manifest lower adipose tissue insulin resistance, inflammation, glucose, and free fatty acids: a pilot study," *Diabetes Care*, vol. 39, no. 1, pp. 39–42, 2016.

[6] F. Santilli, N. Vazzana, R. Liani, M. T. Guagnano, and G. Davi, "Platelet activation in obesity and metabolic syndrome," *Obesity Reviews*, vol. 13, no. 1, pp. 27–42, 2012.

[7] I. A. Jagroop, S. Tsiara, and D. P. Mikhailidis, "Mean platelet volume as an indicator of platelet activation: methodological issues," *Platelets*, vol. 14, no. 5, pp. 335-336, 2003.

[8] C. B. Maluf, S. M. Barreto, R. C. dos Reis, and P. G. Vidigal, "Platelet volume is associated with the Framingham risk score for cardiovascular disease in the Brazilian Longitudinal Study of Adult Health (ELSA-Brasil)," *Clinical Chemistry and Laboratory Medicine*, vol. 54, no. 5, pp. 879–887, 2016.

[9] N. Sansanayudh, D. Muntham, S. Yamwong, P. Sritara, T. Akrawichien, and A. Thakkinstian, "The association between mean platelet volume and cardiovascular risk factors," *European Journal of Internal Medicine*, vol. 30, pp. 37–42, 2016.

[10] D. Kadic, S. Hasic, and E. Spahic, "Mean platelet volume predicts the glycemic control deterioration in diabetes mellitus type 2 patients," *Medicinski Glasnik*, vol. 13, no. 1, pp. 1-7, 2016.

[11] L. Gang, Z. Yanyan, Z. Zhongwei, and D. Juan, "Association between mean platelet volume and hypertension incidence," *Hypertension Research*, vol. 40, no. 8, pp. 779–784, 2017.

[12] L. Kebapcilar, A. G. Kebapcilar, T. T. Ilhan et al., "Is the mean platelet volume a predictive marker of a low Apgar score and insulin resistance in gestational diabetes mellitus? A retrospective case-control study," *Journal of Clinical and Diagnostic Research*, vol. 10, no. 10, 2016.

[13] A. Sahbaz, H. Cicekler, O. Aynioglu, H. Isik, and U. Ozmen, "Comparison of the predictive value of plateletcrit with various other blood parameters in gestational diabetes development," *Journal of Obstetrics and Gynaecology*, vol. 36, no. 5, pp. 589–593, 2016.

[14] S. Yıldız, R. Üçler, M. Alay, and E. B. Ekici, "Which hemogram parameter is more cautionary in euthyroid patients with gestational diabetes mellitus," *Eastern Journal of Medicine*, vol. 21, no. 4, pp. 162–167, 2016.

[15] C. Zhu, H. Yang, Q. Geng et al., "Association of oxidative stress biomarkers with gestational diabetes mellitus in pregnant women: a case-control study," *PLoS One*, vol. 10, no. 4, article e0126490, 2015.

[16] S. Gorar, G. B. Abanonu, A. Uysal et al., "Comparison of thyroid function tests and blood count in pregnant women with versus without gestational diabetes mellitus," *Journal of Obstetrics and Gynaecology Research*, vol. 43, no. 5, pp. 848–854, 2017.

[17] H. Yang, C. Zhu, Q. Ma, Y. Long, and Z. Cheng, "Variations of blood cells in prediction of gestational diabetes mellitus," *Journal of Perinatal Medicine*, vol. 43, no. 1, pp. 89–93, 2015.

[18] G. M. van Dijk, M. Maneva, V. Colpani et al., "The association between vasomotor symptoms and metabolic health in peri- and postmenopausal women: a systematic review," *Maturitas*, vol. 80, no. 2, pp. 140–147, 2015.

[19] A. Masi, D. S. Quintana, N. Glozier, A. R. Lloyd, I. B. Hickie, and A. J. Guastella, "Cytokine aberrations in autism spectrum disorder: a systematic review and meta-analysis," *Molecular Psychiatry*, vol. 20, no. 4, pp. 440–446, 2015.

[20] J. P. Ioannidis, N. A. Patsopoulos, and E. Evangelou, "Uncertainty in heterogeneity estimates in meta-analyses," *BMJ*, vol. 335, no. 7626, pp. 914–916, 2007.

[21] S. Baldane, S. H. Ipekci, and A. Kebapcilar, "Relationship between insulin resistance and mean platelet volume in gestational diabetes mellitus," *Journal of Laboratory Physicians*, vol. 7, no. 2, pp. 112–115, 2015.

[22] E. B. Gur, M. Karadeniz, M. Genc et al., "Relationship between mean platelet volume and vitamin D deficiency in gestational diabetes mellitus," *Archives of Endocrinology and Metabolism*, vol. 59, no. 5, pp. 448–454, 2015.

[23] S. Erdogan, O. Ozdemir, H. O. Dogan et al., "Liver enzymes, mean platelet volume, and red cell distribution width in gestational diabetes," *Turkish Journal of Medical Sciences*, vol. 44, no. 1, pp. 121–125, 2014.

[24] O. T. Iyidir, C. K. Degertekin, B. A. Yilmaz, F. B. Toruner, M. Akturk, and M. Arslan, "Elevated mean platelet volume is associated with gestational diabetes mellitus," *Gynecological Endocrinology*, vol. 30, no. 9, pp. 640–643, 2014.

[25] M. Maconi, S. Cardaropoli, and A. M. Cenci, "Platelet parameters in healthy and pathological pregnancy," *Journal of Clinical Laboratory Analysis*, vol. 26, no. 1, pp. 41–44, 2012.

[26] M. E. Sak, H. E. Soydinc, A. Ozler et al., "Platelet profile in patients with gestational diabetes: a retrospective study," *Journal of the Turkish German Gynecological Association*, vol. 13, no. 4, pp. 223–226, 2012.

[27] A. A. Erikci, M. Muhcu, O. Dundar, and A. Ozturk, "Could mean platelet volume be a predictive marker for gestational diabetes mellitus?," *Hematology*, vol. 13, no. 1, pp. 46–48, 2008.

[28] N. Bozkurt, E. Yilmaz, A. Biri, Z. Taner, and O. Himmetoglu, "The mean platelet volume in gestational diabetes," *Journal of Thrombosis and Thrombolysis*, vol. 22, no. 1, pp. 51–54, 2006.

[29] S. M. Yin, Y. Q. Li, S. F. Xie et al., "Study on the variation of platelet function in pregnancy induced hypertension and gestational diabetes mellitus," *Zhonghua Fu Chan Ke Za Zhi*, vol. 40, no. 1, pp. 25–28, 2005.

[30] A. Çeltik, B. Akıncı, and T. Demir, "Mean platelet volume in women with gestational diabetes," *Turkish Journal of Endocrinology and Metabolism*, vol. 20, no. 2, pp. 48–53, 2016.

[31] S. Soydinc, M. Oylumlu, M. Yuksel, A. Turgut, and H. E. Soydinc, "Blood pressure diurnal rhythm is related with hematological indices in gestational diabetes mellitus patients," *Acta Medica Mediterranea*, vol. 29, no. 4, p. 767, 2013.

[32] E. Erdem Çelikel, S. Kurt, E. Töz, A. Arici, T. Gürbüz, and A. Taşyurt, "Mean platelet volume in diagnosis of gestational diabetes," *Journal of Experimental and Clinical Medicine*, vol. 30, no. 4, pp. 291–294, 2013.

[33] A. Köşüş, N. Köşüş, M. Duran, and N. Ö. Turhan, "Assessment of mean platelet volume of pregnant women with gestational diabetes mellitus and impaired glucose tolerance as a marker of future cardiovascular disease risk," *The British Journal of Diabetes & Vascular Disease*, vol. 10, no. 10, pp. 233–237, 2011.

[34] S. Basili, G. Pacini, M. T. Guagnano et al., "Insulin resistance as a determinant of platelet activation in obese women," *Journal of the American College of Cardiology*, vol. 48, no. 12, pp. 2531–2538, 2006.

[35] K. Stanley, R. Fraser, and C. Bruce, "Physiological changes in insulin resistance in human pregnancy: longitudinal study with the hyperinsulinaemic euglycaemic clamp technique," *BJOG*, vol. 105, no. 7, pp. 756–759, 1998.

[36] E. A. Reece, G. Leguizamon, and A. Wiznitzer, "Gestational diabetes: the need for a common ground," *The Lancet*, vol. 373, no. 9677, pp. 1789–1797, 2009.

[37] F. Santilli, P. Simeone, R. Liani, and G. Davi, "Platelets and diabetes mellitus," *Prostaglandins & Other Lipid Mediators*, vol. 120, pp. 28–39, 2015.

[38] D. C. Calverley, M. R. Hacker, K. A. Loda et al., "Increased platelet Fc receptor expression as a potential contributing cause of platelet hypersensitivity to collagen in diabetes mellitus," *British Journal of Haematology*, vol. 121, no. 1, pp. 139–142, 2003.

[39] T. Lekva, E. R. Norwitz, P. Aukrust, and T. Ueland, "Impact of systemic inflammation on the progression of gestational diabetes mellitus," *Current Diabetes Reports*, vol. 16, no. 4, p. 26, 2016.

[40] M. Wolf, J. Sauk, A. Shah et al., "Inflammation and glucose intolerance: a prospective study of gestational diabetes mellitus," *Diabetes Care*, vol. 27, no. 1, pp. 21–27, 2004.

[41] N. Terrin, C. H. Schmid, J. Lau, and I. Olkin, "Adjusting for publication bias in the presence of heterogeneity," *Statistics in Medicine*, vol. 22, no. 13, pp. 2113–2126, 2003.

[42] G. F. Borm, M. den Heijer, and G. A. Zielhuis, "Publication bias was not a good reason to discourage trials with low power," *Journal of Clinical Epidemiology*, vol. 62, no. 1, pp. 47–53.e3, 2009.

[43] P. P. Zwetsloot, M. Van Der Naald, E. S. Sena et al., "Standardized mean differences cause funnel plot distortion in publication bias assessments," *eLife*, vol. 6, 2017.

[44] A. Stang, "Critical evaluation of the Newcastle-Ottawa scale for the assessment of the quality of nonrandomized studies in meta-analyses," *European Journal of Epidemiology*, vol. 25, no. 9, pp. 603–605, 2010.

12

Perceptions on Diet and Dietary Modifications during Postpartum Period Aiming at Attenuating Progression of GDM to DM: A Qualitative Study of Mothers and Health Care Workers

Thamudi D. Sundarapperuma,[1] Champa J. Wijesinghe,[2] Priyadarshika Hettiarachchi,[3] and Sudharshani Wasalathanthri[4]

[1]*Department of Nursing, University of Ruhuna, Galle 80000, Sri Lanka*
[2]*Department of Community Medicine, University of Ruhuna, Galle 80000, Sri Lanka*
[3]*Department of Physiology, University of Sri Jayewardenepura, Nugegoda 11222, Sri Lanka*
[4]*Department of Physiology, University of Colombo, Colombo 00800, Sri Lanka*

Correspondence should be addressed to Sudharshani Wasalathanthri; sudharshaniw@gmail.com

Academic Editor: Ulrike Rothe

Background. Gestational diabetes mellitus (GDM) is a global concern. GDM mothers have a 7-fold relative risk of developing type 2 diabetes mellitus (T2DM) in their later life. User-friendly and culturally acceptable dietary interventions can minimize this risk. Therefore, this study aims at exploring the perceptions of GDM mothers and health care workers regarding factors that influence postpartum dietary practices aimed at attenuating the trajectory from GDM to DM. *Methods.* The study was conducted in selected MOH areas in three districts of Sri Lanka. Six focus group discussions were conducted with thirty mothers with a history of GDM and six in-depth interviews with six health care workers. The phenomenon of interest was to obtain inputs of two stakeholder groups on healthy food habits of GDM mothers during the postpartum period. Framework analysis was used to analyse the data. Data were coded using the analytical framework, abstracted from transcripts, and summarized verbatim in Microsoft Excel in a matrix comprised of one row per participant and one column per code. Finally, the matrix was reviewed intensely and themes were generated. *Results.* Overall, seven themes emerged from both cases: (1) myths and traditions specific to the postpartum period, (2) lack of motivation, (3) time pressure, (4) financial barriers, (5) negligence of mothers and families, (6) lack of awareness regarding GDM and its postpartum dietary recommendations, and (7) cultural barriers. *Conclusions.* This study provides an insight into the existing knowledge, common practices, and attitudes regarding food habits among postpartum mothers with a history of GDM. Since the postpartum period is unique, identifying barriers is crucial when introducing dietary modification protocols in order to prevent or attenuate the progression of GDM to T2DM in these mothers. The knowledge gained will be used to introduce feasible, scientifically sound, and culturally acceptable postpartum dietary recommendations for GDM mothers.

1. Introduction

Gestational diabetes mellitus (GDM) is a state of glucose intolerance commencing with the onset of pregnancy, or first recognized during pregnancy [1]. Due to the current economic, social, and nutritional transition, an increasing prevalence of GDM is noted globally [2]. Women with a previous history of GDM have a high risk of recurrence of the same in subsequent pregnancies [3] and also has a 7.43-fold relative risk of developing type 2 diabetes mellitus (T2DM) compared to women without GDM [4]. Although ethnicity, prepregnancy weight, age, family history of diabetes, and glycaemic indices during pregnancy are nonmodifiable risk factors favouring progression of GDM to overt diabetes [5], increase in BMI is a risk factor [6] modifiable by appropriate intervention.

Life style interventions attenuate the progression of GDM to T2DM [4, 7] delaying or preventing the development by one-sixth times [8]. Weight reduction by increased physical activity and limiting the consumption of calories reduces the risk of diabetes [9]. Previous studies have suggested reducing the postpartum energy intake by limiting the consumption of energy-dense foods such as fast foods, high-fat snacks, fried foods and sugar-sweetened beverages, reducing the portion size, increasing fruit and vegetable intake, and modifying ethnic recipes accordingly [10–12]. Carolan et al. [13] recommended that these interventions should be culturally acceptable to get the optimal benefit.

Postpartum mothers are a special group who face difficulties in maintaining healthy eating patterns and regular physical activities [14]. Therefore, a better understanding of the barriers to behaviour changes is needed when planning out lifestyle interventions. Many factors such as extreme tiredness, time and financial constraints [15], needs of the newborn, and demands of the family [16] act as obstacles for healthy lifestyles. In addition, food preferences of other family members and confidence and skills in cooking healthy food were other psychosocial factors influencing postpartum dietary behaviours [17]. A careful exploration and analysis of these factors is therefore important when designing nutrition interventions for postpartum mothers.

Though several studies have been done to determine the perception of mothers [17–19] and health care workers [20, 21] regarding diet during the postpartum period, there is a dearth of evidence emerging from South Asian cultures. Since postpartum mothers are faced with unique issues, findings of studies on dietary perceptions of diabetic patients [22] are not directly applicable to them. Cultural beliefs, traditions, and social influences can directly affect the food habits of postpartum mothers, and these should be taken into account when implementing dietary guidelines to reduce the risk of diabetes [7, 14, 23]. Therefore, the aim of this study was to explore the perceptions of GDM mothers and healthcare workers regarding factors that influence postpartum dietary practices, for the purpose of attenuating the trajectory from GDM to T2DM.

2. Materials and Methods

2.1. Study Design and Settings. This study was a community-based, phenomenological qualitative study carried out in three selected districts in Sri Lanka, namely, Colombo, Gampaha, and Galle.

Focus group discussions (FGDs) were used to explore the perceptions of mothers regarding postpartum dietary practices in order to allow cross talk between them and to generate ideas freely. Thirty volunteering antenatal mothers with a history of GDM, who spoke the native language, Sinhala, who were not employees of the health sector were recruited. Five to ten mothers were invited for each FGD, as smaller groups are more manageable to obtain optimum results [24].

In-depth interviews (IDIs) were chosen to assess the perspective of healthcare workers as IDIs allow detailed exploration of the reactions of respondents without contamination [25]. Further, IDIs ensured longer speaking time and privacy during information gathering which could be challenging to the health care workers. Three public health midwives and three postnatal nurses were recruited as they were believed to have the closest contact with mothers. All healthcare workers were required to have at least 3 years of experience in maternal and well-baby clinics or in postnatal wards. All eligible mothers and health care workers were verbally invited and written informed consent was obtained thereafter.

2.2. Data Collection. Six FGDs were carried out until new information was no longer generated; that is, data saturation was achieved [24] with each session lasting for 30–60 minutes [25]. Six IDIs were conducted; that is, one for each health care worker, each lasting approximately one hour. Two separate semistructured guides prepared by the research team were used to facilitate the FGDs and IDIs. The guides were developed by using the findings of a literature review, expert advice of a nutritionist, and information obtained through informal discussions carried out with 10 GDM mothers regarding dietary practices. The discussion guides were rephrased and finalized after pilot testing them on 5 mothers and 2 healthcare workers. The discussions and interviews were conducted in comfortable rooms in healthcare institutions in close proximity to the location of the participants. The same moderator, a postgraduate student (TS), facilitated all sessions, while the notetaker recorded all nonverbal and verbal expressions. All sessions were audiorecorded and transcribed verbatim.

2.3. Data Analysis. The framework approach [26] was used for data analysis. The entire research team checked all transcripts for errors by reading them and listening to the audiorecordings simultaneously. After familiarizing further with the transcripts and audiorecorded interviews, the coders (TS and CW) discussed the common and uncommon code categories with the team members. The coders independently coded the data of the 12 transcripts (6 of FGDs and 6 of IDIs) to minimize potential bias. Coding was compared between coders and differences were reviewed and resolved. The process of refining and applying was repeated until no new codes were generated. Once all data had been coded using the analytical framework, the data was abstracted from transcripts and summarized verbatim in Microsoft Excel in a matrix comprised of one row per participant and one column per code. Finally, the matrix was reviewed intensely and themes were generated.

3. Results

3.1. Participant Characteristics. A total of 30 postpartum mothers participated in focus group discussions and 6 healthcare workers (3 postnatal nurses and 3 field midwives) were interviewed. All mothers were either in their second or third pregnancy and had a past history of GDM. Twenty-four mothers (80%) were below 35 years. Sixty-seven percent of the samples have studied up to ordinary level while only 23% and 10% have studied up to advanced level and diploma/degree level, respectively. All midwives and nurses who participated in the study had a work experience of more than ten years. All mothers and health care workers reported that they felt comfortable and relaxed during the procedure.

3.2. Emerging Themes. Seven major themes emerged from focus group discussions and in-depth interviews.

3.2.1. Theme 1: Myths and Traditions Specific to the Postpartum Period. In general, almost all mothers reported negative perceptions on consuming a variety of healthy food. Mothers emphasized the importance of consuming traditional food to maintain their health in the postpartum period. Inclusion or restriction of certain food items in the diet of the mother was influenced by traditional beliefs on top of scientific evidence.

All postpartum mothers believed that traditional foods, especially "thambunhodi" (a Sri Lankan soup made out of water and spices), are an excellent alternative to take with rice after delivery in spite of having curries. In the words of a mother regarding traditional foods,

My mother, mother-in-law, and grandmother asked me to drink thambunhodi every day because it gives lot of energy as it is prepared using garlic, karapincha (curry leaves), and pepper.

We have prepared a special energetic drink which contains "Arrack" (an alcoholic beverage) and garlic. I drank it. It gave me additional energy and also helped to stop my vaginal bleeding.

Restriction of certain food items during the postpartum period was another common practice which is related to the traditional beliefs. Mothers avoided eggs, small bony fish, and green leaves expecting an array of benefits during the postpartum period.

In the words of a mother,

They did not allow me to eat small bony fish and green leaves as the bones can get stuck in my mammary glands obstructing the milk secretion.

My mother told me not to eat eggs as it increases the tendency for placental parts to remain in the womb. She also told to avoid fried meat and fish as if I eat them, demons would follow me.

Health care workers reaffirmed the mothers' views on perceived health benefits of the chosen foods. One midwife stated,

Actually, the mothers believe that "thambunhodi" is the best curry to reduce maternal complications because garlic and pepper have the magical ability to clean the gastrointestinal tract and improve immunity. Traditional alcoholic drink is the best energy source for mothers.

Health care workers also commented that although they have educated the mothers regarding nutritious food, women usually consumed traditional food. One midwife stated,

However much we educate them about healthy food, it's not an easy task to change their traditional views. To tell you the truth, actually we also drank "thambunhodi" during our postpartum period.

Although we advise them to take more proteins and iron-containing food, they like to eat food rich in starch like "kirikos" (mature jack fruit curry) and "polos" (tender jack fruit curry) without a limit as they believe that these foods increase production of milk. Mothers do not consider their food as important after the baby is born.

The healthcare workers indicated that myths regarding food are related to religious beliefs of the community and the social influence on the mothers. One postnatal nurse stated,

The mother, other relatives and neighbours always interfere with their dietary practices. People around them offer food to these mothers and to maintain the goodwill, most mothers consume what is offered.

3.2.2. Theme 2: Lack of Motivation. Mothers did not feel the necessity to restrict carbohydrates in the diet after the baby is born. Almost all mothers attributed restricting carbohydrates to reduced production of breast milk, lack of energy, and gastritis. They were not prepared to accept that they are vulnerable to developing T2DM in their later life. Several mothers stated this during the focus group discussions.

My baby is no longer in my womb; therefore, why should I go for dietary modifications?

After the baby came out, my sugar level became normal. Therefore, there is no harm to me or my baby.

After my first pregnancy, nobody asked me to restrict carbohydrates and none of my friends did so. They did not develop any illness. So why should I do it?

3.2.3. Theme 3: Time Pressure. Time is a limited resource after the baby is born. Mothers mentioned that they do not have time to prepare separate food for themselves. It was observed that they eat anything available at home while attending to the needs of the baby. One mother said,

I have a lot of work at home. I have to fulfil the demands of my baby and my husband. Every time my baby cries, I have to lull him and feed him. My husband also expects me to fulfil some of his duties. Nobody helps me. Hence, I have no time to prepare special food for me. Whole day I work like a machine. Twenty-four hours is not enough for me. I am so tired.

3.2.4. Theme 4: Financial Barriers. Another concern expressed by mothers was the financial difficulties. Twenty-eight mothers out of thirty expressed about their financial problems. As mothers stated, only one person earns in most families. Therefore, they have to choose food which is easily available like jack fruit and manioc (cassava). They consume these high-carbohydrate foods to achieve satiety as these foods were perceived as inexpensive and thus economically viable.

One mother stated,

It is not easy to spend additional money for special food. I prepare common food for all family members. Some foods are very expensive. One hand to earn and many mouths to eat! How can I be selfish to prepare special food for me? It is not practical.

Another mother noted,

My mother-in-law and the unmarried sisters-in-law also depend on my husband's salary. Hence it is difficult to eat food

items like fish or chicken every day. I prepare cheap food that can be obtained from our garden for all three meals.

The healthcare workers confirmed that the families give priority in fulfilling the needs of the babies than the mothers. One postnatal nurse stated,

Only one person earns for the family and this money is not enough to fulfil the family needs. Therefore, they spend money to fulfil baby's needs. Sometimes it is useless giving dietary advice to mothers because they are really poor. They eat cheap, easily available food items preparing one item for the entire family.

3.2.5. Theme 5: Negligence of Mothers and Families. Mothers indicated that they do not have an interest to follow healthy dietary modifications after the baby is born. The baby is the treasure and the focus of the family. Therefore, they are not concerned about the well-being of the mother. According to their point of view, diet does not have any effect after the baby is born.

I have no interest to do it. What is the use of changing my diet? After the baby is born, why should I spend time thinking about my food? Although I have been advised to modify my diet, I am not interested and do not care about it.

Healthcare workers endorsed the statement made by the mothers regarding healthy food practices. They indicated that after the birth of a baby, most mothers and family members do not care about the well-being of the mother. One public health midwife said,

They think that there is no need to change their food habits because the baby is not in the womb any more. However much we try to educate them about healthy food practices, they don't care. When we give them instructions, they nod and seem to agree but when we inquire later whether they practiced, they just smile. Although they neglect themselves, they are willing to practice whatever advices given regarding the newborn.

3.2.6. Theme 6: Lack of Awareness Regarding GDM and Its Postpartum Dietary Recommendations. The healthcare workers indicated that not only the mothers but the healthcare workers themselves have limited knowledge about GDM and are not aware about the importance of postpartum dietary modifications for GDM mothers. In Sri Lankan society, the main focus is given to the antepartum period. As several health care workers explained,

Actually, I am not aware about the relationship between GDM and DM. According to my knowledge, GDM is a disease which appears only during pregnancy and disappears when the baby is born. Therefore, there is no need to worry about GDM in the postpartum period.

To tell you the truth, we also do not have much knowledge about how a GDM mother should be managed in the postpartum period. We are not aware of the government health policy nor of recommendations for proper postpartum follow-up of these mothers. However, as a routine we advise the mothers to get a fasting blood sugar done at six weeks of their delivery.

3.2.7. Theme 7: Cultural Barriers. This theme has emerged mainly from healthcare workers. They explained that some Sri Lankan cultural beliefs are major barriers for a healthy diet.

One postnatal nurse stated,

Our Sinhala culture promotes mothers to move to the maternal home soon after the baby is born. Then, the mature ladies, that is, the grandmother and mother decide what the new mother eats.

One midwife stated,

Our culture gives more priority to the new member who they think will protect their family name. The mothers' health is not so important after the baby is born.

4. Discussion

From our semistructured focus group discussions and in-depth interviews, we identified seven main themes and recognized many factors which act as obstacles for women to practice healthy food habits. Discussions with mothers revealed several themes such as myths and traditions specific to the postpartum period, lack of motivation, time pressure, financial barriers, and negligence of mothers and families that hinder healthy food habits during the postpartum period. Lack of awareness regarding GDM and postpartum dietary recommendations for GDM mothers and cultural barriers surfaced solely from in-depth interviews with healthcare workers.

Careful exploration of the themes shows that as a result of many factors, almost all women end up consuming large portions of high carbohydrates while restricting foods rich in proteins, micronutrients, and fibre such as eggs, small fish, and green leaves. This not only compromises the nutritional needs of the mother who will be possibly lactating but also speed up the trajectory towards development of T2DM. In general, Sri Lankans are shown to consume high levels of carbohydrates and fats and low levels of protein and dietary fibres, which may have detrimental effects on health [27]. Therefore, it is likely that the myths, traditions, and practices even in the postpartum period are aligned with the general trend of food habits in the population. Focus group findings suggest that the myths regarding postpartum diet are perpetuated through generations possibly supported by the health care workers [22]. In addition, almost all women in the present study identified the mismatch between their income and food prices as a main inhibitor for healthy food choices. A previous qualitative study done among mothers with a history of GDM in Atlanta has also reported financial barriers as a major drawback for sustaining healthy eating behaviours [18]. This will further aggravate the situation as carbohydrate-rich foods such as jack fruit that is often consumed by these mothers are easily available even in their home gardens or can be purchased at low cost.

Mothers have identified lack of motivation and negligence as major barriers for healthy eating. Both self-motivation and social motivation appear to be poor among women who participated in focus group discussions. Similarly, studies conducted elsewhere have also shown that the mothers lose the motivation and interest for healthy behaviour after the delivery of the baby [16, 18]. In the present study, "Lack of awareness" has emerged during in-depth interviews with healthcare workers as a factor affecting dietary behaviour in the postpartum period. Similar to our findings, studies conducted elsewhere also reported that most GDM mothers were unaware of their risk of developing T2DM [18, 19] which can be considered as a barrier for lifestyle modifications. Lack of awareness regarding the link between GDM and T2DM may be considered as the root cause for the lack of motivation and negligence.

In the present study, health care workers stated that lack of clear guidelines was one of the main barriers in achieving lifestyle changes among postpartum mothers. Lack of awareness of health care workers seen in this study as well as in studies done in other settings [19] is a major drawback in postpartum management of these mothers. In many settings, women with GDM were found to receive close medical monitoring only during the pregnancy with inadequate postpartum follow-up and support from health professionals [20, 21, 28]. Our study also revealed that mothers get minimum inputs from health professionals during the postpartum period regarding healthy food practices, a finding confirmed even by researchers elsewhere [28, 29]. This suboptimal follow-up has the potential to downplay the significance of GDM as a risk factor for developing T2DM in the future.

The postpartum period is unique globally as these mothers are faced with childcare demands which are tiring [16]. As in other studies [19, 30], the lack of time was also identified by our mothers as a barrier to comply with healthy food choices. Therefore, all these factors should be considered when designing behaviour change strategies to suit this special group of women [14, 17]. Diet modification programmes should be culturally acceptable and aimed at all literacy levels [13] and delivered and followed up in innovative ways. Previous research has suggested home-based programmes [14] delivered and monitored through telephone calls [17, 23] due to time constraints and difficulties in transportation. Since the lack of social support has been identified as a barrier to implement a healthy diet [18], a collective role of all health care professionals catering to these women [19], their partners [30], and other family members [31] is of utmost importance. Although health care workers in the present study reported a lack of proper postpartum dietary guidelines for GDM mothers, a Canadian study reported that even in the presence of guidelines, there is a mismatch between the recommendations and the diet consumed by them [30]. This shows that adherence to guidelines needs continuous support and monitoring. Although the period of pregnancy could be used as an opportunity to increase the awareness of mothers regarding the future risk of DM [20], the support should continue in the postpartum period. Although women in some settings desired to learn strategies to attenuate future diabetes [32], additional efforts by healthcare personnel are needed if mothers do not show interest as in the present study.

Inclusion of two stakeholder groups from the same setting is a strength which enabled pooling of ideas to get a better understanding of the situation. In a multicultural country, inclusion of only one cultural group is considered a limitation as ideas of ethnic minorities would have explored different perceptions and barriers. However, the authors felt that the possibility of not disclosing information during focus group discussions was minimized as these mothers had the same experiences. The study had to be limited to only three districts in the country due to logistic reasons.

5. Conclusions

The findings have paved the way to understand the existing knowledge, common practices, and attitudes of society about dietary behaviours of postpartum mothers with a history of GDM. The information that emerged will be useful in developing culturally acceptable and scientifically valid dietary protocols for postpartum mothers with GDM to attenuate its progression to T2DM. Addressing the concerns of mothers is expected to increase acceptance and long-term adherence.

Lack of optimum awareness of not only mothers, but healthcare workers seen in our study as well as in other studies [19], seems to be a serious issue which needs immediate remedial action. Dissemination of valid information to mothers by health care workers should be ensured by appropriate awareness programmes. Close monitoring of GDM mothers during the postpartum period is a responsibility of all stakeholders. The barriers unique to postpartum mothers have to be considered when planning and monitoring follow-up.

Conflicts of Interest

The authors declare that they have no conflicts of interest.

Acknowledgments

The authors are most grateful to the participating mothers and healthcare workers who made this study possible. Funding for this study was provided by the University of Sri Jayewardenepura, Sri Lanka (ASP/06/RE/MED/2013/39).

References

[1] B. E. Metzger, D. R. Coustan, and Organizing Committee, "Summary and recommendations of the fourth international workshop-conference on gestational diabetes mellitus," *Diabetes Care*, vol. 21, pp. B161–B167, 1998.

[2] International Diabetes Federation, *Diabetes Atlas*, 59, 8th edition, 2017.

[3] D. Getahun, M. J. Fassett, and S. J. Jacobsen, "Gestational diabetes: risk of recurrence in subsequent pregnancies," *American Journal of Obstetrics and Gynecology*, vol. 203, no. 5, pp. 467.e1–467.e6, 2010.

[4] O. Verier-Mine, "Outcomes in women with a history of gestational diabetes. Screening and prevention of type 2 diabetes. Literature review," *Diabetes & Metabolism*, vol. 36, no. 6, pp. 595–616, 2010.

[5] J. H. Moon, S. H. Kwak, and H. C. Jang, "Prevention of type 2 diabetes mellitus in women with previous gestational diabetes mellitus," *Korean Journal of Internal Medicine*, vol. 32, no. 1, pp. 26–41, 2017.

[6] J. Lauenborg, T. Hansen, D. M. Jensen et al., "Increasing incidence of diabetes after gestational diabetes: a long-term follow-up in a Danish population," *Diabetes Care*, vol. 27, no. 5, pp. 1194–1199, 2004.

[7] C. Kim, "Gestational diabetes: risks, management, and treatment options," *International Journal of Women's Health*, vol. 2, p. 339, 2010.

[8] A. Stuebe, J. Ecker, D. W. Bates, C. Zera, R. Bentley-Lewis, and E. Seely, "Barriers to follow-up for women with a history of gestational diabetes," *American Journal of Perinatology*, vol. 27, no. 9, pp. 705–710, 2010.

[9] R. F. Hamman, R. R. Wing, S. L. Edelstein et al., "Effect of weight loss with lifestyle intervention on risk of diabetes," *Diabetes Care*, vol. 29, no. 9, pp. 2102–2107, 2006.

[10] M. J. Franz, J. P. Bantle, C. A. Beebe et al., "Evidence-based nutrition principles and recommendations for the treatment and prevention of diabetes and related complications," *Diabetes Care*, vol. 25, no. 1, pp. 148–198, 2002.

[11] J. Lindström, A. Louheranta, M. Mannelin et al., "The Finnish Diabetes Prevention Study (DPS)," *Diabetes Care*, vol. 26, no. 12, pp. 3230–3236, 2003.

[12] R. E. Ratner, "Prevention of type 2 diabetes in women with previous gestational diabetes," *Diabetes Care*, vol. 30, Supplement 2, pp. S242–S245, 2007.

[13] M. Carolan, G. K. Gill, and C. Steele, "Women's experiences of factors that facilitate or inhibit gestational diabetes self-management," *BMC Pregnancy and Childbirth*, vol. 12, no. 1, p. 99, 2012.

[14] N. W. Cheung, B. J. Smith, H. Henriksen, L. C. Tapsell, M. McLean, and A. Bauman, "A group-based healthy lifestyle program for women with previous gestational diabetes," *Diabetes Research and Clinical Practice*, vol. 77, no. 2, pp. 333-334, 2007.

[15] M. J. Saurel-Cubizolles, P. Romito, N. Lelong, and P. Y. Ancel, "Women's health after childbirth: a longitudinal study in France and Italy," *BJOG: An International Journal of Obstetrics and Gynaecology*, vol. 107, no. 10, pp. 1202–1209, 2000.

[16] M. L. S. Lie, L. Hayes, N. J. Lewis-Barned, C. May, M. White, and R. Bell, "Preventing type 2 diabetes after gestational diabetes: women's experiences and implications for diabetes prevention interventions," *Diabetic Medicine*, vol. 30, no. 8, pp. 986–993, 2013.

[17] K. Zehle, B. J. Smith, T. Chey, M. McLean, A. E. Bauman, and N. Wah Cheung, "Psychosocial factors related to diet among women with recent gestational diabetes opportunities for intervention," *The Diabetes Educator*, vol. 34, no. 5, pp. 807–814, 2008.

[18] S. A. Collier, C. Mulholland, J. Williams, P. Mersereau, K. Turay, and C. Prue, "A qualitative study of perceived barriers to management of diabetes among women with a history of diabetes during pregnancy," *Journal of Women's Health*, vol. 20, no. 9, pp. 1333–1339, 2011.

[19] M. K. Morrison, J. M. Lowe, and C. E. Collins, "Australian women's experiences of living with gestational diabetes," *Women and Birth*, vol. 27, no. 1, pp. 52–57, 2014.

[20] K. Hjelm, K. Bard, and J. Apelqvist, "Gestational diabetes: prospective interview-study of the developing beliefs about health, illness and health care in migrant women," *Journal of Clinical Nursing*, vol. 21, no. 21-22, pp. 3244–3256, 2012.

[21] E. Van Ryswyk, P. Middleton, W. Hague, and C. Crowther, "Clinician views and knowledge regarding healthcare provision in the postpartum period for women with recent gestational diabetes: a systematic review of qualitative/survey studies," *Diabetes Research and Clinical Practice*, vol. 106, no. 3, pp. 401–411, 2014.

[22] P. Ranasinghe, A. S. A. D. Pigera, M. H. Ishara, L. M. D. T. Jayasekara, R. Jayawardena, and P. Katulanda, "Knowledge and perceptions about diet and physical activity among Sri Lankan adults with diabetes mellitus: a qualitative study," *BMC Public Health*, vol. 15, no. 1, pp. 1160–1110, 2015.

[23] A. Ferrara, M. M. Hedderson, C. L. Albright et al., "A pregnancy and postpartum lifestyle intervention in women with gestational diabetes mellitus reduces diabetes risk factors: a feasibility randomized control trial," *Diabetes Care*, vol. 34, no. 7, pp. 1519–1525, 2011.

[24] I. McLafferty, "Focus group interviews as a data collecting strategy," *Journal of Advanced Nursing*, vol. 48, no. 2, pp. 187–194, 2004.

[25] B. DiCicco-Bloom and B. F. Crabtree, "The qualitative research interview," *Medical Education*, vol. 40, no. 4, pp. 314–321, 2006.

[26] N. Mays and C. Pope, "Qualitative research in health care: assessing quality in qualitative research," *BMJ*, vol. 320, no. 7226, pp. 50–52, 2000.

[27] R. Jayawardena, S. Thennakoon, N. Byrne, M. Soares, P. Katulanda, and A. Hills, "Energy and nutrient intakes among Sri Lankan adults," *International Archives of Medicine*, vol. 7, no. 1, pp. 34–11, 2014.

[28] Y. Linné, B. Barkeling, and S. Rössner, "Natural course of gestational diabetes mellitus: long term follow up of women in the SPAWN study," *BJOG: An International Journal of Obstetrics and Gynaecology*, vol. 109, no. 11, pp. 1227–1231, 2002.

[29] A. L. Wennberg, A. Lundqvist, U. Högberg, H. Sandström, and K. Hamberg, "Women's experiences of dietary advice and dietary changes during pregnancy," *Midwifery*, vol. 29, no. 9, pp. 1027–1034, 2013.

[30] M. K. Evans, L. J. Patrick, and C. M. Wellington, "Health behaviours of postpartum women with a history of gestational diabetes," *Canadian Journal of Diabetes*, vol. 34, no. 3, pp. 227–232, 2010.

[31] P. L. Thornton, E. C. Kieffer, Y. Salabarría-Peña et al., "Weight, diet, and physical activity-related beliefs and practices among pregnant and postpartum Latino women: the role of social support," *Maternal and Child Health Journal*, vol. 10, no. 1, pp. 95–104, 2006.

[32] J. A. Nolan, S. McCrone, and I. R. A. Chertok, "The maternal experience of having diabetes in pregnancy," *Journal of the American Academy of Nurse Practitioners*, vol. 23, no. 11, pp. 611–618, 2011.

13

Prevalence and Risk Factors for Glucose Intolerance among Saudi Women with Gestational Diabetes

Hayfaa Wahabi

Chair of Evidence-Based Healthcare and Knowledge Translation, College of Medicine, King Saud University, P.O. Box 2925 Riyadh 11461, Saudi Arabia

Correspondence should be addressed to Hayfaa Wahabi; umlena@yahoo.com

Academic Editor: Daniela Foti

Objectives. The objective of this study was to determine the incidence and risk factors of glucose intolerance one year after delivery in women with gestational diabetes (GDM). *Methods.* All women who had GDM and completed one year since delivery at King Khalid University Hospital were contacted to participate in the study. Based on to the American Diabetes Association criteria and the results of fasting blood glucose (FPG) and HbA1c, participants were classified into three groups: diabetic, impaired glucose tolerance (IGT), and normal. The incidence of diabetes and IGT was calculated. Clinical, biochemical, and sociodemographic predictors of glucose intolerance were compared between the three groups. Odds ratio (OR) for risk factors with P value less than 0.05 was calculated. *Results.* From a total 316 eligible women, 133 fulfilled the inclusion criteria and agreed to participate in the study. From the study participants, 58 (44%) women were normoglycemic, 60 (45%) women had IGT, and 15 (11%) women were diabetic. The odds of developing IGT or diabetes increased to nearly fourfold when women needed insulin for the control of GDM during pregnancy (OR 3.8, 95% CI 0.81–18.3, $P = 0.08$) and to nearly one-and-a-half-fold when they have positive family history of T2DM (OR 1.2, 95% CI 0.74–2.09, $P = 0.40$). Nevertheless, none of the odds ratios was statistically significant. *Conclusion.* The incidence of postpartum hyperglycemia (diabetes and IGT) is very high in Saudi women with GDM. Family history of diabetes and insulin treatment of GDM may be predictors of postpartum hyperglycemia.

1. Introduction

The physiological changes of pregnancy mediate carbohydrate intolerance through pregnancy-specific hormones by increasing the peripheral resistance to insulin and production of glucose; these changes call for more production of insulin to maintain normal blood glucose levels during pregnancy [1].

Gestational diabetes (GDM) is one of the commonest metabolic disorders of pregnancy. It is defined as diabetes diagnosed during pregnancy that is clearly not pregestational in nature [2].

Long follow-up of women with history of GDM showed that they are at increased risk of developing type 2 diabetes mellitus (T2DM) and cardiovascular diseases later in life [3, 4].

The majority of women with GDM convert to normal glycemic status following delivery; however, they have increased risk of developing T2DM compared to women who did not have GDM [5]. The reported rate of progression to T2DM varied considerably in different studies and is dependent on the period of follow-up, the diagnostic criteria for GDM, and the ethnicity of the studied population [6]. Risk factors for progression to T2DM include family history of T2DM, need of insulin treatment, and obesity [7–10].

It has been proven that lifestyle modification and pharmacological interventions can prevent or delay progression to T2DM in women with history of GDM [11–13]. Such interventions should be considered in the management of women with GDM especially that one in four Saudi women develops GDM during pregnancy and is among the high-risk population for developing T2DM [14].

Based on the American Diabetes Association (ADA) guidelines, different tests are equally effective for screening for impaired glucose tolerance (IGT) and diabetes including 75 oral glucose tolerance test (OGTT), fasting plasma glucose (FPG), or glycosylated hemoglobin A1C (HbA1c) [15].

There is paucity of studies on the progression to T2DM among postpartum Saudi women. The objective of this study was to determine the prevalence and risk factors of glucose intolerance one year after delivery in women with GDM.

2. Methods

This is a cross-sectional study conducted at King Khalid University Hospital (KKUH) in Riyadh, Saudi Arabia. KKUH is a tertiary referral hospital with 800 beds. It has all the essential departments including 20 operating theatres, an assisted reproduction unit, and a cardiac center. The hospital provides free medical care to Saudi nationals and the staff of King Saud University. The obstetrics department provides care for 3000–4000 deliveries per year.

2.1. Definitions

(i) GDM was diagnosed based on one abnormal value of 75 g on the oral glucose tolerance test (OGTT) done between 24 and 34 gestation weeks using the following World Health Organization (WHO) cutoff values [16]:

(1) Fasting plasma glucose (FPG): 5.1–6.9 mmol/l (92–125 mg/dl),

(2) 1-Hour plasma glucose ≥ 10.0 mmol/l (180 mg/dl),

(3) 2-Hour plasma glucose: 8.5–11.0 mmol/l (153–199 mg/dl).

(ii) Diabetes and IGT were diagnosed using either fasting plasma glucose and glycosylated hemoglobin A1C (HbA1c) levels according to the following cutoff levels of the ADA [17]:

(1) Fasting plasma glucose (FPG) values:

(a) Normal: <5.6 mmol/l (100 mg/dl)

(b) IGT: 5.6–6.9 mmol/l (100 mg/dl to 125 mg/dl)

(c) Diabetes: ≥7.0 mmol/l (126 mg/dl)

(2) HbA1c values:

(a) Normal: <5.7%

(b) IGT: 5.7%–6.4%

(c) Diabetes: ≥6.5%

(iii) Maternal pre-pregnancy body mass index (BMI) was calculated from maternal recall of weight prior to pregnancy and height measured during the first antenatal clinic. Current BMI was calculated using the current maternal weight and height. Participants were classified according to the following WHO BMI definitions: underweight (<18.5 kg/m^2), normal weight (18.5–24.9 kg/m^2), overweight (25.0–29.9 kg/m^2), and obese (≥30 kg/m^2) [18].

2.2. Participants. Each woman who delivered one year prior to the study period (September 2017–March 2018) and had GDM during the index pregnancy was invited to participate in the study.

The inclusion criteria were as follows:

(1) Gestational age of 37–41 weeks at the time of delivery, calculated from the last menstrual period and/or early ultrasound scan

(2) Singleton pregnancy

(3) History of GDM during the index pregnancy

We excluded women with unknown glycemic status, those with pre-GDM diagnosed before or during pregnancy, women who were pregnant at the time of this study, and those who declined to participate in the study.

All women who fulfilled the inclusion criteria were contacted by phone to participate in this study. Women who agreed to participate were invited to attend a designated outpatient clinic (research clinic) fasting for at least eight hours before their appointment. The objective of the study was explained again face-to-face to each participant who subsequently signed an informed consent form. Data collected from the participants included demographic profile, obstetric history such as parity and pre-pregnancy weight, and the type of treatment of GDM in the index pregnancy (diet or insulin). Clinical data measured in each participant included current weight and height to calculate the BMI. Blood tests done for each participant were fasting blood glucose (FPG) and glycosylated hemoglobin A1c (HbA1c) levels.

Based on the results of blood tests, participants were divided into three groups: diabetic, prediabetic, and normal.

2.3. Statistical Analysis. Statistical analysis was performed using Statistical Package for the Social Sciences (SPSS version 22). The prevalence of diabetes and IGT was calculated. Clinical, biochemical, and sociodemographic characteristics of women who progressed to postpartum glucose intolerance (IGT and diabetes) were compared with women with normal glucose tolerance using univariate analysis. The odds ratio (OR) of the known risk factors and 95% confidence interval (CI) were estimated for factors with significant P value after grouping the IGT and diabetic women together in one group compared to the normoglycemic group. A P value of <0.05 was considered significant.

2.4. Ethical Approval. The study was conducted after the approval of King Saud University review board. It was conducted according to the principles expressed in the Declaration of Helsinki.

3. Results

From a total of 316 women with GDM who delivered one year prior to the study period, 133 met the inclusion criteria and agreed to participate in this study. From the participants, 58 women were normoglycemic, 60 had IGT, and 15 developed diabetes.

Table 1 shows the comparison of the distribution of the risk factors between the three groups. There were no significant differences between the three groups with respect to age and parity. However, there was increased frequency of risk factors when normoglycemic women were compared to those with IGT and those who developed diabetes (Table 1). The current mean BMI of normoglycemic women was significantly lower than that of the IGT and diabetic women (30.9 ± 6.4, 31.1 ± 5.6, 36.2 ± 4.8, resp., $P < 0.01$). In addition, from the women who developed postpartum diabetes, 14 (93%) had pre-pregnancy BMI of $\geq 30\,kg/m^2$, while the corresponding proportions from the IGT group and the normoglycemic group were 24 (40%) and 31 (53%), respectively (Table 1). Significantly more women with IGT and diabetes had a family history of diabetes; in addition, they more frequently needed insulin for control of GDM during pregnancy, compared to normoglycemic women (Table 2).

Table 2 shows the odds of developing IGT or diabetes with different risk factors. The odds of developing IGT or diabetes increased to nearly fourfold when women needed insulin for the control of GDM during pregnancy and to nearly one-and-a-half-fold when they have positive family history of T2DM. On the other hand, pre-pregnancy normal BMI and diet treatment of GDM reduce the odds of developing glucose abnormalities one year postpartum. Nevertheless, none of the odds ratios for these risk factors was statistically significant (Table 2).

4. Discussion

The incidences of IGT and diabetes, in this study, were 45% and 11%, respectively. The results showed that women who developed glucose abnormalities (IGT and diabetes) were significantly more obese, during pregnancy and in the postpartum period. Furthermore, a significantly higher proportion from this group had a family history of T2DM and they needed insulin more frequently, for control of GDM, than the normoglycemic group.

The incidence of IGT reported in this study is higher than that reported in a national survey conducted in Saudi Arabia which showed that 25% of the adult population have prediabetes [19]. Furthermore, the incidence (new cases) of diabetes in this study is higher than the 1.3% estimated previously by Al-Quwaidhi et al. for the general population [20]. These differences may be due to the difference in the distribution of the risk factors between the general population and the participants of this study who are at higher risk of developing glucose abnormalities.

A recent study from Italy on the prevalence of glucose abnormalities in women with a history of GDM showed rates similar to those found in our study (32% and 4% for IGT and diabetes, resp.) [17]. However, a study from Iran showed lower rates than ours for both IGT and diabetes (17.5% IGT and 4.5% T2DM) [21]. These differences in rates can be explained by the variation in the criteria for diagnosing glucose intolerance, the duration of the follow-up period in addition to the ethnic differences between the studied populations [5].

Similar to previous reports, this study showed that the risk factors for developing hyperglycemia were significantly more frequent in women who developed diabetes and IGT compared to those who remained normoglycemic in the postpartum period. These include factors existing before pregnancy such as pre-pregnancy weight and a family history of T2DM, factors which occurred during the index pregnancy such as the need to use insulin to control GDM, and postpartum factors such as obesity. Although the odds for developing hyperglycemia after GDM were not statistically significant in this study, this, however, may be due to the small number of participants.

In many published reports, obesity was a significant predictor of progression to IGT and diabetes in women with GDM [16–18]. Postpartum women who are obese have 1.5-fold increase in the risk of developing diabetes in postpartum period compared to those who have normal BMI [18]. Recent published studies from Saudi Arabia showed that more than 68% of women in the reproductive age group are either overweight or obese [22] and that the prevalence of GDM and pre-GDM increases with the increase in BMI [14].

Based on a recently published systematic review, lifestyle interventions, such as healthy eating and adequate activity, are effective for the control of GDM [23]. The review showed that women who modified their lifestyle were more likely to achieve the target weight in the postnatal period and hence reduce their risk of developing hyperglycemia in the postnatal period [23, 24].

4.1. Strength and Limitations of the Study. This study quantified the problem of glucose intolerance following GDM in a Saudi population and provides valuable information for policymakers and researchers about the risk factors for the progression to T2DM in Saudi women. One of the limitation of this study is the relatively small number of participants compared to the total number of women who had GDM during the study period. This is due to the poor postpartum response to recall for follow-up, a problem faced by other researchers in the Middle East [25].

4.2. Implication to Practice

(i) Establishing a national program for screening women with a history of GDM for diabetes and prediabetes should be a health-service priority in a strategy for controlling the epidemic of diabetes in the country. Such programs were proven to be cost-effective considering the saving in the cost of premature death and treatment of complications of diabetes [26].

(ii) Implementation of evidence-based national guidelines for the treatment of GDM that includes lifestyle

Table 1: Comparison of the characteristics of women with previous gestational diabetes who developed impaired glucose tolerance/diabetes and women who remained normoglycemic.

Characteristic	Normal glucose tolerance ($n = 58$)	Impaired glucose tolerance ($n = 60$)	Diabetes ($n = 15$)	P value
Age (years)				
Less than 30	18 (31)	20 (33)	2 (13)	0.41
30 or more	40 (69)	40 (67)	13 (87)	
Primiparous	15 (26)	12 (20)	2 (13)	0.71
Multiparous	43 (74)	48 (80)	13 (87)	
Family history of DM				
Yes	41 (71)	53 (88)	13 (87)	0.04
No	17 (29)	7 (12)	2 (13)	
Pre-pregnancy BMI (mean ± SD)	28.2 ± 6.4	28.4 ± 5.2	34.3 ± 5.5	<0.01
BMI ≤ 25 kg/m^2	14 (24)	14 (23)	0 (0.0)	
BMI = 25.1–29.9 kg/m^2	13 (22)	15 (25)	1 (7)	0.01
BMI ≥ 30 kg/m^2	31 (53)	31 (52)	14 (93)	
Pregnancy fasting glucose level (mmol/l)	5.19 ± 0.98	5.19 ± 0.71	5.5 ± 0.7	0.35
Treatment of GDM				
Diet only	56 (97)	56 (93)	9 (60)	<0.01
Insulin	2 (3)	4 (7)	6 (40)	
Current BMI (kg/m^2)				
BMI ≤ 25 kg/m^2	11 (19)	7 (12)	0 (0.0)	
BMI = 25.1–29.9 kg/m^2	15 (26)	15 (25)	2 (13)	0.22
BMI ≥ 30 kg/m^2	32 (55)	38 (63)	13 (87)	
BMI (mean ± SD)	30.9 ± 6.4	31.4 ± 5.6	36.2 ± 4.8	<0.01

Table 2: Risk factors associated with the development of impaired glucose tolerance and diabetes in women with previous gestational diabetes.

Characteristic	Normoglycemic, $N = 58$ (44%)	Impaired glucose tolerance and diabetes, $N = 75$ (56%)	Odds ratio (95% CI)	P value
Pre-pregnancy BMI ≥ 30 kg/m^2	31 (53%)	38 (51%)	0.94 (0.52–1.7)	0.8
Pre-pregnancy BMI < 25 kg/m^2	14 (24%)	14 (23%)	0.78 (0.34–1.75)	0.5
Insulin treatment of GDM	2 (3%)	10 (13%)	3.8 (0.81–18.3)	0.08
Diet treatment of GDM	56 (97%)	65 (87%)	o.89 (0.54–1.47)	0.66
Family history of T2DM	41 (71%)	66 (88%)	1.2 (0.74–2.09)	0.40

modification is an essential step in the control of postpartum progression to T2DM.

4.3. Implication to Research. Research should be directed towards effective interventions to reduce the burden of obesity in Saudi pregnant and postpartum women.

4.4. Conclusion. The incidence of postpartum IGT and diabetes is very high in Saudi women with GDM. Treatment of GDM with insulin and a family history of T2DM may be predictors of the progression to IGT and T2DM.

Disclosure

The funders had no role in study design, data collection, data analysis, decision to publish, or preparation of the manuscript.

Conflicts of Interest

The author declares that she has no conflict of interest for the publication of this research.

Acknowledgments

This study is funded by the Deanship of Scientific Research at King Saud University. Thanks are due to all women who participated in the study and to Mrs. Ruba Elawad and all the laboratory technicians for their efforts and detection.

References

[1] E. A. Ryan and L. Enns, "Role of gestational hormones in the induction of insulin resistance," *The Journal of Clinical Endocrinology and Metabolism*, vol. 67, no. 2, pp. 341–347, 1988.

[2] American Diabetes Association, "Management of diabetes in pregnancy," *Diabetes Care*, vol. 39, Supplement 1, pp. S94–S98, 2016.

[3] L. Bellamy, J. P. Casas, A. D. Hingorani, and D. Williams, "Type 2 diabetes mellitus after gestational diabetes: a systematic review and meta-analysis," *The Lancet*, vol. 373, no. 9677, pp. 1773–1779, 2009.

[4] E. P. Gunderson, V. Chiang, M. J. Pletcher et al., "History of gestational diabetes mellitus and future risk of atherosclerosis in mid-life: the coronary artery risk development in young adults study," *Journal of the American Heart Association*, vol. 3, no. 2, article e000490, 2014.

[5] A. Tovar, L. Chasan-Taber, E. Eggleston, and E. Oken, "Postpartum screening for diabetes among women with a history of gestational diabetes mellitus," *Preventing Chronic Disease*, vol. 8, no. 6, article A124, 2011.

[6] L. Leuridan, J. Wens, R. Devlieger, J. Verhaeghe, C. Mathieu, and K. Benhalima, "Glucose intolerance in early postpartum in women with gestational diabetes: who is at increased risk?," *Primary Care Diabetes*, vol. 9, no. 4, pp. 244–252, 2015.

[7] K. Baptiste-Roberts, B. B. Barone, T. L. Gary et al., "Risk factors for type 2 diabetes among women with gestational diabetes: a systematic review," *The American Journal of Medicine*, vol. 122, no. 3, pp. 207–214.e4, 2009.

[8] C. E. Eades, M. Styles, G. P. Leese, H. Cheyne, and J. M. Evans, "Progression from gestational diabetes to type 2 diabetes in one region of Scotland: an observational follow-up study," *BMC Pregnancy and Childbirth*, vol. 15, no. 1, p. 11, 2015.

[9] D. S. Feig, B. Zinman, X. Wang, and J. E. Hux, "Risk of development of diabetes mellitus after diagnosis of gestational diabetes," *CMAJ*, vol. 179, no. 3, pp. 229–234, 2008.

[10] G. Rayanagoudar, A. A. Hashi, J. Zamora, K. S. Khan, G. A. Hitman, and S. Thangaratinam, "Quantification of the type 2 diabetes risk in women with gestational diabetes: a systematic review and meta-analysis of 95,750 women," *Diabetologia*, vol. 59, no. 7, pp. 1403–1411, 2016.

[11] M. Hod, E. Hadar, and L. Cabero-Roura, "Prevention of type 2 diabetes among women with prior gestational diabetes mellitus," *International Journal of Gynaecology and Obstetrics*, vol. 131, pp. S16–S18, 2015.

[12] S. L. O'Reilly, J. A. Dunbar, V. Versace et al., "Mothers after gestational diabetes in Australia (MAGDA): a randomised controlled trial of a postnatal diabetes prevention program," *PLoS Medicine*, vol. 13, no. 7, article e1002092, 2016.

[13] A. S. Peacock, F. Bogossian, H. D. McIntyre, and S. Wilkinson, "A review of interventions to prevent type 2 diabetes after gestational diabetes," *Women and Birth*, vol. 27, no. 4, pp. e7–e15, 2014.

[14] H. Wahabi, A. Fayed, S. Esmaeil, H. Mamdouh, and R. Kotb, "Prevalence and complications of pregestational and gestational diabetes in Saudi women: analysis from Riyadh mother and baby cohort study (RAHMA)," *BioMed Research International*, vol. 2017, Article ID 6878263, 9 pages, 2017.

[15] American Diabetes Association, "Glycemic targets: standards of medical care in diabetes—2018," *Diabetes Care*, vol. 41, Supplement 1, pp. S55–S64, 2018.

[16] N. W. Cheung and D. Helmink, "Gestational diabetes: the significance of persistent fasting hyperglycemia for the subsequent development of diabetes mellitus," *Journal of Diabetes and its Complications*, vol. 20, no. 1, pp. 21–25, 2006.

[17] C. Capula, E. Chiefari, A. Vero, D. P. Foti, A. Brunetti, and R. Vero, "Prevalence and predictors of postpartum glucose intolerance in Italian women with gestational diabetes mellitus," *Diabetes Research and Clinical Practice*, vol. 105, no. 2, pp. 223–230, 2014.

[18] K. Lobner, A. Knopff, A. Baumgarten et al., "Predictors of postpartum diabetes in women with gestational diabetes mellitus," *Diabetes*, vol. 55, no. 3, pp. 792–797, 2006.

[19] K. Al-Rubeaan, H. A. Al-Manaa, T. A. Khoja et al., "Epidemiology of abnormal glucose metabolism in a country facing Its epidemic: SAUDI-DM study," *Journal of Diabetes*, vol. 7, no. 5, pp. 622–632, 2015.

[20] A. J. Al-Quwaidhi, M. S. Pearce, E. Sobngwi, J. A. Critchley, and M. O'Flaherty, "Comparison of type 2 diabetes prevalence estimates in Saudi Arabia from a validated Markov model against the international diabetes federation and other modelling studies," *Diabetes Research and Clinical Practice*, vol. 103, no. 3, pp. 496–503, 2014.

[21] S. Nouhjah, H. Shahbazian, N. Shahbazian, A. Jahanshahi, S. Jahanfar, and B. Cheraghian, "Incidence and contributing factors of persistent hyperglycemia at 6-12 weeks postpartum in Iranian women with gestational diabetes: results from LAGA cohort study," *Journal of Diabetes Research*, vol. 2017, 9 pages, 2017.

[22] H. Wahabi, A. Fayed, S. Esmaeil et al., "Riyadh mother and baby multicenter cohort study: the cohort profile," *PLoS One*, vol. 11, no. 3, article e0150297, 2016.

[23] J. Brown, N. A. Alwan, J. West et al., "Lifestyle interventions for the treatment of women with gestational diabetes," *Cochrane Database of Systematic Reviews*, vol. 5, article CD011970, 2017.

[24] V. R. Aroda, C. A. Christophi, S. L. Edelstein et al., "The effect of lifestyle intervention and metformin on preventing or delaying diabetes among women with and without gestational diabetes: the diabetes prevention program outcomes study 10-year follow-up," *The Journal of Clinical Endocrinology & Metabolism*, vol. 100, no. 4, pp. 1646–1653, 2015.

[25] H. Shahbazian, S. Nouhjah, S. Jahanfar, and M. Nasiri, "Recall for postpartum follow-up of women with gestational diabetes mellitus: climbing a mountain," *Journal of Diabetes and Metabolic Disorders*, vol. 15, no. 1, p. 20, 2015.

[26] E. Marseille, N. Lohse, A. Jiwani et al., "The cost-effectiveness of gestational diabetes screening including prevention of type 2 diabetes: application of a new model in India and Israel," *The Journal of Maternal-Fetal & Neonatal Medicine*, vol. 26, no. 8, pp. 802–810, 2013.

14

Joint Effect of Maternal Tobacco Smoking and Pregestational Diabetes on Preterm Births and Congenital Anomalies: A Population-Based Study in Northern Italy

Lucia Borsari,[1] **Carlotta Malagoli**,[1] **Martha M. Werler**,[2,3] **Kenneth J. Rothman**,[2,3,4] **Marcella Malavolti**,[1] **Rossella Rodolfi**,[5] **Gianfranco De Girolamo**,[6] **Fausto Nicolini**,[5] **and Marco Vinceti**[1,2,3]

[1]*Department of Biomedical, Metabolic and Neural Sciences, Environmental, Genetic and Nutritional Epidemiology Research Center (CREAGEN), University of Modena and Reggio Emilia, Modena 41125, Italy*
[2]*Clinical and Experimental Medicine PhD Program, University of Modena and Reggio Emilia, Modena, Italy*
[3]*Department of Epidemiology, Boston University School of Public Health, Boston, MA 02118, USA*
[4]*Research Triangle Institute, Research Triangle Park, NC 27709, USA*
[5]*Local Health Authority of Reggio Emilia, Reggio Emilia 42122, Italy*
[6]*Department of Public Health, Unit of Epidemiology and Risk Communication, Local Health Authority of Modena, Modena 41126, Italy*

Correspondence should be addressed to Marco Vinceti; marco.vinceti@unimore.it

Academic Editor: Andrea Scaramuzza

Smoking and pregestational diabetes (PGD) are recognized risk factors for adverse pregnancy outcomes, but to date, no population-based study has investigated their joint effects. Using hospital discharges, we identified all women with PGD delivering in Emilia-Romagna region during 2007–2010 matched 1 : 5 with parturients without diabetes. Our study endpoints were preterm births and congenital anomalies. We measured interaction between PGD and maternal smoking, by calculating excess prevalence and prevalence ratio due to interaction, relative excess risk due to interaction (RERI), attributable proportion (AP), and the synergy index (S). Analyses were performed in the overall study population and in the subgroup whose PGD was validated through diabetes registers. The study included 992 women with PGD (10.5% smokers) and 4788 comparison women (11.9% smokers). The effects of PGD and maternal tobacco smoking were greater than additive for both preterm birth (excess prevalence due to interaction = 11.7%, excess ratio due to interaction = 1.5, RERI = 2.39, AP = 0.51, S = 2.82) and congenital anomalies (excess prevalence due to interaction = 2.2%, excess ratio due to interaction = 1.3, RERI = 1.33, AP = 0.49, S = 5.03). Joint effect on both endpoints was confirmed in the subgroup whose PGD status was validated. In conclusion, we found that maternal tobacco smoking and PGD intensify each other's effect on preterm birth and congenital anomalies.

1. Introduction

Tobacco smoking during pregnancy is one of the main modifiable risk factors associated with adverse maternal and fetal outcomes, including intrauterine growth restriction, ectopic pregnancy, premature birth, and congenital anomalies [1–4]. Pregnancy therefore represents a unique motivation for smoking cessation, and more women quit smoking during pregnancy than at any other time in their lives [5]. However, despite the known risks, the majority of women smoking at conception continue to smoke. More than 10% of women smoke during pregnancy in many high-income countries [6, 7]. In Italy, epidemiologic studies and routinely collected health data show that tobacco smoking prevalence among pregnant population varies from 6.7% to 22.3%. Tobacco smoking is associated with young maternal age and low economic status or education level [8–11].

Pregestational diabetes (PGD) represents the most common chronic condition complicating pregnancy. The number of affected pregnancies has been increasing, largely due to the obesity epidemic and consequent increase in type 2 diabetes in younger women [12, 13]. Several studies showed that PGD is an important risk factor for adverse pregnancy outcomes. In particular, women with existing diabetes have a risk of pregnancy resulting in major structural congenital anomaly up to fourfold greater than women without PGD [14–18]. In addition, the risk of preterm delivery, either spontaneous or indicated, was increased in women with pregnancies complicated by PGD, with studies reporting rates up to sevenfold higher than that among women not affected [19–21].

While maternal smoking and diabetes have been both recognized as independent relevant risk factors for adverse pregnancy outcomes, little is known about their interaction. Nicotine, one of the major bioactive substances in cigarettes, has been shown to alter glucose homeostasis, implying an important role for this agent in the development of cardiometabolic and other complications in diabetic patients [22]. Moreover, tobacco smoking seems able to amplify the effect of some risk factors on outcomes such as cardiovascular mortality or diseases, disability, and gestational diabetes, implying synergism between smoking and other factors [23–27].

The aim of this study was to investigate the joint effect of smoking and PGD on the risk of preterm birth and congenital anomalies in a population-based cohort of Italian pregnant women.

2. Materials and Methods

2.1. Study Population. Following approval by the Modena Province Ethics Committee, we conducted a retrospective cohort study by identifying all deliveries in Emilia-Romagna region (Northern Italy, population about 4,000,000) in the 2007–2010 period through the Hospital Discharge (HD) database (International Classification of Diseases version 9 Clinical Medicine (ICD-9-CM) codes V27.0-V27.9). We selected parturients with PGD through the presence of ICD-9-CM codes 250.xx or 648.0x listed anywhere on the HD records. For each selected HD record, we matched five comparison mothers without diabetes, according to year of birth and delivery, province of residence, and referral hospital. Among all mothers who matched the index mother by these criteria, we randomly selected the five comparators. To carry out this sampling of matched comparison women, we used the STATA-12 optmatch2 routine. If five women without diabetes were not available to match a woman with diabetes, we accepted a lower number. No matched woman was available for 2.3% of the women with diabetes. For these women, we relaxed the matching criteria first for province of residence, then for hospital of delivery, and finally for year of delivery. Women who experienced more than one delivery during the 4-year study period were included as multiple observations. Twin pregnancies were excluded.

We used the birth certificates to collect information on tobacco smoking habits of the mother, as well as on other sociodemographic and clinical characteristics used as covariates in the analysis (nationality, maternal age at the time of delivery, and education level of both parents). Smoking habits during pregnancy were therefore self-reported by mothers. Maternal smoking was defined as smoking for any period during pregnancy. Thus, it includes both women smoking only in early pregnancy and women smoking throughout pregnancy, regardless of the number of cigarettes smoked. Women who never smoked or who quit smoking before pregnancy were considered nonsmokers. Missing data on smoking habit during pregnancy was considered as an exclusion criterion in the selection of the study population. Method for selecting the study population is shown in Figure 1.

Lastly, through the population-based diabetes registers recently established in two out of nine provinces of the Emilia-Romagna region [28], Modena and Reggio-Emilia, we validated PGD diagnosis for the subgroup of women residing in these two provinces. Diabetes registers are based on case identification algorithms involving both administrative and clinical data, so their data tend to be more complete and accurate than data from other sources [29].

2.2. Pregnancy Adverse Outcomes. We focused on two adverse pregnancy outcomes, preterm births and congenital anomalies. We defined preterm birth as gestational age at delivery, according to the birth certificate, of <37 weeks. We detected congenital anomalies by matching each selected birth certificate to the Registry of Birth Defects of the Emilia-Romagna Region named IMER (*Indagine sulle Malformazioni congenite in Emilia Romagna*). This registry, established in 1978, is part of the European Network for the Surveillance of Congenital Anomalies EUROCAT [30].

2.3. Data Analysis. We measured the interaction between tobacco smoking and PGD as the excess over additivity of effects, comparing the combined effect of the two exposures with the sum of their individual effects. Firstly, we computed prevalence difference (PD) and prevalence ratio (PR) with associated 95% confidence interval (CI) of preterm birth and congenital anomalies using Episheet statistical software (version of April 10, 2017, downloaded from http://krothman.org/Episheet.xls). Women without PGD and nonsmokers represented the reference category. Excess prevalence of preterm birth and congenital anomalies due to interaction was calculated as the difference between PD in women exposed to both smoking and PGD (PD_{11}) and the sum of PD in women exposed to only smoking (PD_{01}) or only PGD (PD_{10}) (excess prevalence due to interaction $= PD_{11} - (PD_{01} + PD_{10})$). Excess ratio due to interaction was calculated as $PR_{11} - PR_{01} - PR_{10} + 1$ [31].

Then, we measured departures from additivity using appropriately defined relative measures of effect derived from multiplicative regression models. We estimated relative risks (RRs) from the odds ratios generated by logistic regression models, introducing PGD and maternal smoking in the models as a product term. In this model, we included

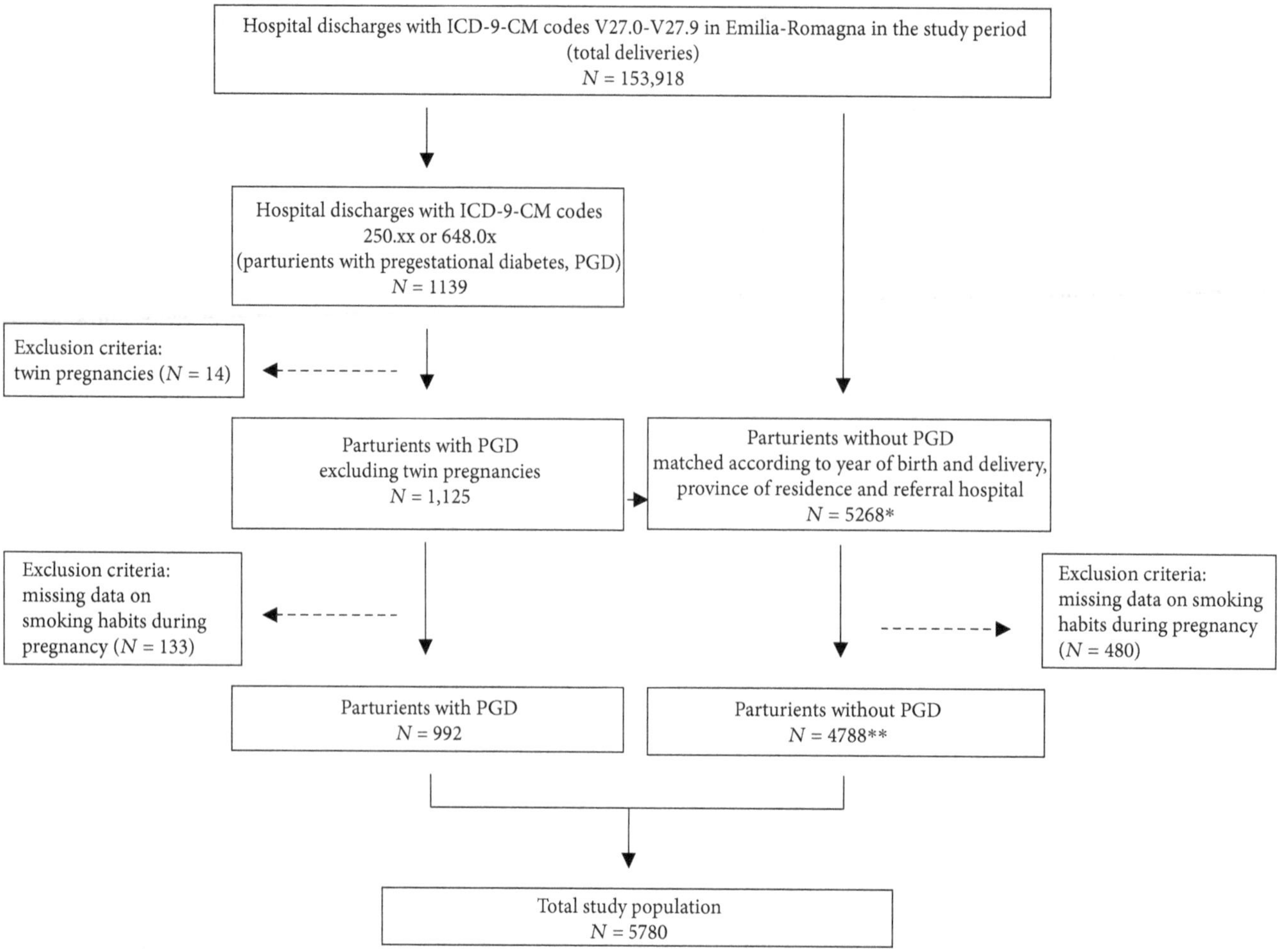

FIGURE 1: Flowchart of the study population. * 954 cases matched 5 controls, 66 cases matched 4 controls, 49 cases matched 3 controls, 31 cases matched 2 controls and 25 cases matched 1 control. ** 921 cases matched 5 controls, 22 cases matched 4 controls, 17 cases matched 3 controls, 12 cases matched 2 controls and 20 cases matched 1 control.

maternal age at delivery, nationality, and parents' education as confounding variables. We used the estimates from logistic regression models to calculate the relative excess risk due to interaction (RERI), the attributable proportion due to interaction (AP), and the synergy index (S), using an Excel spreadsheet by Andersson et al. [32]. RERI should be interpreted as the relative excess risk (RR-1) in those with both exposures minus that expected on the basis of the sum of the relative excess risks for the individual exposures. The AP represents the proportion of disease that is due to interaction among persons with both exposures. The synergy index S measures the extent to which the joint effect for both factors together, expressed as the relative excess risk, which exceeds the sum of the relative excess risk for each of the two factors' separate effect [33, 34].

Statistical analyses were performed by using Stata 15 statistical software (StataCorp LP, College Station, TX).

3. Results

The study included 5780 pregnant women, among them 992 with PGD and 4788 without PGD (Figure 1). The prevalence of tobacco smoking was similar among women with and without PGD (10.5% and 11.9%, resp.). General characteristics of the study population are presented in Table 1. Overall, we identified 536 (9.3%) preterm births and 118 (2.1%) newborns with one or more congenital anomalies.

Prevalence differences, PRs and RRs of preterm birth and congenital anomalies are reported in Table 2. We used these results to calculate measures of interaction between PGD and tobacco smoking, and we found that the effects were greater than additive for both preterm birth and congenital anomalies. The excess prevalence of preterm birth due to interaction was 11.7%, and the excess ratio of preterm birth due to interaction was 1.5. The joint effects on preterm birth were confirmed also when confounding variables were considered, with RERI = 2.39 (95% CI: 0.25, 4.53), AP = 0.51 (95% CI: 0.26, 0.75), and S = 2.82 (95% CI: 1.39, 5.79). An AP of 0.51 for preterm birth means that we estimate that 51% of the preterm births occurring to women who had diabetes and were smokers is attributable to the interaction between these two risk factors, assuming all the effects are causal and biases are controlled. As for congenital anomalies, we found excess prevalence due to interaction = 2.2%, excess ratio due to interaction = 1.3, RERI = 1.33 (95% CI: −1.19, 3.88), AP = 0.49 (95% CI: 0, 1.05), and S = 5.03 (95% CI: 0.23, 42.25). The AP

TABLE 1: Demographic characteristics of the study population, according to maternal pregestational diabetes and smoking habits.

	Women with PGD					Women without PGD				
	Nonsmoking		Smoking		Total	Nonsmoking		Smoking		Total
	n	(%)	*n*	(%)	*n*	*n*	(%)	*n*	(%)	*n*
Age at delivery										
<35 years	502	(56.5)	68	(65.4)	**570**	2469	(58.5)	337	(59.1)	**2806**
≥35 years	386	(43.5)	36	(34.6)	**422**	1749	(41.5)	233	(40.9)	**1982**
Nationality										
Italian	465	(52.4)	89	(85.6)	**554**	3157	(74.8)	511	(89.6)	**3668**
Other	423	(47.6)	15	(14.4)	**438**	1061	(25.2)	59	(10.4)	**1120**
Education										
Elementary/middle school	383	(43.1)	42	(40.4)	**425**	1129	(26.8)	181	(31.8)	**1310**
High school	360	(40.5)	42	(40.4)	**402**	1883	(44.6)	288	(50.5)	**2171**
University	145	(16.3)	20	(19.2)	**165**	1206	(28.6)	101	(17.7)	**1307**
Father's education										
Elementary/middle school	423	(47.6)	49	(47.1)	**472**	1362	(32.3)	236	(41.4)	**1598**
High school	314	(35.4)	44	(42.3)	**358**	1734	(41.1)	240	(42.1)	**1974**
University	110	(12.4)	10	(9.6)	**120**	903	(21.4)	72	(12.6)	**975**
Missing	41	(4.6)	1	(1.0)	**42**	219	(5.2)	22	(3.9)	**241**
Total	888	(100.0)	104	(100.0)	**992**	4218	(100.0)	570	(100.0)	**4788**

PGD = pregestational diabetes.

TABLE 2: Prevalence difference per 100, prevalence ratio and relative risk of preterm birth, and congenital anomalies associated with pregestational diabetes and/or tobacco smoking, Emilia-Romagna region, 2007–2010.

PGD	Smoking	Total	*n*	(%)	PD* 100	(95% CI)	PR	(95% CI)	RR*	(95% CI)
						Preterm birth				
No	No	4218	317	(7.51)	Ref.		Ref.		Ref.	
No	Yes	570	39	(6.84)	−0.67	(−2.89, 1.54)	0.91	(0.66, 1.25)	0.89	(0.63, 1.27)
Yes	No	888	151	(17.01)	9.48	(6.89, 12.08)	2.26	(1.89, 2.70)	2.41	(1.93, 3.02)
Yes	Yes	104	29	(27.88)	20.36	(11.67, 29.06)	3.71	(2.67, 5.15)	4.69	(2.97, 7.41)
						Congenital anomalies				
No	No	4218	79	(1.87)	Ref.		Ref.		Ref.	
No	Yes	570	10	(1.75)	−0.12	(−1.27, 1.03)	0.93	(0.49, 1.79)	0.92	(0.47, 1.79)
Yes	No	888	24	(2.70)	0.83	(0.31, 1.97)	1.44	(0.92, 2.26)	1.41	(0.88, 2.25)
Yes	Yes	104	5	(4.81)	2.93	(−1.22, 7.08)	2.57	(1.06, 6.23)	2.66	(1.05, 6.71)

*Adjusted for maternal age at delivery, nationality, and parents' education level. PGD = pregestational diabetes; PD = prevalence difference; PR = prevalence ratio; RR = relative risk.

of 0.49 indicates again that about half of the occurrence of births with congenital anomalies can be attributed to the interaction of tobacco smoking with pregestational diabetes.

Effect estimates for major categories of congenital anomalies were statistically unstable because of the small number of subjects. The congenital anomalies for which prevalence was considerably increased among diabetic women who also smoked during pregnancy were those affecting the cardiovascular system (RR = 2.88, 95% CI: 0.67–12.37), the genitourinary system (RR = 3.46, 95% CI: 0.43–27.62), and cleft palate/lip (RR = 7.42, 95% CI: 0.85–64.71), with RERI = 2.70 (95% CI: −1.52–6.91), 0.58 (95% CI: −6.88–8.05), and 4.96 (95% CI: −10.73–20.64), respectively. Concerning only anomalies of the cardiovascular system, which accounted for the highest number of congenital anomalies, we assessed the single anomalies, and we found that the increased risk in the offspring of women both smoking and affected by diabetes involved mainly atrial septal defects (RR = 9.29, 95% CI: 1.04–83.13), with RERI = 8.02 (95% CI: −12.05–28.09).

The analysis restricted to the subgroup of women validated through provincial diabetes registers of Modena and Reggio-Emilia included 108 women with PGD and 513 comparison women. Prevalence differences, PRs and RRs of preterm birth, and congenital anomalies among these women are reported in Table 3. Patterns were similar among these validated cases, but subject to more variation as a consequence of the small number of validated cases (for preterm birth, excess prevalence due to interaction = 5.3%, excess ratio due to interaction = 0.6, RERI = 1.75 (95% CI: −7.14, 10.63), AP = 0.29 (95% CI: 0, 1.37), S = 1.54 (95% CI: 0.24, 9.75) and

Table 3: Prevalence difference per 100, prevalence ratio and relative risk of preterm birth, and congenital anomalies associated with pregestational diabetes and/or tobacco smoking, Provinces of Modena and Reggio Emilia, 2007–2010.

PGD	Smoking	Total	n	(%)	PD*100	(95% CI)	PR	(95% CI)	RR	(95% CI)
						Preterm birth				
No	No	449	40	(8.91)	Ref.		Ref.		Ref.	
No	Yes	64	7	(10.94)	2.02	(−6.12, 10.17)	1.23	(0.57, 2.64)	1.30	(0.55, 3.08)
Yes	No	100	30	(30.01)	21.09	(11.68, 30.49)	3.37	(2.21, 5.14)	3.94	(2.25, 6.92)
Yes	Yes	8	3	(37.50)	28.6	(−7.37, 64.55)	4.21	(1.55, 11.51)	5.99	(1.37, 26.29)
						Congenital anomalies				
No	No	449	6	(1.34)	Ref.		Ref.		Ref.	
No	Yes	64	3	(4.69)	3.35	(−1.97, 8.67)	3.51	(0.89, 13.81)	4.46	(1.04, 19.09)
Yes	No	100	6	(6.01)	4.66	(−0.13, 9.46)	4.49	(1.47, 13.71)	4.01	(1.22, 13.18)
Yes	Yes	8	1	(12.50)	11.16	(−13.36, 35.68)	9.35	(1.13, 77.62)	12.91	(1.30, 127.75)

*Adjusted for maternal age at delivery, nationality, and parents' education level. PGD = pregestational diabetes; PD = prevalence difference; PR = prevalence ratio; RR = relative risk.

for congenital anomalies, excess prevalence due to interaction = 3%, excess ratio due to interaction = 2.2, RERI = 5.44 (95% CI: −23.03, 33.91), AP = 0.42 (95% CI: 0, 1.75), S = 1.84 (95% CI: 0.14, 21.19)).

4. Discussion

This is the first population-based study evaluating the interaction between diabetes and tobacco smoking in the specific population of pregnant women. Among women with both PGD and smoking, we found 11 preterm births and 2 congenital anomalies per 100 newborns more than we would expect on the basis of the sum of the separate effects of PGD and smoking, consistent with the presence of causal interaction between the two factors. In particular, calculation of AP showed that 51% of preterm births and 49% of congenital anomalies that occurred in the offspring of women with PGD and tobacco smoking habit were attributable to the interaction of the two exposures. This excess risk over additivity of effects was confirmed in the analysis performed on the subpopulation validated through the provincial diabetes registers. Despite the limited statistical stability from small numbers in this subgroup, the analysis of the provincial Diabetes Registers is reassuring, considering the higher accuracy in identifying cases of diabetes mellitus in this data source. Indeed, two Canadian and American studies [35, 36] have already highlighted that the use of only administrative data to identify diabetes in populations such as pregnant women could involve substantial misclassifications, mainly due to a limited ability to distinguish between pregestational and gestational diabetes.

These results are consistent with the hypothesis that PGD has effects that make offspring of affected women more susceptible to the effects of tobacco smoke. The negative effect of tobacco smoking on glycemic control, which has been already demonstrated [37], could partially explain the joint effect between the two risk factors. In fact, poor glycemic control at preconception or during pregnancy has been identified as one of the main factors associated with adverse pregnancy outcomes in women with diabetes [37–39].

Among the limitations of our study are considerable statistical variability of some estimates and lack of information about the metabolic status of the diabetic women. In addition, there are the possible confounding effects of concomitant obesity, folic acid consumption, and drug prescription at the time of pregnancy. We could not retrieve information about these variables for both parturients with and without diabetes. In addition, some exposure misclassification may have occurred for tobacco smoking during pregnancy, because of possible underreporting in studies relying on self-report [40]. Lack of availability of individual data, however, is frequently an inherent limitation of studies based on administrative or registry databases like the present one. On the other hand, administrative data affords much larger study sizes and may reduce selection bias. Lastly, given the high prevalence of preterm births in the doubly exposed group, the adjusted odds ratios derived from the logistic regression are slight overestimates of the prevalence ratios.

These results have greater importance because the prevalence of tobacco smoking during pregnancy remains high, as we found here, and was also reported in previous studies [8–11]. This is the first study reporting the prevalence of tobacco smoking among Italian pregnant women with PGD, and we unexpectedly found that it was similar to that found among pregnant women without PGD (more than 10%). This finding is concerning in view of the adverse risks related to diabetes and more so as a result of the interaction between the two factors.

5. Conclusions

In conclusion, our results indicate an interaction between maternal tobacco smoking and pregestational diabetes in increasing the risk of preterm birth and congenital anomalies. Given the still high prevalence of smokers among pregnant women, including those with PGD, and the interactive relation with PGD, further efforts to discourage smoking during pregnancy among women with diabetes would have a considerable public-health benefit. Further studies, including larger samples of pregnant women, would help to clarify the extent of this benefit as well as to deeply understand the relation between smoking and diabetes on adverse pregnancy outcomes.

Abbreviations

PGD: Pregestational diabetes
HD: Hospital discharge
ICD: International Classification of Diseases
IMER: Indagine sulle Malformazioni congenite in Emilia Romagna (Registry of Birth Defects of the Emilia-Romagna Region)
PD: Prevalence difference
PR: Prevalence ratio
RR: Relative risk
RERI: Relative excess risk due to interaction
AP: Attributable proportion due to interaction
S: Synergy index.

Conflicts of Interest

The authors declare that there is no conflict of interest regarding the publication of this paper.

Acknowledgments

This work was supported by the Lega Italiana per la Lotta contro i Tumori (LILT) of Reggio Emilia and the Local Health Authority of Reggio Emilia (Italy). The authors thank Dr. Eleonora Verdini (Emilia Romagna Region Health Authority) for her cooperation in retrieving hospital discharge records.

References

[1] S. Baba, A. K. Wikstrom, O. Stephansson, and S. Cnattingius, "Influence of smoking and snuff cessation on risk of preterm birth," *European Journal of Epidemiology*, vol. 27, no. 4, pp. 297–304, 2012.

[2] C. I. Vardavas, L. Chatzi, E. Patelarou et al., "Smoking and smoking cessation during early pregnancy and its effect on adverse pregnancy outcomes and fetal growth," *European Journal of Pediatrics*, vol. 169, no. 6, pp. 741–748, 2010.

[3] A. Hackshaw, C. Rodeck, and S. Boniface, "Maternal smoking in pregnancy and birth defects: a systematic review based on 173 687 malformed cases and 11.7 million controls," *Human Reproduction Update*, vol. 17, no. 5, pp. 589–604, 2011.

[4] S. Räisänen, U. Sankilampi, M. Gissler et al., "Smoking cessation in the first trimester reduces most obstetric risks, but not the risks of major congenital anomalies and admission to neonatal care: a population-based cohort study of 1,164,953 singleton pregnancies in Finland," *Journal of Epidemiology and Community Health*, vol. 68, no. 2, pp. 159–164, 2014.

[5] S. R. Crozier, S. M. Robinson, S. E. Borland et al., "Do women change their health behaviours in pregnancy? Findings from the Southampton Women's Survey," *Paediatric and Perinatal Epidemiology*, vol. 23, no. 5, pp. 446–453, 2009.

[6] "Statistics on women's smoking status at time of delivery (SATOD), England 2014. The Health and Social Care Information Centre 2014," Febuary 2018, http://www.hscic.gov.uk/searchcatalogue?productid=14841&returnid=3945.

[7] "European Perinatal Health Report. Health and care of pregnant women and babies in Europe in 2010," 2010, Febuary 2018, http://www.europeristat.com/reports/european-perinatal-health-report-2010.html.

[8] G. Esposito, R. Ambrosio, F. Napolitano, and G. Di Giuseppe, "Women's knowledge, attitudes and behavior about maternal risk factors in pregnancy," *PLoS One*, vol. 10, no. 12, article e0145873, 2015.

[9] XI Rapporto sui dati del Certificato di Assistenza al Parto (CedAP), "Regione Emilia Romagna," 2013, August 2018, http://salute.regione.emiliaromagna.it/siseps/sanita/cedap/files/RAPPORTO_CEDAP_2013.pdf.

[10] P. Mastroiacovo, R. M. Nilsen, E. Leoncini et al., "Prevalence of maternal preconception risk factors: an Italian multicenter survey," *Italian Journal of Pediatrics*, vol. 40, no. 1, p. 91, 2014.

[11] S. Nutini, L. Carrozzi, A. Melani et al., "Cigarette smoking in pregnancy: observational prospective study in three towns of Tuscany Region (Central Italy)," *Epidemiologia e Prevenzione*, vol. 37, no. 2-3, pp. 145–152, 2013.

[12] R. Bell, K. Bailey, T. Cresswell et al., "Trends in prevalence and outcomes of pregnancy in women with pre-existing type I and type II diabetes," *BJOG : An International Journal of Obstetrics and Gynaecology*, vol. 115, no. 4, pp. 445–452, 2008.

[13] D. S. Feig, J. Hwee, B. R. Shah, G. L. Booth, A. S. Bierman, and L. L. Lipscombe, "Trends in incidence of diabetes in pregnancy and serious perinatal outcomes: a large, population-based study in Ontario, Canada, 1996-2010," *Diabetes Care*, vol. 37, no. 6, pp. 1590–1596, 2014.

[14] E. Garne, M. Loane, H. Dolk et al., "Spectrum of congenital anomalies in pregnancies with pregestational diabetes," *Birth Defects Research. Part A, Clinical and Molecular Teratology*, vol. 94, no. 3, pp. 134–140, 2012.

[15] J. J. Newham, S. V. Glinianaia, P. W. G. Tennant, J. Rankin, and R. Bell, "Improved antenatal detection of congenital anomalies in women with pre-gestational diabetes: population-based cohort study," *Diabetic Medicine*, vol. 30, no. 12, pp. 1442–1448, 2013.

[16] M. Vinceti, C. Malagoli, K. J. Rothman et al., "Risk of birth defects associated with maternal pregestational diabetes," *European Journal of Epidemiology*, vol. 29, no. 6, pp. 411–418, 2014.

[17] M. Balsells, A. Garcia-Patterson, I. Gich, and R. Corcoy, "Maternal and fetal outcome in women with type 2 versus type 1 diabetes mellitus: a systematic review and metaanalysis," *The Journal of Clinical Endocrinology and Metabolism*, vol. 94, no. 11, pp. 4284–4291, 2009.

[18] R. M. Simeone, O. J. Devine, J. A. Marcinkevage et al., "Diabetes and congenital heart defects: a systematic review, meta-analysis, and modeling project," *American Journal of Preventive Medicine*, vol. 48, no. 2, pp. 195–204, 2015.

[19] B. M. Sibai, S. N. Caritis, J. C. Hauth et al., "Preterm delivery in women with pregestational diabetes mellitus or chronic hypertension relative to women with uncomplicated pregnancies. The National institute of Child health and Human Development Maternal- Fetal Medicine Units Network," *American Journal of Obstetrics & Gynecology*, vol. 183, no. 6, pp. 1520–1524, 2000.

[20] F. Mimouni, M. Miodovnik, T. A. Siddiqi, M. A. Berk, C. Wittekind, and R. C. Tsang, "High spontaneous premature labor rate in insulin-dependent diabetic pregnant women: an association with poor glycemic control and urogenital infection," *Obstetrics and Gynecology*, vol. 72, no. 2, pp. 175–180, 1988.

[21] M. F. Greene, J. W. Hare, M. Krache et al., "Prematurity among insulin-requiring diabetic gravid women," *American Journal of Obstetrics and Gynecology*, vol. 161, no. 1, pp. 106–111, 1989.

[22] D. Kar, C. Gillies, F. Zaccardi et al., "Relationship of cardiometabolic parameters in non-smokers, current smokers, and quitters in diabetes: a systematic review and meta-analysis," *Cardiovascular Diabetology*, vol. 15, no. 1, p. 158, 2016.

[23] E. T. Roos, T. Lallukka, E. Lahelma, and O. Rahkonen, "Joint associations between smoking and obesity as determinants of premature mortality among midlife employees," *European Journal of Public Health*, vol. 27, no. 1, pp. 135–139, 2017.

[24] T. Lallukka, O. Rahkonen, E. Lahelma, and J. Lahti, "Joint associations of smoking and physical activity with disability retirement: a register-linked cohort study," *BMJ Open*, vol. 5, no. 7, article e006988, 2015.

[25] M. C. Turner, A. Cohen, R. T. Burnett et al., "Interactions between cigarette smoking and ambient PM2.5 for cardiovascular mortality," *Environmental Research*, vol. 154, pp. 304–310, 2017.

[26] H. R. Banack and J. S. Kaufman, "Estimating the time-varying joint effects of obesity and smoking on all-cause mortality using marginal structural models," *American Journal of Epidemiology*, vol. 183, no. 2, pp. 122–129, 2016.

[27] M. Nishiyama, M. Kimijima, T. Muto, and K. Kimura, "Presence of an interaction between smoking and being overweight increases risks of hypertension, diabetes, and cardiovascular disease in outpatients with mood disorders," *Environmental Health and Preventive Medicine*, vol. 17, no. 4, pp. 285–291, 2012.

[28] P. Ballotari, S. Chiatamone Ranieri, M. Vicentini et al., "Building a population-based diabetes register: an Italian experience," *Diabetes Research and Clinical Practice*, vol. 103, no. 1, pp. 79–87, 2014.

[29] L. Borsari, C. Malagoli, P. Ballotari et al., "Validity of hospital discharge records to identify pregestational diabetes in an Italian population," *Diabetes Research and Clinical Practice*, vol. 123, pp. 106–111, 2017.

[30] P. A. Boyd, M. Haeusler, I. Barisic, M. Loane, E. Garne, and H. Dolk, "Paper 1: the EUROCAT network—organization and processes," *Birth Defects Research Part A, Clinical and Molecular Teratology*, vol. 91, Supplement 1, pp. S2–15, 2011.

[31] K. J. Rothman, *Epidemiology. An Introduction*, Oxford University Press, New York, NY, USA, 2002.

[32] T. Andersson, L. Alfredsson, H. Kallberg, S. Zdravkovic, and A. Ahlbom, "Calculating measures of biological interaction," *European Journal of Epidemiology*, vol. 20, no. 7, pp. 575–579, 2005.

[33] K. J. Rothman, S. Greenland, and A. M. Walker, "Concepts of interaction," *American Journal of Epidemiology*, vol. 112, no. 4, pp. 467–470, 1980.

[34] M. J. Knol, T. J. VanderWeele, R. H. H. Groenwold, O. H. Klungel, M. M. Rovers, and D. E. Grobbee, "Estimating measures of interaction on an additive scale for preventive exposures," *European Journal of Epidemiology*, vol. 26, no. 6, pp. 433–438, 2011.

[35] V. M. Allen, L. Dodds, A. Spencer, E. A. Cummings, N. MacDonald, and G. Kephart, "Application of a national administrative case definition for the identification of pre-existing diabetes mellitus in pregnancy," *Chronic Diseases and Injuries in Canada*, vol. 32, no. 3, pp. 113–120, 2012.

[36] M. T. Lydon-Rochelle, V. L. Holt, V. Cárdenas et al., "The reporting of pre-existing maternal medical conditions and complications of pregnancy on birth certificates and in hospital discharge data," *American Journal of Obstetrics and Gynecology*, vol. 193, no. 1, pp. 125–134, 2005.

[37] P. M. Nilsson, S. Gudbjörnsdottir, B. Eliasson, J. Cederholm, and Steering Committee of the Swedish National Diabetes Register, "Smoking is associated with increased HbA_{1c} values and microalbuminuria in patients with diabetes — data from the National Diabetes Register in Sweden," *Diabetes & Metabolism*, vol. 30, no. 3, pp. 261–268, 2004.

[38] A. Lapolla, M. G. Dalfra, and D. Fedele, "Pregnancy complicated by diabetes: what is the best level of HbA1c for conception?," *Acta Diabetologica*, vol. 47, no. 3, pp. 187–192, 2010.

[39] M. E. Inkster, T. P. Fahey, P. T. Donnan, G. P. Leese, G. J. Mires, and D. J. Murphy, "Poor glycated haemoglobin control and adverse pregnancy outcomes in type 1 and type 2 diabetes mellitus: systematic review of observational studies," *BMC Pregnancy and Childbirth*, vol. 6, no. 1, p. 30, 2006.

[40] S. C. Gorber, S. Schofield-Hurwitz, J. Hardt, G. Levasseur, and M. Tremblay, "The accuracy of self-reported smoking: a systematic review of the relationship between self-reported and cotinine-assessed smoking status," *Nicotine & Tobacco Research*, vol. 11, no. 1, pp. 12–24, 2009.

15

Inflammatory Markers in Older Women with a History of Gestational Diabetes and the Effects of Weight Loss

Alice S. Ryan

VA Maryland Health Care System, Research Service, Department of Medicine, Division of Gerontology and Geriatric Medicine, University of Maryland School of Medicine and Baltimore Geriatric Research Education and Clinical Center (GRECC), Baltimore, MD 21201, USA

Correspondence should be addressed to Alice S. Ryan; aryan@som.umaryland.edu

Academic Editor: Daniela Foti

The purpose of this study was to compare systemic inflammation in older women with a history of gestational diabetes (GDM) who developed impaired glucose tolerance (IGT) or type 2 diabetes (T2DM) to that in those with normal glucose tolerance (NGT) and to determine, in these women, the effect of weight loss (WL) induced by diet and exercise training on systemic inflammation and adipokine levels. This was a longitudinal clinical investigation of overweight/obese (BMI: 32 ± 1 kg/m^2) women (59 ± 1 years) with a GDM history ($n = 19$) who had normal glucose tolerance (NGT, $n = 7$) or IGT/T2DM ($n = 12$). Women completed 6 months of weight loss induced by diet and exercise and underwent VO_2max, body composition, blood draw, glucose tolerance testing, and 2-hour hyperinsulinemic-euglycemic clamps (40 mU·m^{-2}·min^{-1}). Glucose utilization (M) was 42% higher in the NGT group ($P < 0.05$). CRP was two-fold higher in the IGT/T2DM group than that in the NGT group ($P < 0.01$). Adiponectin levels were 59% higher in the NGT group than those in the IGT/T2DM group ($P < 0.01$). IL-6sR was higher in the NGT group ($P < 0.01$). The women lost body weight, body fat, visceral fat, and subcutaneous abdominal fat ($P < 0.001$). Fasting glucose ($P < 0.05$), fasting insulin, glucose, and insulin AUC decreased (all $P < 0.005$) after the intervention. M increased by 21% ($P < 0.05$). CRP (−16%) and TNFR1 (−6%) tended to decrease, whereas TNFα, IL-6, SAA, and adiponectin did not change in the group. In conclusion, older women with a history of GDM who have developed IGT or T2DM have higher CRP and reduced adiponectin levels despite similar BMI and total and abdominal obesity to those with NGT. Six months WL induced by diet and exercise improves body composition and increases insulin sensitivity without a significant modification of inflammatory markers and adiponectin levels.

1. Introduction

The global prevalence estimate of total diabetes in pregnancy (e.g., both known diabetes in pregnancy and previously undiagnosed diabetes in pregnancy) is nearly 17% [1]. Gestational diabetes mellitus (GDM) carries a long-term risk of developing type 2 diabetes for the mother with estimates reported as an overall relative risk of 6.0 [2] and a 7–12-fold greater lifetime risk for subsequent development of type 2 diabetes [3]. Our results indicate that postmenopausal women with prior GDM are more insulin resistant than postmenopausal women controls of similar age, adiposity, and fitness levels and are as insulin resistant as women with T2DM [4] further supporting conclusions that women with GDM are at risk for diabetes.

Inflammation is associated with increased risk for cardiovascular disease, and inflammatory markers are elevated in obesity and diabetes. Inflammatory markers are, for the most part, elevated during pregnancy in GDM women compared to those in non-GDM women [5]. Furthermore in a systematic meta-analysis, maternal adiponectin levels are significantly lower and TNFα and leptin are higher in GDM patients than those in controls [6]. It is, therefore, reasonable to hypothesize that inflammation may play a part in the heightened insulin resistance observed in older women with a history of GDM.

In a recent meta-analysis of approximately 30 randomized controlled trials of either diet, physical activity, or both, lifestyle interventions during pregnancy resulted in an 18% reduction in the risk of GDM, but a lifestyle intervention initiated at or after the 16th week of gestation did not reduce the risk of GDM [7]. Lifestyle programs may also be beneficial postpartum in women with a history of GDM, wherein an increase in physical activity can halve the risk of developing type 2 diabetes mellitus [8], and even a small amount of postpartum weight loss is associated with improved glucose metabolism [9]. In older women with a history of GDM, we reported that aerobic exercise with moderate weight loss reduces body weight and visceral and subcutaneous abdominal fat and improves insulin sensitivity [10]. Yet, the effects of lifestyle modification on adipokines were not investigated in older women with a history of GDM. However, in a broad context, modest weight loss alone or with exercise reduces inflammatory markers in overweight and obese adults [11–14].

Although our data suggest that older overweight and sedentary women with a history of GDM are insulin resistant, the role of inflammation in this context is unknown. The hypothesis tested was that inflammatory markers would be higher and adiponectin levels would be lower in women with a history of gestational diabetes who later developed impaired glucose tolerance (IGT) or type 2 diabetes than in women with a history of GDM who have normal glucose tolerance and that lifestyle modification would reduce inflammatory profiles. Therefore, the aim of this study was to compare systemic inflammation in older women with a history of GDM who developed IGT or type 2 diabetes to that in those with NGT and to determine, in these women, the effect of weight loss induced by diet and exercise training on systemic inflammation and adipokine levels.

2. Materials and Methods

2.1. Study Sample and Study Intervention. Women were recruited from the Baltimore metropolitan area for participation in this study. Each had a history of GDM between 5 and 32 years prior as confirmed by a physician or healthcare provider. Women were overweight and obese with a body mass index (BMI) between 26 and 38 kg/m^2 and were 41–68 years of age. They were weight stable, defined as <2.0 kg weight change in past year, as well as sedentary, defined as performing aerobic exercise for <20 min twice per week. The University of Maryland Institutional Review Board approved the study. Each woman provided written informed consent. Subjects underwent a screening process, which included a medical history and physical exam, fasting blood chemistries, a 12-lead resting electrocardiogram, and graded exercise treadmill test. Exclusion criteria included hormone replacement therapy; smoking; cancer; or any indication of liver, renal or hematological disease, or other medical disorders.

Nineteen eligible women completed a 6-month weight loss program induced by diet and aerobic exercise. The effects of weight loss on body composition and insulin sensitivity were reported in a larger sample size ($n = 25$); however, the influence of glucose tolerance on inflammatory cytokines and adiponectin levels were not examined. All women attended weekly weight loss classes led by a registered dietitian for instruction in the American Heart Association (AHA) Step I [15] guidelines for weight loss. They were instructed to restrict their caloric intake by 250–350 kcal/d. Some women exercised on motorized treadmills and cycle ergometers 3 times/week, 45 min/session, for 6 months. Exercise intensity was prescribed as ~50–60% heart rate reserve and gradually progressed in duration and intensity to >60% VO_2max for 45 minutes. The heart rate was monitored during exercise using heart rate monitors (Polar Electro Inc., Lake Success, NY).

2.2. Research Testing. Before and after 6 months of weight loss, subjects underwent research testing consisting of body composition measurements, maximal exercise tests, oral glucose tolerance tests, and blood draws. Height (cm) and weight (kg) were determined for BMI (kg/m^2). Subjects underwent dual-energy X-ray absorptiometry (DXA) (Model DPX-L, Lunar Radiation Corp., Madison, WI) scan to measure fat mass, lean tissue mass, and bone mineral content (BMC) and to calculate fat-free mass (FFM = lean tissue + BMC). Women also had an L_4-L_5 abdominal computed tomography (CT) scan (PQ 6000 Scanner General Electric Hi-Light, Cleveland, Ohio) for determination of visceral (VAT) and subcutaneous abdominal adipose tissue (SAT) areas [10]. A continuous treadmill test protocol [16] was used to determine VO_2max, whereby subjects met two of three following criteria including a plateau in oxygen uptake with an increased work load as evidenced by a difference in the oxygen uptake of <2 mL·kg^{-1}·min^{-1}, a respiratory exchange ratio of >1.10, or a maximal heart rate within 10 beats/min of the age-predicted maximal value.

All testing was performed in the morning after a 12-hr overnight fast. All subjects were weight stabilized (<1 kg) for at least two weeks prior to testing. Subjects underwent a 75-g, 2-h oral glucose tolerance test (OGTT) [17] with blood samples drawn every 30 min for measurement of plasma glucose and insulin levels. For two days prior to the glucose clamps, the RD provided the subjects with two days of an isocaloric diet (55–60% carbohydrates, 15–20% protein, and <30% fat). The number of calories given to each woman was estimated from the 7-day food records, and estimates of energy expenditure were based on the Harris-Benedict equation [18]. Peripheral tissue sensitivity to exogenous insulin was measured using the hyperinsulinemic-euglycemic clamp technique [19] with a priming and continuous infusion of insulin for two hours (240 pmol·m^{-2}·min^{1}, Humulin, Eli Lilly Co., Indianapolis, IN). The infusion of glucose and insulin was made through an intravenous catheter, and blood samples were drawn from a dorsal hand or wrist vein in which the hand was warmed to "arterialize" [20] the blood through the use of a warmed chamber. The amount of glucose infused after glucose space correction determined glucose utilization or M. One woman in the NGT group and five women in the IGT/T2DM did not undergo the glucose clamp because of venous access difficulty or scheduling conflict.

2.3. Blood Sample Analyses (Cytokines, Adiponectin, Glucose, and Insulin). Blood samples were transferred into chilled tubes containing 1 mg of EDTA per cc of blood. The plasma was separated by centrifugation at 4°C for 15 min at 2000 ×g. Plasma IL-6, TNFα, their soluble receptors (sIL-6R, TNFR1), adiponectin, glucose, and insulin were measured in duplicate, and the average of the two values was used for data analyses. Duplicate samples that did not provide a coefficient of variation less than 15% were reanalyzed, and all values were averaged for data analyses. All cytokines and cytokine-soluble receptors were measured using Quantikine ELISA kits (R&D Systems, Minneapolis, MN). The inter- and intra-assay CVs were 6% for IL-6 and sIL-6R and 12% for TNFα and TNFR1. The CRP was measured in triplicate using an automated immunoanalyzer (Immulite, Diagnostics Products Corp., Los Angeles, CA) with inter- and intra-assay CVs of 7.5 and 4.4%, respectively. SAA levels were measured in triplicate with an ELISA kit according to the manufacturer's instructions (BioSource, Camarillo, CA, USA) with the intra-assay CV of 4%. Adiponectin was determined by RIA (Millipore, St. Charles, MO) with the inter- and intra-assay coefficient of variations of <10% at ED20, ED50, and ED80 concentrations of the standard range. Plasma insulin and leptin were measured by RIA (Millipore, St. Charles, MO) and glucose with the glucose oxidase method (2300 STAT Plus; YSI, Yellow Springs, OH).

3. Statistical Analyses

The statistical significance between glucose tolerance groups was determined by unpaired t-tests. Changes with the treatment were determined by paired t-test. Relationships between variables were determined by linear regression analyses and calculation of Pearson correlation coefficients. Data were analyzed using SPSS (PASW Statistics 18, SPSS Inc., Chicago, IL) and expressed as mean ± standard error of the mean (SEM). Statistical significance was set at the $P < 0.05$.

4. Results

4.1. Baseline Characteristics. Of the 19 women with a history of GDM, seven women had NGT and 12 women had IGT ($n = 5$) or T2DM ($n = 7$). Only one woman was on an oral agent for T2DM, and the remaining six were untreated. The NGT and IGT/T2DM groups did not differ in age, body weight, BMI, VO_2max, percent body fat, fat mass, or FFM (Table 1). The visceral adipose tissue area was higher in the NGT group ($P < 0.05$), but the SAT was not different between groups. Fasting glucose and insulin levels were not significantly different between groups, but as expected, G_{120} and glucose AUC was higher in the IGT/T2DM group than that in the NGT group ($P < 0.0001$). Glucose utilization (M) was 42% higher in the NGT group ($P < 0.01$). CRP was over twofold higher in the IGT/T2DM group than that in the NGT group ($P < 0.01$, Figure 1(a)). Fasting plasma SAA, TNFα, TNFR1, and IL-6 did not differ between groups at baseline (Table 1). IL-6sR was higher in the NGT group ($P < 0.01$, Figure 1(b)). Adiponectin levels were 59% higher in the NGT group than those in the IGT/T2DM group ($P < 0.01$, Figure 2). Insulin AUC increased with age ($r = 0.56$, $P < 0.05$). VO_2max ($r = -0.47$, $P < 0.05$) and M ($r = -0.59$, $P < 0.05$) decreased with age.

Table 1: Baseline body composition, glucose metabolism, and inflammation.

	NGT ($n = 7$)	IGT/T2DM ($n = 12$)
Age (year)	50 (2)	52 (2)
Weight (kg)	85.9 (4.4)	85.1 (3.0)
Body mass index (kg/m^2)	32.2 (1.5)	32.0 (0.9)
Percent body fat	46.1 (1.7)	45.4 (1.4)
Fat mass (kg)	39.5 (2.7)	38.3 (2.5)
Fat-free mass (kg)	45.9 (2.2)	47.3 (2.6)
VO_2max (L/min)	1.93 (0.10)	1.72 (0.09)
Visceral fat (cm^2)	150.2 (22.9)	127.7 (10.9)[a]
Subcutaneous abdominal fat (cm^2)	457.3 (38.2)	484.9 (42.6)
Fasting glucose (mmol/L)	5.2 (0.1)	6.3 (0.4)
Glucose at 120 min (mmol/L)	5.9 (0.5)	11.1 (0.6)[c]
Fasting insulin (pmol/L)	76 (13)	107 (15)
G_{AUC} (mmol/L/120 min)	862 (25)	1231 (57)[c]
I_{AUC} (pmol/L/120 min)	55,700 (9209)	56,794 (9954)
Glucose utilization (μmol/kg/min)	31.9 (4.6)	17.7 (2.4)[b]
Glucose utilization (μmol/kg$_{FFM}$/min)	57.9 (7.2)	63.8 (3.1)[a]
TNFα (pg/mL)	2.93 (1.92)	1.51 (0.36)
TNFR1(μg/mL)	808.9 (84.7)	744.9 (48.5)
IL-6 (pg/mL)	2.08 (0.30)	2.38 (0.52)
SAA (μg/mL)	43.1 (9.65)	64.7 (37.1)

Values are mean (SEM). Baseline differences tested between groups: [a]$P < 0.05$, [b]$P < 0.01$, and [c]$P < 0.001$. NGT: normal glucose tolerance; IGT/T2DM: impaired glucose tolerance/type 2 diabetes mellitus; VO_2max: maximum oxygen uptake; G_{AUC}: glucose area under the curve; I_{AUC}: insulin area under the curve.

4.2. Relationships with Inflammation. Relationships between cytokines and clinical phenotypes indicate that IL-6sR was negatively associated with G_{120} ($r = -0.62$, $P < 0.05$) and glucose AUC ($r = -0.72$, $P < 0.01$) but not insulin AUC. The CRP was negatively associated with M ($r = -0.56$, $P < 0.05$). Adiponectin was negatively associated with fasting glucose ($r = -0.50$, $P < 0.05$), G_{120} ($r = -0.65$, $P < 0.01$), and fasting insulin ($r = -0.59$, $P < 0.05$) and positively with M ($r = 0.63$, $P < 0.05$). Of all the cytokines, only IL-6 increased with age ($r = 0.52$, $P < 0.05$). There were some relationships with total and abdominal adiposity such that the percent body fat was associated with higher CRP ($r = 0.64$, $P < 0.01$) and SAA ($r = 0.49$, $P < 0.05$). VAT predicted TNFR1 ($r = 0.67$, $P < 0.01$) and IL-6sR ($r = 0.55$, $P < 0.05$) and approached significance for SAA ($r = 0.47$, $P = 0.08$). SAT predicted SAA ($r = 0.53$, $P < 0.05$). Relationships between cytokines indicate that TNFR1 is related to IL-6sR ($r = 0.68$, $P < 0.01$) and CRP is related to SAA ($r = 0.51$, $P < 0.05$).

4.3. Effects of Interventions (Table 2). In the total group or in the NGT and IGT/T2DM groups, there were significant losses of body weight (total group: $-7.4 \pm 1.0\%$,

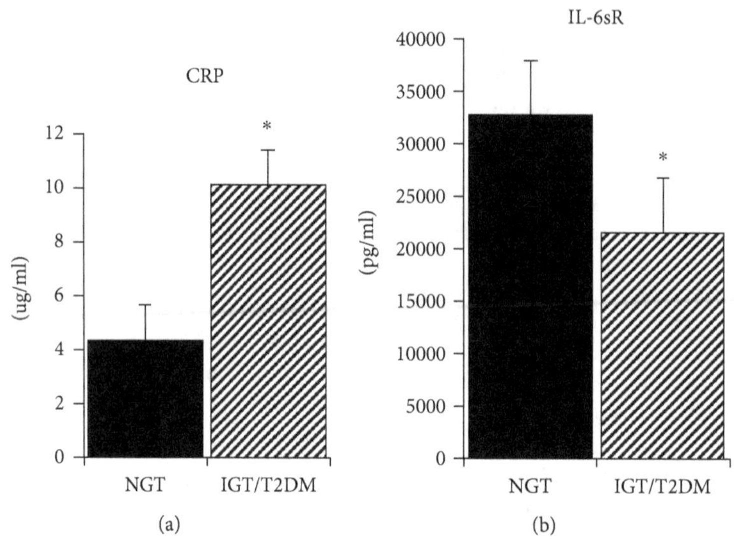

FIGURE 1: (a) CRP levels in NGT and IGT/T2DM groups. Values are mean ± SEM. Significantly different between groups, $^*P < 0.01$. (b). IL-6sR levels in NGT and IGT/T2DM groups. Values are mean ± SEM. Significantly different between groups, $^*P < 0.01$.

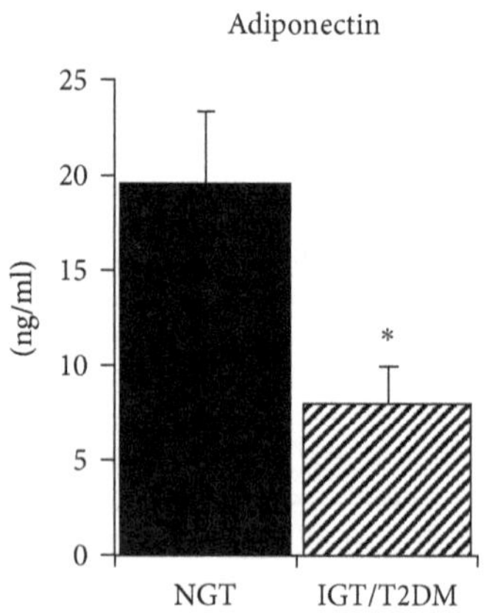

FIGURE 2: Adiponectin levels in NGT and IGT/T2DM groups. Values are mean ± SEM. Significantly different between groups, $^*P < 0.01$.

NGT: −7.1 ± 1.7%, IGT/T2DM: −7.6 ± 1.4%, all $P < 0.005$). There were also significant reductions in BMI, body fat, visceral fat, and subcutaneous abdominal fat ($P = 0.01$ – <0.0001). There was a 7% increase in VO_2max (l/min) in the total group ($P < 0.05$) and VO_2max increased in both the NGT group and the IGT/T2DM group ($P < 0.05$). Fasting glucose ($P < 0.05$), fasting insulin ($P < 0.005$), and 120-min glucose ($P < 0.01$) decreased along with a 14 and 31% reduction in glucose AUC ($P < 0.0001$) and insulin AUC ($P < 0.005$), respectively, after WL treatments in the total group. Fasting, 120 min glucose, and glucose AUC did not significantly change but fasting insulin and insulin AUC decreased in the NGT group ($P < 0.05$). Fasting, 120-min glucose, glucose, and insulin AUC decreased in the IGT/T2DM group (P's < 0.05). M increased by 21% ($P = 0.05$) in the total group and increased in the NGT group ($P < 0.05$). Plasma leptin decreased by 31% ($P < 0.01$) in the total group and decreased in the IGT/T2DM group ($P < 0.0001$). There were no significant changes in CRP, TNFα, TNFR1, IL-6, SAA, and adiponectin after WL in the total group or NGT and IGT/T2DM groups.

5. Discussion

In studies that have examined inflammatory markers *during* pregnancy, results are somewhat conflicting. Women with GDM ($n = 200$) had higher TNFα but not CRP in the first trimester than 800 unaffected women [21], whereas higher CRP levels were observed in another case-control study of GDM women ($n = 36$) [22]. Adiponectin levels are reported as lower in 30 GDM women compared to the same number of healthy pregnant women [23]. In another study, CRP and TNFα levels were higher in GDM than those in NGT pregnant women, but differences disappeared when adjusting for age, family history of T2DM, and previous GDM history and prepregnancy BMI [24]. It is possible that differences in the timing of measurements (trimester), adjustment for confounders, sample sizes, and ethnicity may help explain these disparate results. However, a systematic review and meta-analysis concluded from 27 trials that maternal TNFα and leptin levels are higher in GDM women than those in controls, and adiponectin concentrations are lower [6], which would support that some inflammatory markers are altered during pregnancy.

There is limited information regarding inflammatory markers in women with a prior *history* of GDM. In young women who had GDM about seven years prior to enrolment, soluble TNFαR2 and IL-6 levels were higher than those in young women without a history of GDM [25]. In another cross-sectional study of predictors of inflammatory markers in young women ~three years after pregnancy complicated by GDM, higher waist circumference was significantly associated with higher CRP, leptin, and resistin and negatively with adiponectin [26]. Although the majority of women

Table 2: Effects of the interventions on body composition, glucose metabolism, and inflammation.

	NGT/IGT/T2DM (n = 19)		NGT (n = 7)		IGT/T2DM (n = 12)	
	Before	After	Before	After	Before	After
Age (yr)	52 ± 2		50 ± 2		52 ± 2	
Weight (kg)	85.4 ± 2.4	79.2 ± 2.6^{d}	85.9 ± 4.4	79.6 ± 3.7^{b}	85.1 ± 3.0	78.9 ± 3.6^{d}
Body mass index (kg/m^2)	32.0 ± 0.7	29.9 ± 0.9^{d}	32.2 ± 1.5	29.9 ± 1.4^{b}	31.9 ± 0.9	29.9 ± 1.2^{b}
Percent body fat	45.6 ± 1.1	42.2 ± 1.5^{d}	46.1 ± 1.7	42.2 ± 2.1^{c}	45.4 ± 1.4	42.1 ± 2.1^{b}
Fat mass (kg)	38.7 ± 1.8	33.9 ± 2.1^{d}	39.5 ± 2.7	33.6 ± 2.8^{c}	38.3 ± 2.5	34.0 ± 3.0^{c}
Fat-free mass (kg)	46.8 ± 1.8	44.9 ± 1.1	45.9 ± 2.2	45.4 ± 1.9	47.3 ± 2.6	44.7 ± 1.3
VO_2max (L/min)	1.80 ± 0.07	1.92 ± 0.07^{c}	1.92 ± 0.09	1.91 ± 0.09	1.72 ± 0.09	1.92 ± 0.09^{c}
Waist circumference (cm)	93.4 ± 1.9	88.1 ± 2.1^{d}	92.8 ± 4.4	88.6 ± 4.1^{b}	93.7 ± 1.6	87.8 ± 2.5^{c}
Hip circumference (cm)	112.2 ± 1.5	105.7 ± 1.6^{d}	114.8 ± 2.3	106.8 ± 1.8^{a}	110.5 ± 1.9	104.9 ± 2.5^{c}
Visceral fat (cm^2)	137.5 ± 11.6	110.0 ± 10.1^{d}	150.2 ± 22.9	121.8 ± 20.1^{a}	127.7 ± 10.9	100.9 ± 8.9^{c}
Subcutaneous abdominal fat (cm^2)	472.8 ± 28.5	414.5 ± 31.2^{d}	457.3 ± 38.2	399.1 ± 40.4^{a}	484.9 ± 42.6	426.5 ± 47.4^{c}
Sagittal diameter (cm)	25.9 ± 0.7	24.8 ± 0.7^{d}	25.3 ± 1.1	23.7 ± 1.0^{a}	26.3 ± 0.9	24.6 ± 1.0^{c}
Fasting glucose (mmol/L)	5.9 ± 0.3	5.6 ± 0.2^{a}	5.2 ± 0.1	5.1 ± 0.2	6.3 ± 0.4	5.9 ± 0.3^{a}
Glucose at 120 min (mmol/L)	9.4 ± 0.7	7.9 ± 0.6^{b}	6.2 ± 0.3	5.9 ± 0.5	11.1 ± 0.6	9.0 ± 0.6^{a}
Fasting insulin (pmol/L)	93 ± 11	68 ± 8^{c}	76 ± 13	68 ± 11	107 ± 15	67 ± 11^{c}
G_{AUC} (mmol/L/120 min)	1092 ± 58	941 ± 46^{d}	862 ± 25	779 ± 51	1231 ± 57	1037 ± 45^{d}
I_{AUC} (pmol/L/120 min)	56,289 ± 6558	38,821 ± 4868^{c}	55,700 ± 9209	45,816 ± 8108^{a}	56,794 ± 9954	32,825 ± 5300^{a}
Glucose utilization (μmol/kg/min)	23.9 ± 3.3	28.9 ± 3.3^{a}	32.0 ± 4.6	37.5 ± 3.9^{a}	17.1 ± 2.9	21.4 ± 3.2
Glucose utilization (μmol/kg$_{FFM}$/min)	43.3 ± 5.9	49.9 ± 5.5	57.9 ± 7.2	64.8 ± 6.2	30.8 ± 5.9	37.1 ± 5.2
CRP (μg/mL)	7.24 ± 1.11	7.10 ± 1.18	4.87 ± 1.26	4.40 ± 1.25	9.08 ± 1.49	9.10 ± 1.60
TNFα (pg/mL)	2.13 ± 0.85	2.08 ± 0.51	2.93 ± 1.92	1.91 ± 0.98	1.51 ± 0.36	2.21 ± 0.54
TNFR1 (μg/mL)	772.9 ± 45.1	724.3 ± 42.5	808.9 ± 84.7	675.6 ± 73.5	744.9 ± 48.5	762.1 ± 49.7
IL-6 (pg/mL)	2.25 ± 0.31	2.09 ± 0.24	2.08 ± 0.30	2.01 ± 0.42	2.38 ± 0.52	2.15 ± 0.29
IL-6sR (pg/mL)	26,301 ± 2144	27,521 ± 2169	32,994 ± 3406	31,612 ± 4044	21,839 ± 1533	24,793 ± 2142
Adiponectin (ng/mL)	12.6 ± 2.4	12.8 ± 2.6	19.6 ± 3.8	20.1 ± 5.0	8.34 ± 2.2	8.42 ± 2.1
Leptin (pmol/L)	26.0 ± 2.3	19.9 ± 2.1^{b}	23.7 ± 4.0	20.3 ± 3.5	27.8 ± 2.6	19.7 ± 2.7^{d}
SAA (μg/mL)	55.4 ± 21.2	29.5 ± 4.6	43.1 ± 9.6	28.4 ± 7.9	64.7 ± 37.1	30.3 ± 5.9

Values are mean (SEM). Significantly different before and after the intervention: $^{a}P < .05$, $^{b}P < .01$, $^{c}P < 0.005$, and $^{d}P < 0.001$. VO_2max: maximum oxygen uptake; G_{AUC}: glucose area under the curve; I_{AUC}: insulin area under the curve.

(~70%) did not meet recommended weekly levels of physical activity, participation in physical activity lowered cardiometabolic risk in women with prior GDM. In young women with GDM, the skeletal muscle TNFα gene expression was not only 5–6 times higher than that in women with NGT during late pregnancy but also remained threefold higher than that in NGT women at one year postpartum follow-up visit [27]. Further, circulating TNFα did not change postpartum in the GDM women compared to a significant decline in the NGT women suggesting that inflammation persists after GDM.

The current study is unique in its examination of older women with a history of GDM. Although our study did not compare older women with and without a history of GDM, results from our previous study of postmenopausal women (n = 58) without a history of GDM [13], levels of CRP, TNFα, TNFR1, IL-6, and IL-6sR do not appear different from those of the women in the current study with a history of GDM. In the current study, where all women had a history of GDM, those who developed IGT or type 2 diabetes had higher CRP levels, but TNFα, TNFR1, IL-6, and SAA were not significantly different between groups. We have shown that the total body fat mass and subcutaneous abdominal fat are associated with insulin resistance in women with a history of GDM [4] and now add that increased CRP is related to reduced insulin sensitivity. We are also unaware of any studies that have examined adiponectin concentrations in older women with a history of GDM. Our results indicate that the IGT/T2DM group had lower adiponectin levels than the NGT women with a history of GDM. Further, higher adiponectin levels were associated with insulin sensitivity by the glucose clamp in this group of women with a history of GDM, which is similar to our previous study in women without a history of GDM [28]. Thus, inflammation as indicated by high CRP and low adiponectin may alter the risk for the development of type 2 diabetes after pregnancy complicated by GDM.

In overweight and obese postmenopausal women without a history of GDM, we have previously demonstrated a reduction in CRP [11, 13], IL-6 and sTNFR1 [13], and SAA [11, 12, 29] levels with either weight loss or aerobic training plus weight loss. We also previously reported a decrease in plasma leptin after weight loss alone and with aerobic exercise in women with a history of GDM [10], which is consistent with the reduction in plasma leptin in the current study. High plasma leptin predicted low insulin sensitivity in a young group of women with recent GDM, suggesting that leptin signaling may be more important than low-grade inflammation as a contributor to type 2 diabetes [30]. Yet, changes in cytokines were not significant during the same interventions in the current study. Although these studies were conducted with very similar designs and methods for the interventions and had similar reductions in body weight, sample sizes were two to three times larger in our earlier work so it is possible that we did not have a sufficient sample size to detect a change with the interventions. In addition, we were unable to distinguish differences in changes in cytokines between women who developed IGT and those who developed type 2 diabetes. It is possible that the magnitude of the effect would be vary between these groups.

The literature is lacking in terms of long-term follow-up of middle-aged and older women with prior history of GDM and the identification of mechanisms for the persistent insulin resistance. It is also possible that different inflammatory sources such as adipose tissue or endothelial cells could contribute to the inflammation observed after GDM. Future work could be directed to investigating these gaps while the results herein provide support for higher inflammation and insulin resistance in older women with a history of GDM.

6. Conclusions

Results of this study indicate that older women with a history of GDM who had developed IGT or T2DM have higher CRP and lower adiponectin levels than women who had NGT despite similar fitness and adiposity, which was related to insulin resistance and insulin sensitivity, respectively, by the glucose clamp. Yet, changes in inflammation were modest with a lifestyle intervention in this group of older women. Thus, in older women with a history of GDM, inflammation appears to play a role in the insulin resistance, although other factors may be more influential for the metabolic improvements observed with weight loss and exercise.

Conflicts of Interest

The author has no conflict of interest.

Acknowledgments

Appreciation is extended to those women who participated in this study and to the medical team and research laboratory assistants for technical assistance. This study was supported by funds from the Baltimore VA Medical Research Service, Senior Research Career Scientist Award, and NIH grants K01-AG00747, RO1-AG19310, P30-AG028747, and P30-DK072488 and the Baltimore Veterans Affairs Medical Center Geriatric Research Education, and Clinical Center (GRECC).

References

[1] L. Guariguata, U. Linnenkamp, J. Beagley, D. R. Whiting, and N. H. Cho, "Global estimates of the prevalence of hyperglycaemia in pregnancy," *Diabetes Research and Clinical Practice*, vol. 103, no. 2, pp. 176–185, 2014.

[2] N. W. Cheung and K. Byth, "Population health significance of gestational diabetes," *Diabetes Care*, vol. 26, no. 7, pp. 2005–2009, 2003.

[3] L. Bellamy, J. P. Casas, A. D. Hingorani, and D. Williams, "Type 2 diabetes mellitus after gestational diabetes: a systematic review and meta-analysis," *The Lancet*, vol. 373, no. 9677, pp. 1773–1779, 2009.

[4] A. S. Ryan, J. C. McLenithan, and G. M. Zietowski, "Accelerated metabolic susceptibility to type 2 diabetes in older women with a history of gestational diabetes," *Endocrine Connections*, vol. 2, no. 2, pp. 79–86, 2013.

[5] T. Lekva, E. R. Norwitz, P. Aukrust, and T. Ueland, "Impact of systemic inflammation on the progression of gestational diabetes mellitus," *Current Diabetes Reports*, vol. 16, no. 4, p. 26, 2016.

[6] J. Xu, Y. H. Zhao, Y. P. Chen et al., "Maternal circulating concentrations of tumor necrosis factor-alpha, leptin, and adiponectin in gestational diabetes mellitus: a systematic review and meta-analysis," *The Scientific World Journal*, vol. 2014, Article ID 926932, 12 pages, 2014.

[7] C. Song, J. Li, J. Leng, R. C. Ma, and X. Yang, "Lifestyle intervention can reduce the risk of gestational diabetes: a meta-analysis of randomized controlled trials," *Obesity Reviews*, vol. 17, no. 10, pp. 960–969, 2016.

[8] W. Bao, D. K. Tobias, K. Bowers et al., "Physical activity and sedentary behaviors associated with risk of progression from gestational diabetes mellitus to type 2 diabetes mellitus: a prospective cohort study," *JAMA Internal Medicine*, vol. 174, no. 7, pp. 1047–1055, 2014.

[9] S. F. Ehrlich, M. M. Hedderson, C. P. Quesenberry Jr. et al., "Post-partum weight loss and glucose metabolism in women with gestational diabetes: the DEBI study," *Diabetic Medicine*, vol. 31, no. 7, pp. 862–867, 2014.

[10] A. S. Ryan, "Improvements in insulin sensitivity after aerobic exercise and weight loss in older women with a history of gestational diabetes and type 2 diabetes mellitus," *Endocrine Research*, vol. 41, no. 2, pp. 132–141, 2016.

[11] A. S. Ryan, S. Ge, J. B. Blumenthal, M. C. Serra, S. J. Prior, and A. P. Goldberg, "Aerobic exercise and weight loss reduce vascular markers of inflammation and improve insulin sensitivity in obese women," *Journal of the American Geriatrics Society*, vol. 62, no. 4, pp. 607–614, 2014.

[12] R. Z. Yang, J. B. Blumenthal, N. M. Glynn et al., "Decrease of circulating SAA is correlated with reduction of abdominal SAA secretion during weight loss," *Obesity*, vol. 22, no. 4, pp. 1085–1090, 2014.

[13] A. S. Ryan and B. J. Nicklas, "Reductions in plasma cytokine levels with weight loss improve insulin sensitivity in overweight and obese postmenopausal women," *Diabetes Care*, vol. 27, no. 7, pp. 1699–1705, 2004.

[14] E. Heggen, T. O. Klemsdal, F. Haugen, I. Holme, and S. Tonstad, "Effect of a low-fat versus a low-gycemic-load diet on inflammatory biomarker and adipokine concentrations," *Metabolic Syndrome and Related Disorders*, vol. 10, no. 6, pp. 437–442, 2012.

[15] American Heart Association, *Heart and Stroke Facts*, AHA, Dallas, TX, 1997.

[16] A. S. Ryan and B. J. Nicklas, "Age-related changes in fat deposition in mid-thigh muscle in women: relationships with metabolic cardiovascular disease risk factors," *International Journal of Obesity*, vol. 23, no. 2, pp. 126–132, 1999.

[17] American Diabetes Association, "Diagnosis and classification of diabetes mellitus," *Diabetes Care*, vol. 32, Supplement_1, pp. S62–S67, 2009.

[18] J. A. Harris, "A biometric study of basal metabolism in man," Carnegie Institute of Washington, Washington, 1919.

[19] R. A. DeFronzo, J. D. Tobin, and R. Andres, "Glucose clamp technique: a method for quantifying insulin secretion and resistance," *American Journal of Physiology-Endocrinology and Metabolism*, vol. 237, no. 3, pp. E214–E223, 1979.

[20] E. A. McGuire, J. H. Helderman, J. D. Tobin, R. Andres, and M. Berman, "Effects of arterial versus venous sampling on analysis of glucose kinetics in man," *Journal of Applied Physiology*, vol. 41, no. 4, pp. 565–573, 1976.

[21] A. Syngelaki, G. H. A. Visser, K. Krithinakis, A. Wright, and K. H. Nicolaides, "First trimester screening for gestational diabetes mellitus by maternal factors and markers of inflammation," *Metabolism*, vol. 65, no. 3, pp. 131–137, 2016.

[22] C. Zhu, H. Yang, Q. Geng et al., "Association of oxidative stress biomarkers with gestational diabetes mellitus in pregnant women: a case-control study," *PLoS One*, vol. 10, no. 4, article e0126490, 2015.

[23] A. Khosrowbeygi, N. Shiamizadeh, and N. Taghizadeh, "Maternal circulating levels of some metabolic syndrome biomarkers in gestational diabetes mellitus," *Endocrine*, vol. 51, no. 2, pp. 245–255, 2016.

[24] F. Haidari, M. T. Jalali, N. Shahbazian, M. H. Haghighizadeh, and E. Azadegan, "Comparison of serum levels of vitamin D and inflammatory markers between women with gestational diabetes mellitus and healthy pregnant control," *Journal of Family & Reproductive Health*, vol. 10, no. 1, pp. 1–8, 2016.

[25] P. Molęda, A. Fronczyk, K. Safranow, and L. Majkowska, "Adipokines and β-cell dysfunction in normoglycemic women with previous gestational diabetes mellitus," *Polish Archives of Internal Medicine*, vol. 125, no. 9, pp. 641–648, 2015.

[26] V. Gingras, J. Vigneault, S. J. Weisnagel, A. Tchernof, and J. Robitaille, "Accelerometry-measured physical activity and inflammation after gestational diabetes," *Medicine & Science in Sports & Exercise*, vol. 45, no. 7, pp. 1307–1312, 2013.

[27] J. E. Friedman, J. P. Kirwan, M. Jing, L. Presley, and P. M. Catalano, "Increased skeletal muscle tumor necrosis factor-α and impaired insulin signaling persist in obese women with gestational diabetes mellitus 1 year postpartum," *Diabetes*, vol. 57, no. 3, pp. 606–613, 2008.

[28] A. S. Ryan, D. M. Berman, B. J. Nicklas et al., "Plasma adiponectin and leptin levels, body composition, and glucose utilization in adult women with wide ranges of age and obesity," *Diabetes Care*, vol. 26, no. 8, pp. 2383–2388, 2003.

[29] R. Z. Yang, M. J. Lee, H. Hu et al., "Acute-phase serum amyloid A: an inflammatory adipokine and potential link between obesity and its metabolic complications," *PLoS Medicine*, vol. 3, no. 6, article e287, 2006.

[30] M. Rottenkolber, U. Ferrari, L. Holland et al., "The diabetes risk phenotype of young women with recent gestational diabetes," *The Journal of Clinical Endocrinology & Metabolism*, vol. 100, no. 6, pp. E910–E918, 2015.

16

Selective Screening Strategies for Gestational Diabetes

Sumaiya Adam[1] and Paul Rheeder[2]

[1]*Department of Obstetrics and Gynecology, University of Pretoria, Pretoria, South Africa*
[2]*Department of Internal Medicine, University of Pretoria, Pretoria, South Africa*

Correspondence should be addressed to Sumaiya Adam; sumaiya.adam@up.ac.za

Academic Editor: Daniela Foti

Aim. We aimed to develop a prediction model for the diagnosis of gestational diabetes and to evaluate the performance of published prediction tools on our population. *Methods.* We conducted a cohort study on nondiabetic women < 26 weeks gestation at a level 1 clinic in Johannesburg, South Africa. At recruitment, participants completed a questionnaire and random basal glucose and HbA1c were evaluated. A 75 g 2-hour OGTT was scheduled between 24–28 weeks gestation, as per FIGO guidelines. A score was derived using multivariate logistic regression. Published scoring systems were tested by deriving ROC curves. *Results.* In 554 women, RBG, BMI, and previous baby ≥ 4000 g were significant risk factors included for GDM, which were used to derive a nomogram-based score. The logistic regression model for prediction of GDM had R^2 0.143, Somer's Dxy rank correlation 0.407, and Harrell's c-score 0.703. HbA1c did not improve predictive value of the nomogram at any threshold (e.g,. at probability > 10%, 25.6% of cases were detected without the HbA1c, and 25.8% of cases would have been detected with the HbA1c). The 9 published scoring systems performed poorly. *Conclusion.* We propose a nomogram-based score that can be used at first antenatal visit to identify women at high risk of GDM.

1. Introduction

Gestational diabetes mellitus (GDM) is regarded as glucose intolerance with first onset in pregnancy. The diagnosis of GDM infers an increased risk of both short- and long-term adverse outcomes for the mother and fetus [1]. The current guidelines of the International Federation of Gynecology and Obstetrics (FIGO) recommend universal screening of pregnant women for GDM with a 75 g 2-hour oral glucose tolerance test (OGTT) [2]. The lower thresholds recommended by FIGO are derived from the findings of the Hyperglycemia and Adverse Pregnancy Outcomes (HAPO) study. The HAPO study found that the adverse events associated with GDM increase along a continuum with increasing hyperglycemia [3]. The estimated prevalence of GDM based on the FIGO guidelines varies between 11.1–44.3% [4, 5].

Universal screening for GDM has the advantage that all pregnant women are screened as part of routine antenatal care. However, this will place an added burden, both financial and personnel, on the health care system. Selective screening based on risk factors such as advanced maternal age, obesity, family history of diabetes, and previous adverse pregnancy outcomes such as recurrent or unexplained pregnancy losses, large-for-gestational-age babies, or congenital abnormalities has been proposed as a screening strategy for GDM. Selective screening based on risk factors performs poorly as a screening tool with up to one-sixth of women with GDM diabetes being missed [6]. Furthermore, recall of historical risk factors is poor, medical records are often incomplete or unavailable, or the recorded history is not often considered by the clinical staff to trigger screening for GDM. Thus, the current risk factor-based screening is ineffective.

Whilst the traditional risk factor-based screening program performs poorly for the screening of GDM, there are several published risk-scoring systems that hold promise. These models combine maternal characteristics and medical history into a simple clinical prediction tool. This may assist in identifying women who require an OGTT with greater efficacy, accuracy, and efficiency [7–15]. However, these models were developed on non-African populations in tertiary centres using data obtained from a selective screening approach in most instances [7–15].

The purpose of this study was to develop a clinical prediction model for GDM in a South African population and to evaluate the performance of the published prediction tools on our study population. The introduction of such a prediction tool would reduce the number of OGTTs, hence decreasing the workload and financial burden on an overburdened healthcare system.

2. Materials and Methods

This paper forms part of a larger study investigating screening strategies for GDM in a South African population. We carried out a prospective cohort observational study at a level 1 primary healthcare clinic in Johannesburg. One thousand consecutive pregnant women that were less than 26 weeks pregnant were recruited. Patients known with diabetes mellitus or greater than 26 weeks pregnant were excluded [16].

At recruitment, each patient completed a questionnaire including demographic data and an evaluation of risk factors for GDM. Risk factors considered were obesity, that is, a body mass index (BMI) ≥ 30 kg/m^2, age ≥ 35 years, a family history of diabetes mellitus, a history of a delivery of a baby ≥ 4000 g in a prior pregnancy, glycosuria, a history of GDM in a prior pregnancy or a history of a baby with a congenital abnormality, and an unexplained stillbirth or recurrent pregnancy losses. Gestational age was based on the patient's last normal menstrual period, ultrasound-determined gestation, or by measuring of the symphysis to fundal height.

A random blood glucose (RBG) and glycated hemoglobin (HbA1c) levels were measured at recruitment on a Roche Accu-check Active point-of-care device and at the laboratory. The glucometer was regularly calibrated as per manufacturer guidelines, and glucose was measured on whole capillary blood. Measurements on the glucometer were not affected by haematocrit. If the random glucose was greater than 11.1 mmol/l or HbA1c was greater than 6.5%, the patient was referred to the local hospital for further management of overt diabetes mellitus. Else, a 75 g two hour oral glucose tolerance test (OGTT) was scheduled for between 24 and 28 weeks gestation. GDM was diagnosed based on the FIGO criteria [2]. All blood was drawn by a registered nurse and was stored on ice until it was delivered to the laboratory on the same day. Point-of-care tests were performed on-site.

We used R version 3.3.0 [17] with packages PredictABEL [18] and rms [19]. In order to compare the different prediction models, we imputed missing values using multivariate imputation by chained equations [20]. Because our dataset is large enough, we used all clinically relevant predictors in a logistic regression model [17]. Random serum glucose demonstrated a nonlinear relationship with the log odds of the outcome, and we used a restricted cubic spline with two knots in the model. The other continuous variables were not transformed in the model. In order to determine the degree of optimism with this model, we validated and calibrated the model with 200 bootstrap samples according to Harrell [19].

To reduce the number of variables for a more parsimonious model, we used the method of approximation as suggested by Harrell (to remove the variables that would have the smallest effect on the R^2 coefficient of determination of the linear regression model of variables on the linear predictor of the logistic regression model as the outcome) [19]. We tested the interaction of HIV with the other variables.

We then investigated the effect of having a model with and without HbA1c as some centres may and some may not have HbA1c testing readily available. These models were compared using Harrell's c-index, Somer's Dxy rank correlation, the Brier score, R^2, and the net reclassification index (NRI) (at probabilities of 10, 50 and 100%) as well as the integration discrimination improvement (IDI) [17]. Harrell's c-index (c-index > 0.5 shows good predictive ability) and Somer's Dxy (where Dxy = 1 when the model is perfectly discriminating) are measures of the general predictive power of a regression model. In effect, they are a natural extension of ROC curve areas. The Brier score (where the best possible score is 0 for total accuracy) measures the accuracy of probabilistic predictions, that is, it is the average gap between the calculated probability and the actual outcome. R^2 (where 1 fits the regression line perfectly) provides information on the goodness of fit of the model. The NRI is an index of how well a new model classifies subjects (in this case how well does our prediction model identify patients at high risk of GDM). The IDI similarly is a tool that evaluates the capacity of a marker or model to predict the outcome (i.e., how well can the prediction model identify patients with GDM).

Categorical NRI equal to x% means that compared with individuals without outcome, individuals with outcome were almost x% more likely to move up a category than down. The function also computes continuous NRI, which does not require any discrete risk categories and relies on the proportions of individuals with outcome correctly assigned a higher probability and individuals without outcome correctly assigned a lower probability by an updated model compared with the initial model. IDI equal to x% signifies that the difference in average predicted risks between the individuals with and without the outcome increased by x% in the updated model. Finally, for ease of use, nomograms were generated for the model with and without HbA1c [19].

Furthermore, nine published risk prediction models for GDM were identified [7–15]. The risk prediction model from each study was applied to our study population, and a receiver operating curve (ROC) was generated to evaluate its performance as a screening tool. We thereafter compared the two ROC curves derived from independent samples to assess if there was a significant difference in the area under the curve.

Approval for this study was obtained from the University of Pretoria, Faculty of Health Sciences Ethics Committee (Protocol 180/2012) and was performed in accordance with the 1964 Declaration of Helsinki and its amendments.

Informed consent was obtained from every patient prior to entry into the study.

3. Results

One thousand (1000) pregnant women were recruited. Eighty-two (8.2%) women had fetal losses and did not continue with the study, 163 (16.3%) women moved away from the area and were thus lost to follow-up, 194 (19.4%) women were unreachable, and seven (0.7%) women withdrew consent for the study. Thus, 554 (55.4%) women had complete data available for analysis. One hundred and forty-four (25.8%) women had GDM.

The mean age of the population was 27.2 years (IR 13–42 ± 5.8), parity 1.1 (IR 0–5 ± 1), BMI 26.7 kg/m^2 (IR 22.7–47.2 ± 5.4), random glucose 4.5 mmol/l (2.9–9.3 ± 0.7), and HbA1c 5.2% (33.3 mmol/mol) (IR 3.8–6.5% ± 0.4; 18–47.5 mmol/mol). One hundred and sixty (28.9%) women were HIV positive of which 59 (36.9%) were on highly active antiretroviral therapy (HAART), 78 (14.1%) women had a positive family history of diabetes mellitus, 55 (9.9%) had a history of a previous stillborn or congenitally abnormal baby, and 44 (7.8%) women had previously delivered a baby > 4000 g.

We considered the role of the random glucose (AUROC 0.63, 95% CI 0.58–0.68) as a screening tool. Furthermore, we included clinically relevant predictors, namely, delivery of a previous baby ≥ 4000 g, random glucose, BMI, family history of diabetes mellitus, HbA1c, history of a previous stillbirth, or previous baby with a congenital abnormality and age, in a logistic regression model [2]. The odds ratio of the full model is illustrated in Supplementary Figure 1 (S1 odds ratio of full model (continuous variables: 75th versus 25th percentile) available online at https://doi.org/10.1155/2017/2849346). The performance of this model including all clinical variables is illustrated in Table 1.

The model was then validated and calibrated with 200 bootstrap samples according to Harrell [19]. One can observe that at higher predicted probabilities the actual probabilities are less in the optimism-corrected model indicating a fair degree of optimism as demonstrated in Supplementary Figure 2 (S2 correcting the model for optimism). At higher predicted probabilities, the actual probabilities are less in the optimism-corrected model indicating a fair degree of optimism. The discriminatory indices for the validated model are illustrated in Table 1. The quantile absolute error was 0.029. The slope of the bias-corrected model was 0.870, it has a 0.130 difference when corrected for optimism.

In order to get a smaller model, we used an approximation method as suggested by Harrell [19] to remove variables that would have the smallest effect on R^2 of the linear regression model (Table 2). We removed family history of diabetes mellitus, history of a previous stillbirth or previous baby with a congenital abnormality, and age and still maintained 95.7% of R^2.

We analysed the interaction of HIV and HAART with the clinical variables. HIV nor the HAART had any interaction with a history of a delivery of a previous baby greater than 4000 g ($p = 0.066$), the random glucose ($p = 0.835$), or BMI ($p = 0.801$). Overall, HIV nor HAART had an effect on our proposed model ($p = 0.974$)

Table 1: Discrimination indices of the full predictive model including all clinical risk factors.

Discrimination index	Full model with all variables	Validated model
R^2	0.143	0.109
Harrell's c-index	0.703	
Somer's Dxy rank correlation	0.407	0.362
Brier score	0.173	0.178

Table 2: β-Coefficient of predictive variables in the model with and without HbA1c.

	Model without HbA1c[1]	Model with HBA1c[1]
Previous baby ≥ 4 kg	102	1.01
Rgluc[2] Rgluc[3]	1.99/ −2.1709	2.17/ −2.28
BMI[4]	0.05	0.05
HbA1c[1]	0.6464	
R^2 coefficient of determination	0.135	0.122
Somer's Dxy rank correlation	0.38	0.36
Harrell's c-index	0.69	0.68
Brier score	0.176	0.174
NRI[5]		
Categorical	0.0355 ($p = 0.06034$)	
Continuous	0.253 ($p = 0.01607$)	
IDI[6]	0.108 ($p = 0.002$)	

HbA1c[1]: glycated haemoglobin; Rgluc[2]: random glucose first spline; Rgluc[3]: random glucose second spline; BMI[4]: body mass index; NRI[5]: net reclassification index; IDI[6]: integrated discrimination improvement.

We thereafter used a smaller model to determine whether adding HbA1c would add any predictive value to the model as demonstrated in Supplementary Figure 3 (S3 comparison of predictive value of model with and without HbA1c). We found that adding an HbA1c did not significantly improve the predictive value of the model (Table 2). The slope of the bias-corrected model was 0.933, and it has a 0.0.067 difference when corrected for optimism.

By adding the HbA1c to the model 12%, 4%, and 9% of patients will be downclassified to being at low risk of GDM at 10, 50, and 100%, respectively. Similarly, 0%, 4%, and 0% will be upclassified to being at high risk of GDM at 10, 50, and 100%, respectively. The integrated discrimination improvement (IDI) shows that the discrimination slope of the updated model with the added HbA1c was 10.8% higher than the original model.

The le Cessie-van Houwelingen-Copas-Hosmer unweighted sum of squares test for global goodness of fit

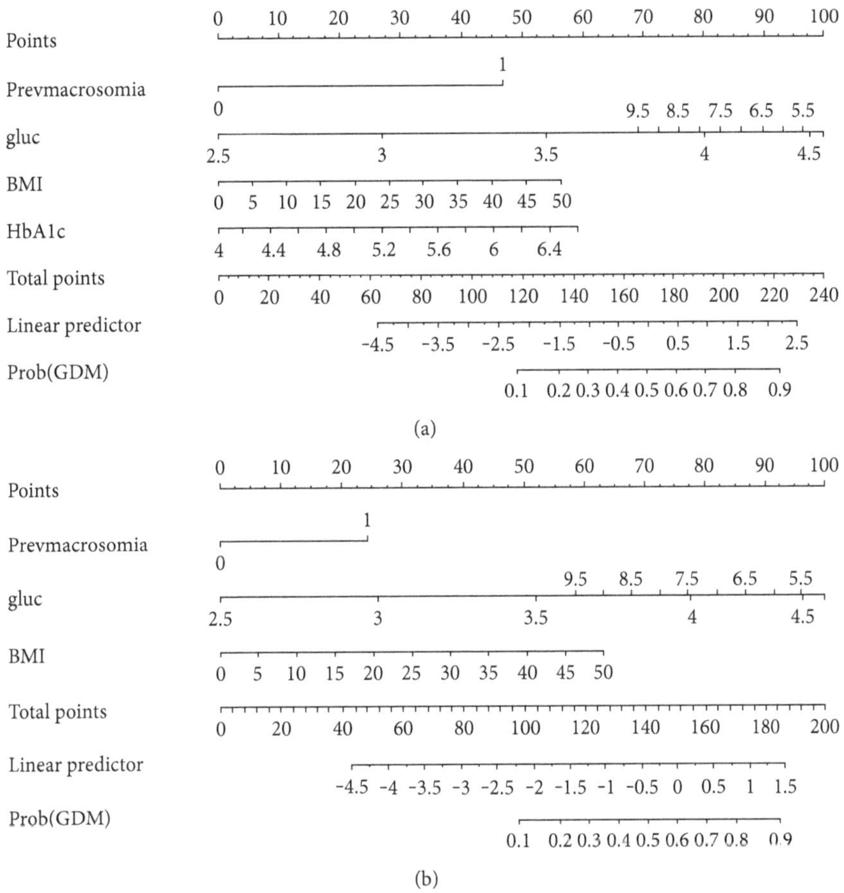

FIGURE 1: Nomograms (a) with HbA1c and (b) without HbA1c. The nomograms consider the history of delivery of a previous baby > 4000 g (prevmacrosomia: 0 = no, 1 = yes), random glucose (gluc: measurement in mmol/l), and BMI (BMI: mass in kilograms/height in metre^2). Two nomograms are illustrated to show the difference with and without and HbA1c measurement being included. The score is derived by aligning the points on each number line with the "points" line at the top. The total score is then calculated and plotted on the "total points" line. When this total score is compared to the prob(GDM) line, the probability of developing GDM is derived. For example, a 30-year-old woman who is now para 2 gravida 3, with a BMI of 35 kg/m2, who previously delivered a 4.3 kg baby, has an HbA1c of 5.8% and now has a random glucose of 6.7 mmol/l will have a score of 155 and thus a 50% chance of developing GDM in this pregnancy based on the nomogram without the HbA1c. Her score is 182 and thus a 52% risk of developing GDM if the HbA1c is incorporated into the prediction model. Prevmacrosomia: history of delivering a baby > 4000 g; gluc: random glucose; BMI: body mass index; HbA1c: glycated hemoglobin; Prob(GDM): probability of developing gestational diabetes.

TABLE 3: Comparison of the efficacy of nomograms at probabilities of 10 and 15%.

Nomogram	With HbA1c[1]				Without HbA1c[1]			
	High risk		Low risk		High risk		Low risk	
Probability of GDM[2]	GDM[2]	No GDM[2]	GDM[2]	No GDM[2]	GDM[2]	No GDM[2]	GDM[2]	No GDM[2]
>10%	142 (25.6%)	354 (63.9%)	2 (0.4%)	56 (10.1%)	143 (25.8%)	361 (62.5%)	1 (0.2%)	49 (8.8%)
>15%	135 (24.3%)	304 (54.9%)	9 (1.6%)	115 (20.8%)	135 (24.3%)	316 (57.0%)	9 (1.6%)	94 (17%)

HbA1c[1]: glycated haemoglobin; GDM[2]: gestational diabetes.

for the model with HbA1c gave a p value of 0.87 and for the model without HbA1c 0.81.

Finally, for ease of use, nomograms were generated for the model with and without the HbA1c (Figure 1).

We then compared the efficacy of the nomograms at >10% and >15% probabilities of GDM (Table 3) as we will need to establish the cutoff risk above which a woman is deemed at high risk of developing GDM. At a cutoff of 10%, 58 (10.5%) and 50 (9.0%) fewer OGTTs would be carried out if HbA1c was or was not incorporated into the nomogram, respectively. Two (0.4%) and one (0.2%) cases of GDM would be missed if the nomogram with and without the HbA1c was applied, respectively. Similarly, at a 15% cutoff, 125 (22.6%) and 103 (18.6%) fewer OGTTs would be carried out if HbA1c was or was not incorporated into the nomogram, respectively. Nine (1.6%) cases of GDM would be missed whether or not HbA1c was incorporated into the nomogram.

Table 4 demonstrates the performance of each published prediction model for GDM once it was applied to our study population as compared to the population that it was derived from.

4. Discussion

This study aimed to evaluate the use of risk indicators to develop a statistical prediction model for GDM. Traditionally identified risk factors such as BMI, age, or family history of diabetes mellitus have been associated with GDM in other populations [21–24]. Data on GDM in Africa, especially since the introduction of the FIGO criteria, is scant. Available data found an association with GDM and obesity, family history of diabetes mellitus, previous stillbirth, previous macrosomic child, and age > 30 years in some sub-Saharan African populations [23].

The fasting glucose appears to be a very attractive tool for screening pregnant women for GDM. However, this would necessitate that all pregnant women present in a fasted state for screening, thus this can only take place on the second antenatal visit and would require all pregnant women to be tested. While this may not seem unrealistic, it can prove to be challenging in a low-income country where women have to travel a great distance to the healthcare facility and they often do not have funds for transport. Thus, we investigated an alternate screening tool that could be used easily on the first antenatal visit to stratify a women's risk for GDM in the current pregnancy.

We found that a previous history of delivering a baby weighing ≥4000 g and an elevated random blood glucose were independent predictors of developing GDM. Church et al. and Meek et al. found that the random glucose was a promising screening tool for GDM with AUROC of 0.8 and 0.86, respectively [25, 26]. By comparison, these retrospective studies employed a 2-stage screening protocol for GDM and did not use the currently widely accepted FIGO diagnostic criteria. By comparison, the basal random glucose alone was a poor predictor of women likely to develop GDM in our study. Thus, we propose that our scoring system, by adding other variables to the random blood glucose, will better identify women at risk at GDM compared to the random blood glucose alone. This premise requires prospective validation.

Other studies have also identified risk factors [19–24]. Only nine of these studies summarised this into a score or a clinical prediction model, of which we were able to test eight on our study population (Table 4). These tests performed poorly as a screening tool in our study population compared with their derivation populations. This may be a result of us testing these scores on a low-risk pregnant population. Risk factors may play a less significant role in predicting GDM when universal screening is applied, and the FIGO diagnostic criteria are used. By contrast, most of the aforementioned scoring systems used a selective screening approach and used criteria other than that recommended by FIGO for the diagnosis of GDM in the derivation and the validation of their scores [7–14]. Furthermore, many of these scores use logarithmic equations in their calculations, thus necessitating a computer in the clinic, which is not always available in South African antenatal clinics [9, 13–15].

As South Africa is a resource-restricted country that faces a dual burden of disease, that is, communicable and noncommunicable diseases, a selective screening approach is an attractive option for the diagnosis of GDM as it seems the more cost-effective approach. As a risk-factor-based approach performs inconsistently, a scoring system that incorporates the more significant risk factors in a population may be a better option. We have proposed a nomogram that incorporates the significant factors in a South African population. The BMI and history of previous deliveries are currently part of routine antenatal practice. The random blood glucose can easily be tested at the first antenatal visit, making this a clinically applicable tool for early pregnancy. In some settings, an HbA1c may be available. However, we have demonstrated that including the HbA1c into the risk stratification tool does not significantly affect the patient's risk of GDM. South Africa has a high burden of HIV. In our study, HIV did not affect the incidence nor did it contribute as a predictive marker of GDM.

The risk stratification system proposed by Harrison et al. performed well in our study population [12]. This score is based on the patient's age in years, BMI, race, family history of diabetes mellitus, a history of GDM in a prior pregnancy, and fasting plasma glucose. The advantage of this system is that it is a scoring system rather than a logarithmic equation, and it incorporates information that is routinely obtained on the first antenatal visit. However, it will require the patient to present to the clinic in a fasted state for a second visit before the risk stratification can be completed. This may be problematic in our setting of a low-middle income population that may not live close to the clinic. In addition, this selective screening approach may not be complied with if it requires the healthcare worker to recalculate the risk on multiple visits. Our proposed nomogram incorporates only two historical factors and a random glucose, thus making it quick and easy to use at the first antenatal visit.

There is an increasing health burden related to obesity and type 2 diabetes mellitus in sub-Saharan Africa, yet little is known about the prevalence of GDM [27]. In South Africa and many other countries worldwide, screening programs are based on risk factors. However, it has been demonstrated that this approach shows a low compliance to guidelines. Hence, many women are not screened and GDM remains underdiagnosed [28]. The FIGO criteria have been criticised for its low diagnostic thresholds. Several studies have shown that women diagnosed with GDM based on the IADPSG criteria had higher adverse outcomes such as fetal macrosomia, risk of primary caesarean delivery, and preeclampsia compared with women with no GDM [29, 30].

Screening for GDM is necessary as it has both short- and long-term implications for the mother and child. The FIGO diagnostic criteria have been adopted almost universally [2]. We have proposed a simple nomogram that can be used for predicting the probability of developing GDM at the first antenatal visit. A limitation of this study is that the prediction model needs to be tested prospectively in the screening and

Table 4: Comparison of the performance of scoring systems for the screening of GDM in our population.

Study	Risk factors	Risk calculation	AUROC[a] (study population)	AUROC[a] (original)	P[20]
Caliskan et al. [7]	(i) Age (years) (ii) Body mass index (BMI) (iii) Family history of diabetes mellitus (DM) (iv) Previous baby > 4000 g (v) Previous adverse pregnancy outcome	(i) <25 = 0; >25 = 1 (ii) <25 = 0; >25 = 1 (iii) No = 0; yes = 1 (iv) No = 0; yes = 1 (v) No = 0; yes = 1	0.5936 (0.5370–0.6504)	0.832 (0.793–0.867)	0.0005
Naylor et al. [8]	(i) Age (years) (ii) Body mass index (BMI) (iii) Race	(i) <30 = 0; 31–34 = 1; >35 = 2 (ii) <22 = 0; 22.1–25 = 2; >25.1 = 3 (iii) White/Black = 0; East Asian = 5; South Asian = 2	0.5897 (0.53214–0.64730)	0.733 (0.711–0.755)	0.0007
Van Leeuwen et al. [9]	(i) Body mass index (BMI) (ii) Race (iii) Family history of diabetes mellitus (FamHx) (iv) Gestational diabetes in previous pregnancy (GDMHx)	$= 1/[1 + \exp(-\beta)]$ $\beta = [-6.1 + (0.83 \times \text{non-Caucasian}) + (0.57 \times \text{FamHx}) - (0.67 \times \text{multipara no GDMhx}) + (0.5 \times \text{multipara GDMhx}) + (0.13 \times \text{BMI})]$ (Non-Caucasian: no = 0; yes = 1 Famhx: no = 0; yes = 1 Nullipara = 0; multiparaNoGDMhx = 1; multiparaGDMhx = 2)	0.5675 (0.51–0.63)	0.770 (0.690–0.850)	0.0015
Phaloprakarn et al. [10]	(i) Age (years) (ii) Body mass index (BMI) (iii) Family history of diabetes mellitus (FH) (iv) Previous baby > 4000 g (v) Previous adverse pregnancy outcome	6 age + 11 BMI + 109FH + 42 baby > 4000 g + 49 adverse pregnancy outcome ≥380 is positive screen	0.5182 (0.48664–0.54972)	0.769 (0.746–0.792)	<0.001
Teede et al. [11]	(i) Age (years) (ii) Body mass index (BMI) (iii) Race (iv) Family history of diabetes mellitus (v) Gestational diabetes in previous pregnancy	(i) <25 = 0; 25–34 = 1; >35 = 2 (ii) <20 = 0; 20–34.9 = 1; >35 = 2 (iii) White = 0; East Asian/South Asian/ African = 1 (iv) No = 0; yes = 1 (v) No = 0; yes = 2	0.5863 (0.52934–0.64334)	0.703 (0.679–0.727)	0.0003
Harrison et al. [12]	(i) Age (years) (ii) Body mass index (BMI) (iii) Race (iv) Family history of diabetes mellitus (v) Gestational diabetes in previous pregnancies (vi) Fasting plasma glucose (FPG)	(i) <25 = 0; 25–34 = 1; >35 = 2 (ii) <20 = 0; 20–34.9 = 1; >35 = 2 (iii) White = 0; East Asian/South Asian/ African = 1 (iv) No = 0; yes = 1 (v) No = 0; yes = 2 (vi) If score ≥ 3 assesses FPG			
Model 1		FPG 4.61–4.89 mmol/l	0.4751 (0.451–0.4995)	0.753 (0.675–0.832)	<0.001
Model 2		FPG ≥ 4.9 mmol/l	0.8662 (0.8336–0.89869)	0.83 (0.77–0.90)	0.1846

Table 4: Continued.

Study	Risk factors	Risk calculation	AUROC[a] (study population)	AUROC[a] (original)	P[20]
Syngekali et al. [13]	(i) Gestational diabetes in previous pregnancy (ii) Family history of DM (iii) Age (years) (iv) Weight (kg) (v) Height (cm) (vi) Race (vii) Method of conception (viii) Birth weight of previous pregnancy	No formula available in article	Could not be calculated as inadequate information on last pregnancy birth weight available	0.823 (0.820–0.826)	
Nanda et al. [14]	(i) Age (years) (ii) Body mass index (BMI) (iii) Race (iv) Gestational diabetes in previous pregnancy (v) Previous baby's birth weight > 90th centile (prevBW)	$=1/[1+\exp(-\beta)]$ $\beta=\{-8.68947+(0.05365\times \text{age})+(0.10852\times \text{BMI})+(1.00312\times \text{South Asian})+(0.88785\times \text{East Asian})+(3.72259\times \text{previous GDM})+(0.67673\times \text{prevBW}>90\text{th centile})\}$	0.6218 (0.56301–0.68058)	0.788 (0.759–0.817)	<0.001
Capula et al. [15]	(i) Age (years) (ii) Pregravid body mass index (BMI) (iii) Previous gestational diabetes (GDM), polycystic ovarian syndrome (PCOS) (iv) Fasting plasma glucose (FPG) 5.6–6.9 mmol/l before pregnancy	$= \text{Constant} - 2.2532\times(\text{age}/10)+0.4128\times(\text{age}/10)^2+0.0795\times \text{pregravid BMI}$ Constant is intercept depending on previous GDM, PCOS, FPG 5.6–6.9 mmol/l before pregnancy	0.5337 (0.48 0.59)	(Information not available)	

[a]AUROC: area under receiver operating curve.

diagnosis of GDM so that it can be validated, and a threshold of clinical usefulness can be determined before it can be widely implemented.

Disclosure

The funders played no part in conducting the research or in the compilation of this manuscript.

Conflicts of Interest

The authors declare that there is no conflict of interest regarding the publication of this article.

Acknowledgments

The authors would like to acknowledge all research assistants who assisted in this study. This study was partly supported by funding from the Society for Endocrinology, Metabolism and Diabetes of South Africa (SEMDSA), the South African Sugar Association (SASA), and Roche. The SASA and SEMDSA grants were awarded following peer review for scientific quality and priority assessment.

References

[1] L. Hiersch and Y. Yogev, "Impact on gestational hyperglycaemia on maternal and child health," *Current Opinion in Clinical Nutrition and Metabolic Care*, vol. 17, pp. 255–260, 2014.

[2] M. Hod, A. Kapur, D. A. Sacks et al., "The International Federation of Gynecology and Obstetrics (FIGO) initiative on gestational diabetes mellitus: a pragmatic guide for diagnosis, management, and care," *International Journal of Gynecology & Obstetrics*, vol. 131, no. S3, pp. S173–S211, 2015.

[3] The HAPO Study Cooperative Research Group, "Hyperglycemia and adverse pregnancy outcomes," *The New England Journal of Medicine*, vol. 358, pp. 1991–2002, 2008.

[4] D. Karcaaltincaba, P. Calis, N. Ocal, A. Ozek, M. Altug Inan, and M. Bayram, "Prevalence of gestational diabetes mellitus evaluated by universal screening with a 75-g, 2-hour oral glucose tolerance test and IADPSG criteria," *International Journal of Gynecology & Obstetrics*, vol. 138, pp. 148–151, 2017.

[5] M. I. March, A. M. Modest, S. J. Ralston, M. R. Hacker, M. Gupta, and F. M. Brown, "The effect of adopting the IADPSG screening guidelines on the risk profile and outcomes of the gestational diabetes population," *The Journal of Maternal-Fetal & Neonatal Medicine*, vol. 29, no. 7, pp. 1141–1145, 2016.

[6] G. Miailhea, G. Kayema, G. Girarda, H. Legardeura, and L. Mandelbrot, "Selective rather than universal screening for gestational diabetes mellitus?," *European Journal of Obstetrics & Gynecology and Reproductive Biology*, vol. 191, pp. 95–100, 2015.

[7] E. Caliskan, F. Kayikcioglu, N. Ozturk, S. Koc, and A. Haberal, "A population-based risk factor scoring will decrease unnecessary testing for the diagnosis of gestational diabetes mellitus," *Acta Obstetricia et Gynecologica Scandinavica*, vol. 83, pp. 524–530, 2004.

[8] C. D. Naylor, M. Sermer, E. Chen, and D. Farine, "Selective screening for gestational diabetes mellitus," *The New England Journal of Medicine*, vol. 337, no. 2, pp. 1591–1596, 1997.

[9] M. Van Leeuwen, B. C. Opmeer, E. J. K. Zweers et al., "Estimating the risk of gestational diabetes mellitus: a clinical prediction model based on patient characteristics and medical history," *BJOG*, vol. 117, pp. 69–75, 2010.

[10] C. Phaloprakarn, S. Tangjitgamol, and S. Manusirivithaya, "A risk score for selective screening for gestational diabetes mellitus," *European Journal of Obstetrics & Gynecology and Reproductive Biology*, vol. 145, pp. 71–75, 2009.

[11] J. H. Teede, C. L. Harrison, W. T. The, E. Paul, and C. A. Allan, "Gestational diabetes: development of an early risk prediction tool to facilitate opportunities for prevention," *Australian and New Zealand Journal of Obstetrics and Gynaecology*, vol. 51, pp. 499–504, 2011.

[12] C. L. Harrison, C. B. Lombard, C. East, J. Boyle, and H. J. Teede, "Risk stratification in early pregnancy for women at increased risk of gestational diabetes," *Diabetes Research and Clinical Practice*, vol. 107, pp. 61–68, 2015.

[13] A. Syngekali, A. Pastides, R. Kotecha, A. Wright, R. Akolekar, and K. H. Nicolaides, "First-trimester screening for gestational diabetes mellitus based on maternal characteristics and history," *Fetal Diagnosis and Therapy*, vol. 35, pp. 14–21, 2015.

[14] S. Nanda, M. Savvidou, A. Syngekali, R. Akolekar, and K. H. Nicolaides, "Prediction of gestational diabetes mellitus by maternal factors and biomarkers at 11 to 13 weeks," *Prenatal Diagnosis*, vol. 31, pp. 135–141, 2011.

[15] C. Capula, E. Chiefari, M. Borelli et al., "A new predictive tool for the early risk assessment of gestational diabetes mellitus," *Primary Care Diabetes*, vol. 10, pp. 31–323, 2016.

[16] S. Adam and P. Rheeder, "Screening for gestational diabetes mellitus in a South African population: prevalence, comparison of diagnostic criteria and the role of risk factors," *South African Medical Journal*, vol. 107, no. 6, pp. 523–527, 2017.

[17] R. Core Team, *R: A Language and Environment for Statistical Computing*, R Foundation for Statistical Computing, Vienna, Austria, 2016, https://www.R-project.org/.

[18] S. Kundu, Y. S. Aulchenko, and A. C. J. W. Janssens, "PredictABEL: assessment of risk prediction models. R package version 1.2-2," 2014, https://CRAN.R-project.org/package=PredictABEL.

[19] F. E. Harrell Jr, "rms: regression modeling strategies. R package version 5.0-0," 2016, https://CRAN.R-project.org/package=rms.

[20] S. van Buuren and K. Groothuis-Oudshoorn, "mice: multivariate imputation by chained equations in R," *Journal of Statistical Software*, vol. 45, no. 3, pp. 1–67, 2011, http://www.jstatsoft.org/v45/i03/.

[21] B. N. Olagbuji, A. S. Atiba, B. A. Olofinbiyi et al., "Prevalence of and risk factors for gestational diabetes using 1999, 2013 WHO and IADPSG criteria upon implementation of a universal one-step screening and diagnostic strategy in a sub-Saharan African population," *European Journal of Obstetrics and Gynecology and Reproductive Biology*, vol. 189, pp. 27–32, 2015.

[22] W. T. The, H. J. Teede, E. Paul, C. L. Harrison, E. M. Wallace, and C. Allan, "Risk factors for gestational diabetes mellitus: implications for the application of screening guidelines," *Australian and New Zealand Journal of Obstetrics and Gynaecology*, vol. 51, pp. 26–30, 2011.

[23] A. W. Mwanri, J. Kinabo, K. Ramaiya, and E. J. M. Feskens, "Gestational diabetes mellitus in sub-Saharan Africa: systemic review and metaregression on prevalence and risk factors,"

Tropical Medicine and International Health, vol. 20, no. 8, pp. 983–1002, 2015.

[24] A. W. Mwanri, J. Kinabo, K. Ramaiya, and E. J. M. Feskens, "Prevalence of gestational diabetes mellitus in urban and rural Tanzania," *Diabetes Research and Clinical Practice*, vol. 103, pp. 71–78, 2014.

[25] C. L. Meek, H. R. Murphy, and D. Simmons, "Random plasma glucose in early pregnancy is a better predictor of gestational diabetes diagnosis than maternal obesity," *Diabetologia*, vol. 59, pp. 445–452, 2016.

[26] D. Church, D. Halsall, C. Meek, R. A. Parker, H. R. Murphy, and D. Simmons, "Random blood glucose measurement at antenatal booking to screen for overt diabetes in pregnancy: a retrospective study," *Diabetes Care*, vol. 34, no. 10, pp. 2217–2219, 2011.

[27] S. Macaulay, D. B. Dunger, and S. A. Norris, "Gestational diabetes mellitus in Africa: a systematic review," *PLoS One*, vol. 9, no. 6, article e97871, 2014.

[28] M. Persson, A. Winkvist, and I. Mogren, "Surprisingly low compliance to local guidelines for risk factor based screening for gestational diabetes mellitus - a population-based study," *BMC Pregnancy and Childbirth*, vol. 9, p. 53, 2009.

[29] C. L. Meek, H. B. Lewis, C. Patient, H. R. Murphy, and D. Simmons, "Diagnosis of gestational diabetes mellitus: falling through the net," *Diabetologia*, vol. 58, pp. 2003–2012, 2015.

[30] T. P. Waters, A. R. Dyer, D. M. Scholtens et al., "Maternal and neonatal morbidity for women who would be added to the diagnosis of GDM using IADPSG criteria: a secondary analysis of the hyperglycaemia and adverse pregnancy outcome study," *Diabetes Care*, vol. 39, no. 12, pp. 2204–2210, 2016.

17

Prevalence of Gestational Diabetes Mellitus in Eastern and Southeastern Asia

Cong Luat Nguyen,[1,2] **Ngoc Minh Pham**,[1,3] **Colin W. Binns**,[1] **Dat Van Duong**,[4] **and Andy H. Lee**[1]

[1]*School of Public Health, Curtin University, Perth, WA, Australia*
[2]*National Institute of Hygiene and Epidemiology, Hanoi, Vietnam*
[3]*Thai Nguyen University of Medicine and Pharmacy, Thai Nguyen, Vietnam*
[4]*United Nations Population Fund, Hanoi, Vietnam*

Correspondence should be addressed to Ngoc Minh Pham; minh.pn@tnu.edu.vn

Academic Editor: Daniela Foti

Aim. To review the prevalence of gestational diabetes mellitus (GDM) in Eastern and Southeastern Asia. *Methods.* We systematically searched for observational studies on GDM prevalence from January 2000 to December 2016. Inclusion criteria were original English papers, with full texts published in peer-reviewed journals. The quality of included studies was evaluated using the guidelines of the National Health and Medical Research Council, Australia. Fixed effects and random effects models were used to estimate the summary prevalence of GDM and the corresponding 95% confidence intervals (CI). *Results.* A total of 4415 papers were screened, and 48 studies with 63 GDM prevalence observations were included in the final review. The pooled prevalence of GDM was 10.1% (95% CI: 6.5%–15.7%), despite substantial variations across nations. The prevalence of GDM in lower- or upper-middle income countries was about 64% higher than in their high-income counterparts. Moreover, the one-step screening method was twice more likely to be used in diagnosing GDM when compared to the two-step screening procedure. *Conclusions.* The prevalence of GDM in Eastern and Southeastern Asia was high and varied among and within countries. There is a need for international uniformity in screening strategies and diagnostic criteria for GDM.

1. Introduction

Gestational diabetes mellitus (GDM), which is defined as diabetes diagnosed in the second and third trimesters of pregnancy [1], has emerged as a global public health concern [2]. It has been associated with short-term and long-term adverse health outcomes for both mothers and their newborns [3]. Women with GDM are known to have decreased quality of life and increased risks of caesarean section, gestational hypertension, preeclampsia, and type 2 diabetes [4–7]. In babies, GDM has been found to be associated with macrosomia or larger than normal gestational-aged infants, neonatal hypoglycemia, and type 2 diabetes mellitus later in life [6, 8, 9]. As such, it is important to understand the burden of GDM in various parts of the world to provide country-specific information to help inform on policy and planning.

The global prevalence of GDM varies widely, from 1% to 28%, depending on population characteristics (e.g., maternal age, socioeconomic status, race/ethnicity, or body composition), screening methods, and diagnostic criteria [10]. In addition, as with the common form of type 2 diabetes [11], GDM can also be influenced by genetic factors, which may differently affect disease prevalence among populations [12]. To date, at least 8 associations have developed their own diagnostic criteria for GDM, namely, the American Diabetes Association (ADA 2004, 2007, 2010, and 2012), Australian Diabetes in Pregnancy Society (ADIPS), Carpenter-Coustan (CC), International Association of the

Diabetes and Pregnancy Study Groups (IADPSG), International Classification of Diseases (ICD), Japan Society of Obstetrics and Gynecology (JSOG), National Diabetes Data Group (NDDG), and World Health Organization (WHO 1998, 1999, 2006, and 2013) [13, 14]. Data in high-income countries (HICs) ranges from 0.6% to 27.5% [15], and those in low- and middle-income countries are in the range of 0.4 and 24.3% [16]. Regional differences exist regarding the distribution of GDM, such as Africa and Asia, after adjusting the data with prevalence reports being 0%–13.9% and 1.6%–17.8%, respectively [17, 18].

Asia is the largest and most populated continent (60% of the world's population), with an increasing prevalence of GDM [19]. While maternal overweight/obesity is an established risk factor for GDM [20], particularly in HICs, recent reviews have found that the prevalence of GDM may be even higher among lean populations than those with a larger body size [2]. This is consistent with the developmental origins of adult disease hypothesis (DOHAD) as undernutrition in the first 1000 days is associated with later diabetes [21–24]. The Eastern and Southeastern subregions include 18 countries, with more than 30% of the Asian population [25] and contributing approximately 80% to the Asian economy [26]. Given the rapid socioeconomic and nutrition transition and the increasing prevalence of GDM in Asia [19, 27], it is of public health importance to provide an overview of this condition in Eastern and Southeastern Asia. However, accessible and systematically organized estimates of GDM prevalence in this subregion are lacking. Moreover, the lack of uniformity in screening methods, definition, and diagnostic criteria for GDM makes it difficult to compare the prevalence of GDM between and within countries. The aim of this study was to undertake a systematic review and meta-analysis of the prevalence and associated risk factors of GDM in selected countries of Eastern and Southeastern Asia.

2. Methods

The present review was conducted according to the Preferred Reporting Items for Systematic Reviews and Meta-Analyses (PRISMA) statement [28] and the Meta-analysis Of Observational Studies in Epidemiology (MOOSE) protocols [29].

2.1. Search Strategy. The databases (PubMed, Embase, and Scopus) were used to search relevant articles with the following key words: "gestational diabetes mellitus," "GDM," "hyperglycemia in pregnancy," "gestational hyperglycemia," or "diabetes in pregnancy" as well as "name of country" in Eastern and Southeastern Asia. The websites of the World Health Organization (WHO) and International Diabetes Federation were also reviewed to extend our search results. Then the reference lists of included articles were assessed to identify further relevant studies.

2.2. Inclusion Criteria. Studies that met the following criteria were retrieved for assessment: (1) being conducted in Eastern and Southeastern Asian countries classified by the United Nations Statistics Division [30]; (2) being published in English language journals between January 1, 2000, and December 31, 2016; (3) reported primary results (i.e., original studies); (4) provided the prevalence of GDM and associated 95% confidence interval (CI) or total of participants and number of GDM events; and (5) had a sample size of at least 1000 and 50 GDM cases. When multiple publications were derived from analyses of the same or overlapping samples, we used data from the largest or most recent results only.

2.3. Study Selection. Relevant papers identified from the aforementioned databases and websites were imported into an EndNote X7.5, and duplicates were removed. Two reviewers independently screened the titles and abstracts for potentially eligible articles based on the inclusion criteria. If a paper contained insufficient information on GDM in the title and/or abstract, the full text was retrieved for further assessment and any disagreement between the two reviewers was resolved through discussion. Finally, the full text of relevant studies was reviewed.

2.4. Quality Assessment and Data Extraction. The guidelines of the National Health and Medical Research Council were used to assess the quality of searched articles by two independent investigators [31]. Only articles that meet the level III of evidence were included and analysed in this review. An extraction form was developed in Excel to record data from selected papers by one reviewer, and the completeness and accuracy of extracted data were verified by a second reviewer. The following characteristics were extracted from each study: first author, country, year of publication, year of survey, setting, gestational age, screening procedure (one and/or two steps), sample size, GDM cases, prevalence of GDM (including percentage and 95% CI), and diagnostic criteria for GDM. If 95% CIs were not reported, they were calculated based on the sample size and observed proportion of GDM in each selected study [32]. Since we only collected published studies, ethical approval was not required for this work.

2.5. Data Analysis. Diagnostic criteria were aggregated into 8 clusters due to some similarities: (1) JSOG, (2) NDDG, (3) ADA 2004/ADA 2010, (4) ICD10, (5) ADA 2007/CC, (6) WHO 1998–2006, (7) ADA 2012/IADPSG/WHO 2013; and (8) ADIPS98. The prevalences of GDM, with 95% CI, were grouped according to the different diagnostic criteria to perform meta-analyses. The summary prevalence (95% CI) regardless of and by each diagnostic criteria was calculated using the random effects model of the DerSimonian and Laird method [33] to allow for the possibility of real differences in the distribution of GDM between studies that are not solely resulted from sampling error. The heterogeneity among studies was tested with the I^2 index (low is <25%, moderate 25%–50%, and high > 50%), which describes the percent of total variation contributed by between-study variations [34]. The overall prevalence of GDM (95% CI) by each group of diagnostic criteria was depicted graphically in forest plots. Statistically significant heterogeneity was considered present at $P < 0.1$ and $I^2 > 50\%$ [35]. In addition, subgroup analysis according to lower- or upper-middle income countries (LMICs) or HICs, type of GDM screening, and individual country under study was performed to understand the

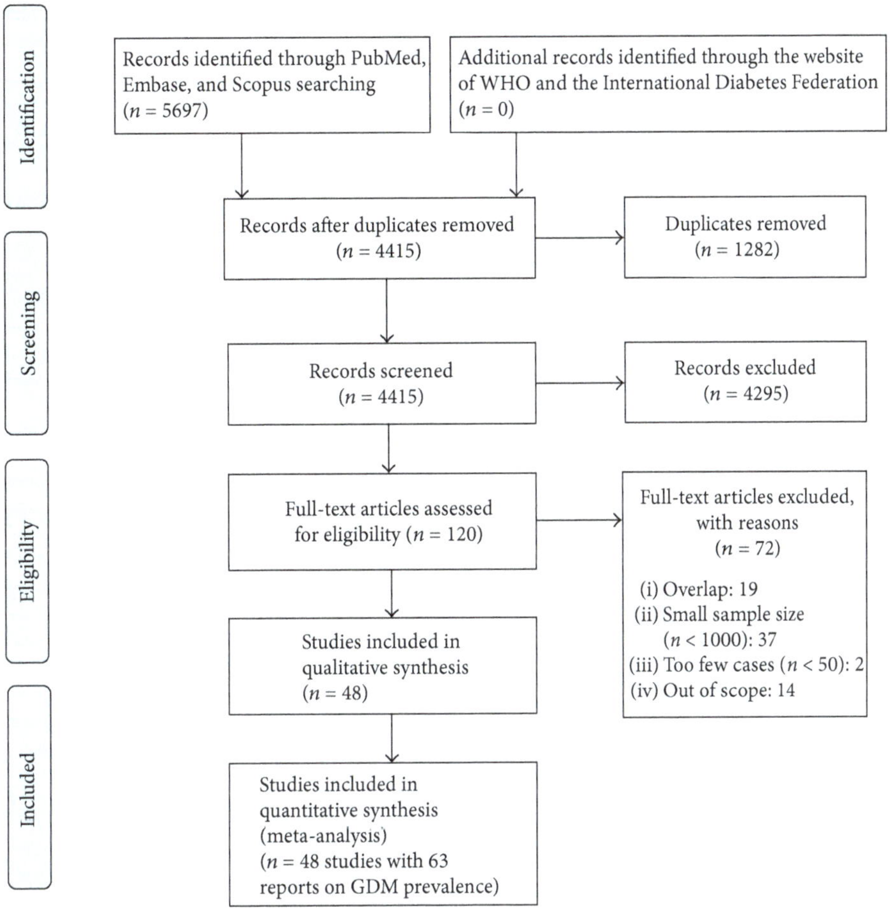

FIGURE 1: PRISMA flow diagram of selected studies.

impact of economic development and geographical location on the prevalence of GDM. The summary prevalence of GDM for each study that used more than one diagnostic criterion was pooled using a fixed effects model. All analyses were performed using Stata 13.1 (StataCorp LP, College Station, TX).

3. Results

3.1. Description of Included Studies. Figure 1 shows the flow diagram of our systematic literature search. The initial search identified 5697 publications, and after the removal of duplicate records ($n = 1282$), 4415 were retrieved for preliminary assessment. Of these, 120 were potentially relevant after title and abstract screening, and thus, their full texts were obtained and evaluated against the inclusion criteria, resulting in 48 studies reported in 63 observations. No papers were retrieved from the reference list. Of 48 studies, one paper reported four values of GDM prevalence by using four diagnostic criteria [36], 12 papers had two values of GDM prevalence by comparing two different diagnostic criteria or screening types [37–48], and 35 papers only used one diagnostic criterion to estimate GDM prevalence [49–83].

3.2. Characteristics of Included Studies. The main characteristics of the included studies are described in the Supplemental Table (available here). Between the years 2000 and 2016, 48 articles were published with a total sample of 3,594,803 pregnant women (range: 1038–1,824,913) in 7 countries. Of the 48 studies, 21 were conducted in China [41–43, 45, 48–64], 8 in the Republic of Korea [65, 68, 70–72, 74, 75, 77], 6 in Thailand [37, 46, 79–81, 83], five in Japan [39, 47, 73, 76, 78], five in Taiwan (China) [38, 44, 66, 67, 69], one in Malaysia [82], one in Singapore [40], and one in Vietnam [36]. Two-thirds of the studies ($n = 32$) used a two-step screening procedure, that is, women underwent a 1-hour glucose challenge test (GCT) and a 3-hour glucose tolerance test (GTT) if GCT were abnormal. To perform these tests, women were required to drink 50 g of glucose and 75 or 100 g of glucose for GCT and GTT, respectively. Over one-quarter of studies ($n = 13$) followed a single-step screening, where all pregnant women were given a 75 g GTT. Three studies did not specify the screening method used [56, 71, 75]. A total of 20 studies used IADPSG, the 2010 ADA, or the 2013 WHO standards as the GDM diagnostic criteria. The number of studies that employed CC or the 2007 ADA, NDDG, WHO (1998, 1999, and 2006) was 13, 12, and 10, respectively. The remaining 8 studies applied other criteria (see Supplemental

TABLE 1: Pooled prevalence and 95% confidence interval of gestational diabetes according to the income group, screening type, and country.

	Studies	Subjects	Prevalence	Lower 95% CI	Upper 95% CI	I^2	$P_{heterogeneity}$
Income level							
High							
JSOG	2	3877	2.80	2.31	3.39	0.00%	0.411
NDDG	4	35,400	4.21	2.15	8.26	99.30%	<0.001
ICD10	1	1,306,281	7.53	7.51	7.56	—	—
ADA 2007/CC	9	1,880,183	7.38	6.03	9.03	98.90%	<0.001
WHO 1999–2006	2	2272	15.37	13.89	17.02	—	—
ADA 2012/IADPSG/WHO 2013	6	16,237	7.48	4.74	11.80	98.60%	<0.001
Subtotal	24	3,244,250	6.66	4.40	10.09	98.30%	<0.001
Lower- or upper-middle							
NDDG	8	79,487	5.83	4.31	7.90	99.10%	<0.001
ADA 2004/ADA 2010	4	28,342	6.59	4.40	9.86	98.50%	<0.001
ADA 2007/CC	4	21,259	11.85	4.94	28.42	99.80%	<0.001
WHO 1999–2006	8	183,545	8.57	5.23	14.06	99.90%	<0.001
ADA 2012/IADPSG/WHO 2013	14	113,656	17.56	15.07	20.47	99.20%	<0.001
ADIPS98	1	2772	20.82	19.34	22.40	—	—
Subtotal	39	429,061	10.84	7.35	15.99	94.40%	<0.001
Type of screening							
One step	13	95,638	15.71	13.88	17.77	98.90%	<0.001
Two-step	32	338,825	7.15	5.63	9.08	99.70%	<0.001
Unspecified	3	3,132,329	7.83	7.39	8.29	99.70%	<0.001
Country							
Mainland China	21	282,086	11.91	8.96	15.83	99.90%	<0.001
Japan	5	12,596	6.08	3.49	10.62	98.70%	<0.001
Korea	8	3,180,515	7.12	6.74	7.53	99.60%	<0.001
Malaysia	1	1538	11.83	10.30	13.60	—	—
Singapore	1	1136	18.93	16.74	21.40	—	—
Taiwan	5	30,944	6.51	4.45	9.54	99.0%	<0.001
Thailand	6	55,205	6.10	4.39	8.48	98.8%	<0.001
Vietnam	1	2772	20.06	19.28	20.87	—	—
All	48	3,566,792	10.07	6.47	15.68	99.3%	<0.001

—: not applicable; ADA: American Diabetes Association; ADIPS: Australian Diabetes in Pregnancy Society; CC: Carpenter-Coustan; IADPSG: International Association of the Diabetes and Pregnancy Study Groups; ICD: International Classification of Diseases; JSOG: Japan Society of Obstetrics and Gynecology; NDDG: National Diabetes Data Group; WHO: World Health Organization.

Table). All studies included in the present review met the level III of evidence of the National Health and Medical Research Council in Australia [31].

3.3. Prevalence of GDM. The overall mean prevalence of GDM, regardless of diagnostic standards, was 10.07 (95% CI: 6.47–15.68) (Table 1). Figure 2 depicts the prevalence of GDM across 8 diagnostic groupings. The highest prevalence of GDM was observed for studies using the IADPSG, ADA 2012, or WHO 2013 criteria (13.77%) while the lowest data was found among Japanese reports that employed JSOG criteria (2.80%). Between that range, the summary prevalence of GDM according to NDDG, ADA 2004 or ADA 2010, ADA 2007 or CC, and WHO (1998, 1999, or 2006) recommendations was 5.24%, 6.59%, 8.54%, and 9.40%, respectively. Only two single data points for GDM prevalence were reported using either ICD 10 [75] or ADIPS 1998 [36], with the respective prevalences being 7.53% and 20.82%, respectively (Table 1). With the exception of studies employing JSOG, there was considerable heterogeneity of GDM prevalence among studies assessed based on various criteria; a measure of heterogeneity varied from 98.5% to 99.8% ($P < 0.001$).

3.4. Prevalence of GDM by Income and Diagnostic Criteria. Overall, the prevalence of GDM was higher in LMICs than HICs, 10.84% versus 6.66%, respectively (Table 1). Except for pooled GDM prevalence according to WHO (1998, 1999, or 2006) criteria, the summary estimates of GDM prevalence based on other diagnostic criteria were greater in LMICs than in HICs. Notably, the prevalence using the most popular criteria, that is, ADA 2012, IADPSG, or WHO 2013, was over twofold higher in the former

Study	Country	Size	Case	Year of data collection	Prevalence (95% CI)
JSOG					
Morikawaet al. 2010 [39]	Japan	1038	25	2002–2006	2.41 (1.56, 3.53)
Nobumoto et al. 2015 [47]	Japan	2839	83	2001–2011	2.92 (2.34, 3.61)
Subtotal ($I^2 = 0.0\%$, $P = 0.411$)					2.80 (2.31, 3.39)
NDDG					
Jang et al. 2003 [65]	Korea	16654	392	1993–1997	2.35 (2.13, 2.60)
Sunsaneevithayakul et al. 2003 [37]	Thailand	9325	235	2000	2.52 (2.21, 2.86)
Chou et al. 2010 [38]	Taiwan	10990	385	2001–2008	3.50 (3.17, 3.86)
Fan et al. 2006 [59]	China	20512	782	1995–2004	3.81 (3.55, 4.08)
Wang et al. 2013 [69]	Taiwan	1387	60	2011	4.33 (3.32, 5.53)
Srichumchit et al. 2015 [83]	Thailand	25255	1350	2002-2012	5.35 (5.07, 5.63)
Ruangvutilert et al. 2010 [81]	Thailand	6812	403	2005-2006	5.92 (5.37, 6.50)
Sunsaneevithayakul et al. 2003 [37]	Thailand	3770	235	2000	6.23 (5.48, 7.05)
Punthumapol et al. 2008 [80]	Thailand	2010	147	2004-2005	7.31 (6.21, 8.54)
Chuang CM et al. 2012 [67]	Taiwan	6369	562	2002-2007	8.82 (8.14, 9.55)
Luengmettakul et al. 2015 [46]	Thailand	10603	1047	2009–2011	9.87 (9.31, 10.46)
Boriboonhirunsarn et al. 2004 [79]	Thailand	1200	119	2001	9.92 (8.28, 11.75)
Subtotal ($I^2 = 99.1\%$, $P = 0.000$)					5.24 (3.98, 6.89)
ADA 2004/ADA 2010					
Yang et al. 2009 [60]	China	16286	708	2006	4.35 (4.04, 4.67)
Tran et al. 2013 [36]	Vietnam	2772	164	2010-2011	5.92 (5.07, 6.86)
Shang et al. 2014 [42]	China	3083	246	2012-2013	7.98 (7.05, 8.99)
Shang et al. 2014 [43]	China	6201	570	2008-2011	9.19 (8.48, 9.94)
Subtotal ($I^2 = 98.5\%$, $P = 0.000$)					6.59 (4.40, 9.86)
ADA 2007/CC					
Luengmettakul et al. 2015 [46]	Thailand	3283	144	2012	4.39 (3.71, 5.14)
Chou et al. 2010 [38]	Taiwan	10990	489	2001–2008	4.45 (4.07, 4.85)
Hung et al. 2015 [44]	Taiwan	3056	141	2009-2010	4.61 (3.90, 5.42)
Park et al. 2013 [68]	Korea	19423	1086	2006–2010	5.59 (5.27, 5.92)
Heo et al. 2015 [72]	Korea	5212	322	2009–2013	6.18 (5.54, 6.87)
Cho et al. 2015 [71]	Korea	1824913	129666	2007–2010	7.11 (7.08, 7.13)
Lin et al. 2009 [66]	Taiwan	8557	636	2001–2006	7.43 (6.89, 8.01)
Jung et al. 2015 [74]	Korea	3435	286	2000–2008	8.33 (7.42, 9.30)
Park et al. 2016 [77]	Korea	3434	306	2001–2013	8.91 (7.98, 9.91)
Chang et al. 2014 [63]	China	10852	1010	2008–2010	9.31 (8.77, 9.87)
Liao et al. 2014 [41]	China	5360	626	2008–2011	11.68 (10.83, 12.57)
Yang et al. 2013 [70]	Korea	1163	269	2004–2006	23.13 (20.73, 25.66)
Wang et al. 2011 [61]	China	1764	725	2006–2010	41.10 (38.79, 43.44)
Subtotal ($I^2 = 99.7\%$, $P = 0.000$)					8.54 (6.21, 11.75)
WHO 1998–2006					
Yang et al. 2002 [58]	China	9471	219	1998-1999	2.31 (2.02, 2.64)
Zhang et al. 2011 [62]	China	105473	5185	1999–2008	4.92 (4.79, 5.05)
Liu et al. 2014 [64]	China	27157	1420	2009–2011	5.23 (4.97, 5.50)
Leng et al. 2015 [45]	China	18589	1506	2010–2012	8.10 (7.71, 8.50)
Chong et al. 2014 [40]	Singapore	1136	111	2009-2010	9.77 (8.11, 11.65)
Tan et al. 2011 [82]	Malaysia	1538	182	Not available	11.83 (10.26, 13.55)
Peng et al. 2015 [51]	China	1359	166	2012	12.21 (10.52, 14.07)
Zhu et al. 2015 [48]	China	17186	2952	2010–2012	17.18 (16.62, 17.75)
Chong et al. 2014 [40]	Singapore	1136	215	2009-2010	18.93 (16.69, 21.33)
Tran et al. 2013 [36]	Vietnam	2772	674	2010-2011	24.31 (22.73, 25.96)
Subtotal ($I^2 = 99.8\%$, $P = 0.000$)					9.40 (6.05, 14.60)
ADA 2012/IADPSG/WHO 2013					
Shimodaira et al. 2016 [78]	Japan	5424	149	2010–2015	2.75 (2.33, 3.22)
Limura et al. 2015 [73]	Japan	1183	53	2010-2011	4.48 (3.37, 5.82)
Morikawa et al. 2010 [39]	Japan	1038	68	2002–2006	6.55 (5.12, 8.23)
Leng et al. 2015 [45]	China	18589	1721	2010–2012	9.26 (8.85, 9.68)
Shang et al. 2014 [43]	China	6201	676	2008–2011	10.90 (10.14, 11.70)
Hung et al. 2015 [44]	Taiwan	3641	453	2012-2013	12.44 (11.39, 13.56)
Nobumoto et al. 2015 [47]	Japan	2839	363	2001–2011	12.79 (11.58, 14.07)
Ohara et al. 2016 [76]	Japan	2112	275	2010–2013	13.02 (11.61, 14.53)
Xu et al. 2016 [56]	China	1135	154	2012-2013	13.57 (11.63, 15.70)
Li et al. 2015 [50]	China	2545	379	2013	14.89 (13.53, 16.34)
Wei et al. 2015 [53]	China	25674	3990	2005–2012	15.54 (15.10, 15.99)
Zhu et al. 2015 [48]	China	17186	3002	2010–2012	17.47 (16.90, 18.04)
He et al. 2015 [49]	China	3063	544	2012–2014	17.76 (16.42, 19.13)
Wang et al. 2015 [52]	China	14168	2750	2013	19.41 (18.76, 20.07)
Shang et al. 2014 [42]	China	3083	612	2012-2013	19.85 (18.46, 21.30)
Tran et al. 2013 [36]	Vietnam	2772	565	2010-2011	20.38 (18.90, 21.93)
Ye et al. 2016 [57]	China	1959	413	2012	21.08 (19.29, 22.96)
Wei et al. 2016 [55]	China	9803	2133	2011–2013	21.76 (20.95, 22.59)
Liao et al. 2014 [41]	China	5360	1314	2008–2011	24.51 (23.37, 25.69)
Li et al. 2016 [54]	China	2118	639	2010–2014	30.17 (28.22, 32.17)
Subtotal ($I^2 = 99.2\%$, $P = 0.000$)					13.77 (11.86, 15.99)

Note: weights are from random effects analysis

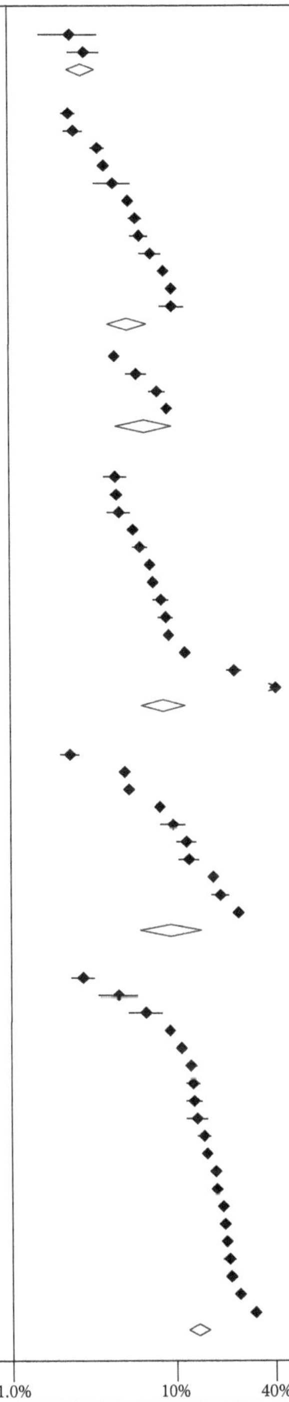

FIGURE 2: Forest plots presenting the prevalence of gestational diabetes for individual studies and the corresponding pooled prevalence for studies combined according to diagnostic criteria in Eastern and Southeastern Asia. Bars and diamonds indicate 95% confidence interval (CI). The size of each square corresponds to the weight of the study in the meta-analysis using the Der Simonian and Laird method. ADA: American Diabetes Association; CC: Carpenter-Coustan; IADPSG: International Association of the Diabetes and Pregnancy Study Groups; JSOG: Japan Society of Obstetrics and Gynecology; NDDG: National Diabetes Data Group; WHO: World Health Organization.

when compared with the corresponding figure in the latter (17.56% versus 7.48%) (Table 1).

3.5. Prevalence of GDM by Screening Method. The mean prevalence of GDM derived using one-step screening and two-step screening was 15.71% (95% CI: 13.88–17.77%) and 7.15% (95%CI: 5.63–9.08%), respectively; there was substantial heterogeneity among studies using either the one-step screening method or the two-step screening method ($I^2 > 98\%$ and $P < 0.001$) (Table 1).

3.6. Prevalence of GDM by Country. There was variation in the overall prevalence of GDM, with Vietnam and Singapore showing the highest rates (20.06% and 18.93%, resp.). While mainland China and Malaysia had a comparable prevalence of GDM (11.91% and 11.83%), the remaining countries (Japan, Korea, Taiwan, and Thailand) had a GDM prevalence of less than 8.0%. It should be noted that mainland China accounted for nearly 50% of the total studies ($n = 21$) (Table 1).

4. Discussion

The present review included 48 studies with more than three and a half million participants from 7 countries in Eastern and Southeastern Asia, showing a wide variation in the overall prevalence of GDM. The pooled prevalence of GDM was approximately 10%, with a higher estimate in LMICs than in HICs. The discrepancy in the overall estimate also existed according to diagnostic criteria and countries. The most widely used criteria were ADA 2012, IADPSG, or WHO 2013, resulting in a pooled prevalence of GDM of 14% while only a limited number of studies used ADIP 1998, ICD 10, JSOG, ADA 2004, or ADA 2010. The highest prevalence of GDM was found in Vietnam and Singapore, where approximately one in five women were diagnosed with GDM, followed by mainland China and Malaysia where about one in 9 women had GDM. The remaining countries had no more than one in 14 women with GDM. To the best of our knowledge, this is the first study that systematically synthesised data on the prevalence of GDM in important subregions of Asia, Eastern and Southeastern, and provided accessible evidence to formulate locally feasible strategies for effective and efficient prevention of GDM in Asia.

Overall, approximately one in 10 pregnant women in Eastern and Southeastern Asia had GDM. This finding is higher than African countries, where the average prevalence of GDM is about 6.0% [17]. Similarly, our data is greater than results reported in Western countries including Europe, US, and Australia, with the prevalence of GDM being 5.4%, 9.2%, and 5.7%, respectively [84–86]. We have no clear reason for such a discrepancy, but we speculate that it may be due to socioeconomic, racial/ethnic, or lifestyle disparities. For instance, Asian women were reportedly having a higher risk of GDM compared with their Caucasian, African-American, and Hispanic counterparts [87]. This observation suggests that the development of GDM may be shaped by early-life exposure to poor nutrition, that is, under- or overnutrition, and/or epigenetics according to the DOHAD theory [88]. Another factor may be the different screening regimes and testing methods that will be discussed below.

The lack of consensus regarding the use of diagnostic criteria for GDM is largely attributable to the heterogeneity of GDM prevalence. Of diverse diagnostic criteria such as NDDG [89], CC [90], ADA [91], and WHO [92], the IADPSG criteria based on the Hyperglycemia and Adverse Pregnancy Outcome Study (HAPO) has recently become more accepted [93]. Indeed, the use of IADPSG criteria may produce an estimated prevalence of GDM two to threefold even up to 7-fold higher than other criteria [13, 94]. In a Brazilian study, for instance, the prevalence of GDM was only 2.3% and 7.1% according to ADA 2010 and WHO 1999, respectively, but it increased to 18.0% following the IADPSG criteria [94]. An alternative explanation for the variation in GDM prevalence may be ascribed to different screening methods, that is, the one-step or two-step approach. Similar to our review, a recent meta-analysis of 40 studies in Europe reported that the one-step screening method resulted in a higher prevalence of GDM compared with the two-step procedure [86]. Although a one-step screening type is simpler, less laborious, and of low lost, it typically overestimates the prevalence of GDM [95]. However a two-step screening method is more accurate and could accordingly reduce personal and societal costs despite its inconvenience for patients and increased workload for healthcare professionals [96]. Given the lack of international consensus in screening and diagnostic methods for GDM, it is imperative to develop a standardised approach to allow for comparison of GDM burdens worldwide.

The high prevalences of GDM in less wealthy countries reviewed here are consistent with studies from other parts of Asia and Africa [17, 18]. Likewise, around 90% of cases of hyperglycemia during pregnancy occur in low- and middle-income nations as reported by the International Diabetes Federation in 2015 [27]. This discrepancy may be associated with limited access to maternal health care and/or low socioeconomic status in low- and middle-income economies [27, 97, 98]. It is evident from this review that the prevalence of GDM in Vietnam, a lower-middle income country, at least tripled the corresponding data in HICs such as Japan, Taiwan, and South Korea. It can also be speculated that the difference in lifestyle factors (e.g., diet and physical activity), acculturation, and urbanisation may explain the variation in GDM prevalence between the two aforementioned country-income groups [99]. This finding implies that improvement of socioeconomic conditions may contribute to the prevention of GDM.

On the other hand, more epidemiological studies on GDM in the remaining countries of Eastern and Southeastern Asian regions including Mongolia, Indonesia, Philippines, Myanmar, Cambodia, and Laos need to be conducted to add information to the current evidence. These studies should be performed in both urban and rural populations in order to compare and evaluate the effects of urbanisation on GDM in particular and public health in general.

The present review has the advantages of a large sample size with studies involving over three and a half million women, using different methods for screening and diagnosis of GDM and consistency of method, quality, and focus. There are several limitations that need to be considered when interpreting the results of this work. Our review indicated substantial heterogeneity of GDM prevalence across studies, making direct comparison difficult. Such variation may be attributable to the potential influence of screening procedures (i.e., selective or universal) for GDM and its diagnostic criteria, population characteristics, or other socioenvironmental factors. Nonetheless, those possible modifiers were not taken into account in this review due to the lack of data available from included studies. In addition, the inclusion of only English publications may have resulted in publication bias. Our review did not address GDM situations in other countries in the region including Indonesia, Philippines, Myanmar, Cambodia, and Laos due to the lack of data, and thus, the findings may not be generalisable to the whole Eastern and Southeastern Asia.

5. Conclusion

A large-scale review of literature shows that around one in 10 pregnant women in Eastern and Southeastern Asia had GDM and the number of women with GDM varied substantially between and within countries. The prevalence of GDM was highest according to ADA 2012, IADPSG, or WHO 2013 criteria, greater following a one-step screening procedure and higher in LMICs. The findings suggest the need for developing an international uniformity regarding screening and diagnostic methods for GDM.

Conflicts of Interest

The authors declare that they have no conflicts of interest.

Authors' Contributions

Cong Luat Nguyen and Ngoc Minh Pham designed the study and wrote the manuscript. Cong Luat Nguyen systematically searched the literature and extracted data. Ngoc Minh Pham reviewed the included studies and conducted statistical analyses. Colin W. Binns and Andy H. Lee critically commented and substantially revised the manuscript. Dat Van Duong contributed to literature review and discussion. All authors participated in drafting the manuscript and approved the final version.

References

[1] American Diabetes Association, "2. Classification and diagnosis of diabetes," *Diabetes Care*, vol. 38, Supplement 1, pp. S8–S16, 2015.

[2] L. Guariguata, U. Linnenkamp, J. Beagley, D. R. Whiting, and N. H. Cho, "Global estimates of the prevalence of hyperglycaemia in pregnancy," *Diabetes Research and Clinical Practice*, vol. 103, no. 2, pp. 176–185, 2014.

[3] D. Farrar, M. Simmonds, M. Bryant et al., "Hyperglycaemia and risk of adverse perinatal outcomes: systematic review and meta-analysis," *BMJ*, vol. 354, article i4694, 2016.

[4] C. Kim, K. M. Newton, and R. H. Knopp, "Gestational diabetes and the incidence of type 2 diabetes: a systematic review," *Diabetes Care*, vol. 25, no. 10, pp. 1862–1868, 2002.

[5] Y. Yogev, E. M. J. Xenakis, and O. Langer, "The association between preeclampsia and the severity of gestational diabetes: the impact of glycemic control," *American Journal of Obstetrics and Gynecology*, vol. 191, no. 5, pp. 1655–1660, 2004.

[6] HAPO Study Cooperative Research Group, B. E. Metzger, L. P. Lowe et al., "Hyperglycemia and adverse pregnancy outcomes," *The New England Journal of Medicine*, vol. 358, no. 19, pp. 1991–2002, 2008.

[7] D. Marchetti, D. Carrozzino, F. Fraticelli, M. Fulcheri, and E. Vitacolonna, "Quality of life in women with gestational diabetes mellitus: a systematic review," *Journal of Diabetes Research*, vol. 2017, Article ID 7058082, 12 pages, 2017.

[8] O. Langer, Y. Yogev, O. Most, and E. M. J. Xenakis, "Gestational diabetes: the consequences of not treating," *American Journal of Obstetrics and Gynecology*, vol. 192, no. 4, pp. 989–997, 2005.

[9] T. D. Clausen, E. R. Mathiesen, T. Hansen et al., "High prevalence of type 2 diabetes and pre-diabetes in adult offspring of women with gestational diabetes mellitus or type 1 diabetes," *Diabetes Care*, vol. 31, no. 2, pp. 340–346, 2008.

[10] A. Jiwani, E. Marseille, N. Lohse, P. Damm, M. Hod, and J. G. Kahn, "Gestational diabetes mellitus: results from a survey of country prevalence and practices," *The Journal of Maternal-Fetal & Neonatal Medicine*, vol. 25, no. 6, pp. 600–610, 2012.

[11] C. R. Pullinger, I. D. Goldfine, S. Tanyolaç et al., "Evidence that an *HMGA1* gene variant associates with type 2 diabetes, body mass index, and high-density lipoprotein cholesterol in a Hispanic-American population," *Metabolic Syndrome and Related Disorders*, vol. 12, no. 1, pp. 25–30, 2014.

[12] J. Yan, R. Su, D. Ao, Y. Wang, H. Wang, and H. Yang, "Genetic variants and clinical relevance associated with gestational diabetes mellitus in Chinese women: a case-control study," *The Journal of Maternal-Fetal & Neonatal Medicine*, pp. 1–7, 2017.

[13] M. M. Agarwal, "Gestational diabetes mellitus: an update on the current international diagnostic criteria," *World Journal of Diabetes*, vol. 6, no. 6, pp. 782–791, 2015.

[14] L. R. Mack and P. G. Tomich, "Gestational diabetes: diagnosis, classification, and clinical care," *Obstetrics and Gynecology Clinics of North America*, vol. 44, no. 2, pp. 207–217, 2017.

[15] E. Chiefari, B. Arcidiacono, D. Foti, and A. Brunetti, "Gestational diabetes mellitus: an updated overview," *Journal of Endocrinological Investigation*, vol. 40, no. 9, pp. 899–909, 2017.

[16] L. Kanguru, N. Bezawada, J. Hussein, and J. Bell, "The burden of diabetes mellitus during pregnancy in low- and middle-income countries: a systematic review," *Global Health Action*, vol. 7, no. 1, article 23987, 2014.

[17] S. Macaulay, D. B. Dunger, and S. A. Norris, "Gestational diabetes mellitus in Africa: a systematic review," *PLoS One*, vol. 9, no. 6, article e97871, 2014.

[18] J. Hirst, C. Raynes-Greenow, and H. Jeffery, "A systematic review of trends of gestational diabetes mellitus in Asia," *Journal of Diabetology*, vol. 3, no. 3, p. 5, 2012.

[19] G. E. Tutino, W. H. Tam, X. Yang, J. C. N. Chan, T. T. H. Lao, and R. C. W. Ma, "Diabetes and pregnancy: perspectives from Asia," *Diabetic Medicine*, vol. 31, no. 3, pp. 302–318, 2014.

[20] S. Y. Chu, W. M. Callaghan, S. Y. Kim et al., "Maternal obesity and risk of gestational diabetes mellitus," *Diabetes Care*, vol. 30, no. 8, pp. 2070–2076, 2007.

[21] A. Vaiserman, "Early-life nutritional programming of type 2 diabetes: experimental and quasi-experimental evidence," *Nutrients*, vol. 9, no. 3, 2017.

[22] I. O. L. Wong, B. J. Cowling, and C. M. Schooling, "Vulnerability to diabetes in Chinese: an age–period–cohort analysis," *Annals of Epidemiology*, vol. 25, no. 1, pp. 34–39, 2015.

[23] X. Jiang, H. Ma, Y. Wang, and Y. Liu, "Early life factors and type 2 diabetes mellitus," *Journal of Diabetes Research*, vol. 2013, Article ID 485082, 11 pages, 2013.

[24] G. V. Krishnaveni and C. S. Yajnik, "Developmental origins of diabetes—an Indian perspective," *European Journal of Clinical Nutrition*, vol. 71, no. 7, pp. 865–869, 2017.

[25] The United Nations, "Demographic yearbook 2015," February 2017, https://unstats.un.org/unsd/demographic/products/dyb/dyb2015/Table01.pdf.

[26] International Monetary Fund, "World economic outlook database," August 2017, https://www.imf.org/external/pubs/ft/weo/2017/01/weodata/index.aspx.

[27] International Diabetes Federation, *IDF Diabetes Atlas*, 2015.

[28] D. Moher, A. Liberati, J. Tetzlaff, D. G. Altman, and PRISMA Group, "Preferred reporting items for systematic reviews and meta-analyses: the PRISMA statement," *International Journal of Surgery*, vol. 8, no. 5, pp. 336–341, 2010.

[29] D. F. Stroup, J. A. Berlin, S. C. Morton et al., "Meta-analysis of observational studies in epidemiology: a proposal for reporting," *JAMA*, vol. 283, no. 15, pp. 2008–2012, 2000.

[30] United Nations Statistics Division, "Geographical region and composition of each region," January 2017, http://unstats.un.org/unsd/methods/m49/m49regin.htm#asia.

[31] National Health and Medical Research Council, "NHMRC additional levels of evidence and grades for recommendations for developers of guidelines," March 2017, https://www.nhmrc.gov.au/_files_nhmrc/file/guidelines/developers/nhmrc_levels_grades_evidence_120423.pdf.

[32] M. J. Gardner and D. G. Altman, "Confidence intervals rather than P values: estimation rather than hypothesis testing," *BMJ*, vol. 292, no. 6522, pp. 746–750, 1986.

[33] R. DerSimonian and N. Laird, "Meta-analysis in clinical trials," *Controlled Clinical Trials*, vol. 7, no. 3, pp. 177–188, 1986.

[34] J. P. Higgins and S. G. Thompson, *Cochrane Handbook for Systematic Reviews of Interventions Version 5.1.0 (Updated March 2011)*, The Cochrane Collaboration, 2011, http://handbook.cochrane.org.

[35] J. P. T. Higgins and S. G. Thompson, "Quantifying heterogeneity in a meta-analysis," *Statistics in Medicine*, vol. 21, no. 11, pp. 1539–1558, 2002.

[36] T. S. Tran, J. E. Hirst, M. A. T. Do, J. M. Morris, and H. E. Jeffery, "Early prediction of gestational diabetes mellitus in Vietnam: clinical impact of currently recommended diagnostic criteria," *Diabetes Care*, vol. 36, no. 3, pp. 618–624, 2013.

[37] P. Sunsaneevithayakul, D. Boriboohirunsarn, A. Sutanthavibul et al., "Risk factor-based selective screening program for gestational diabetes mellitus in Siriraj Hospital: result from clinical practice guideline," *Journal of the Medical Association of Thailand*, vol. 86, no. 8, pp. 708–714, 2003.

[38] C. Y. Chou, C. L. Lin, C. K. Yang, W. C. Yang, F. K. Lee, and M. S. Tsai, "Pregnancy outcomes of Taiwanese women with gestational diabetes mellitus: a comparison of Carpenter-Coustan and National Diabetes Data Group Criteria," *Journal of Women's Health*, vol. 19, no. 5, pp. 935–939, 2010.

[39] M. Morikawa, T. Yamada, T. Yamada et al., "Change in the number of patients after the adoption of IADPSG criteria for hyperglycemia during pregnancy in Japanese women," *Diabetes Research and Clinical Practice*, vol. 90, no. 3, pp. 339–342, 2010.

[40] Y.-S. Chong, S. Cai, H. Lin et al., "Ethnic differences translate to inadequacy of high-risk screening for gestational diabetes mellitus in an Asian population: a cohort study," *BMC Pregnancy and Childbirth*, vol. 14, no. 1, 2014.

[41] S. Liao, J. Mei, W. Song et al., "The impact of the International Association of Diabetes and Pregnancy Study Groups (IADPSG) fasting glucose diagnostic criterion on the prevalence and outcomes of gestational diabetes mellitus in Han Chinese women," *Diabetic Medicine*, vol. 31, no. 3, pp. 341–351, 2014.

[42] M. Shang and L. Lin, "IADPSG criteria for diagnosing gestational diabetes mellitus and predicting adverse pregnancy outcomes," *Journal of Perinatology*, vol. 34, no. 2, pp. 100–104, 2014.

[43] M. Shang, L. Lin, L. Ma, and L. Yin, "Investigation on the suitability of the International Association of Diabetes and Pregnancy Study Group diagnostic criteria for gestational diabetes mellitus in China," *Journal of Obstetrics and Gynaecology*, vol. 34, no. 2, pp. 141–145, 2014.

[44] T. H. Hung and T. T. Hsieh, "The effects of implementing the International Association of Diabetes and Pregnancy Study Groups Criteria for diagnosing gestational diabetes on maternal and neonatal outcomes," *PLoS One*, vol. 10, no. 3, article e0122261, 2015.

[45] J. Leng, P. Shao, C. Zhang et al., "Prevalence of gestational diabetes mellitus and its risk factors in Chinese pregnant women: a prospective population-based study in Tianjin, China," *PLoS One*, vol. 10, no. 3, article e0121029, 2015.

[46] J. Luengmettakul, P. Sunsaneevithayakul, and P. Talungchit, "Pregnancy outcome in women with gestational diabetes mellitus according to the Carpenter–Coustan criteria in Thailand," *The Journal of Obstetrics and Gynaecology Research*, vol. 41, no. 9, pp. 1345–1351, 2015.

[47] E. Nobumoto, H. Masuyama, Y. Hiramatsu, T. Sugiyama, H. Kusaka, and N. Toyoda, "Effect of the new diagnostic criteria for gestational diabetes mellitus among Japanese women," *Diabetology International*, vol. 6, no. 3, pp. 226–231, 2015.

[48] H. Yang, M. Zhang, H. Zhang et al., "Comparing the diagnostic criteria for gestational diabetes mellitus of World Health Organization 2013 with 1999 in Chinese population," *Chinese Medical Journal*, vol. 128, no. 1, pp. 125–127, 2015.

[49] J. R. He, M. Y. Yuan, N. N. Chen et al., "Maternal dietary patterns and gestational diabetes mellitus: a large prospective cohort study in China," *British Journal of Nutrition*, vol. 113, no. 08, pp. 1292–1300, 2015.

[50] G. Li, L. Kong, L. Zhang et al., "Early pregnancy maternal lipid profiles and the risk of gestational diabetes mellitus stratified for body mass index," *Reproductive Sciences*, vol. 22, no. 6, pp. 712–717, 2015.

[51] S. Peng, L. Liu, X. Zhang et al., "A nested case-control study indicating heavy metal residues in meconium associate with maternal gestational diabetes mellitus risk," *Environmental Health*, vol. 14, no. 1, p. 19, 2015.

[52] C. Wang, W. Zhu, Y. Wei, H. Feng, R. Su, and H. Yang, "Exercise intervention during pregnancy can be used to manage weight gain and improve pregnancy outcomes in women with gestational diabetes mellitus," *BMC Pregnancy and Childbirth*, vol. 15, no. 1, 2015.

[53] Y. M. Wei, H. X. Yang, W. W. Zhu, H. Y. Yang, H. X. Li, and A. Kapur, "Effects of intervention to mild GDM on outcomes," *The Journal of Maternal-Fetal & Neonatal Medicine*, vol. 28, no. 8, pp. 928–931, 2015.

[54] H. P. Li, F. H. Wang, M. F. Tao, Y. J. Huang, and W. P. Jia, "Association between glycemic control and birthweight with glycated albumin in Chinese women with gestational diabetes mellitus," *Journal of Diabetes Investigation*, vol. 7, no. 1, pp. 48–55, 2016.

[55] Y. M. Wei, J. Yan, and H. X. Yang, "Identification of severe gestational diabetes mellitus after new criteria used in China," *Journal of Perinatology*, vol. 36, no. 2, pp. 90–94, 2016.

[56] Q. Xu, Z. Y. Gao, L. M. Li et al., "The Association of Maternal Body Composition and Dietary Intake with the risk of gestational diabetes mellitus during the second trimester in a cohort of Chinese pregnant women," *Biomedical and Environmental Sciences*, vol. 29, no. 1, pp. 1–11, 2016.

[57] M. Ye, Y. Liu, X. Cao et al., "The utility of HbA1c for screening gestational diabetes mellitus and its relationship with adverse pregnancy outcomes," *Diabetes Research and Clinical Practice*, vol. 114, pp. 43–49, 2016.

[58] X. Yang, B. Hsu-Hage, H. Zhang et al., "Gestational diabetes mellitus in women of single gravidity in Tianjin City, China," *Diabetes Care*, vol. 25, no. 5, pp. 847–851, 2002.

[59] Z. Fan, H. Yang, X. Gao, H. Lintu, and W. Sun, "Pregnancy outcome in gestational diabetes," *International Journal of Gynecology & Obstetrics*, vol. 94, no. 1, pp. 12–16, 2006.

[60] H. Yang, Y. Wei, X. Gao et al., "Risk factors for gestational diabetes mellitus in Chinese women—a prospective study of 16 286 pregnant women in China," *Diabetic Medicine*, vol. 26, no. 11, pp. 1099–1104, 2009.

[61] Y. Wang, M. Nie, W. Li et al., "Association of six single nucleotide polymorphisms with gestational diabetes mellitus in a Chinese population," *PLoS One*, vol. 6, no. 11, article e26953, 2011.

[62] F. Zhang, L. Dong, C. P. Zhang et al., "Increasing prevalence of gestational diabetes mellitus in Chinese women from 1999 to 2008," *Diabetic Medicine*, vol. 28, no. 6, pp. 652–657, 2011.

[63] Y. Chang, X. Chen, H. Cui, Z. Zhang, and L. Cheng, "Follow-up of postpartum women with gestational diabetes mellitus (GDM)," *Diabetes Research and Clinical Practice*, vol. 106, no. 2, pp. 236–240, 2014.

[64] G. Liu, N. Li, S. Sun et al., "Maternal OGTT glucose levels at 26–30 gestational weeks with offspring growth and development in early infancy," *BioMed Research International*, vol. 2014, Article ID 516980, 11 pages, 2014.

[65] H. C. Jang, C. H. Yim, K. O. Han et al., "Gestational diabetes mellitus in Korea: prevalence and prediction of glucose intolerance at early postpartum," *Diabetes Research and Clinical Practice*, vol. 61, no. 2, pp. 117–124, 2003.

[66] C. H. Lin, S. F. Wen, Y. H. Wu, and M. J. Huang, "Using the 100-g oral glucose tolerance test to predict fetal and maternal outcomes in women with gestational diabetes mellitus," *Chang Gung Medical Journal*, vol. 32, no. 3, pp. 283–289, 2009.

[67] C. M. Chuang, I. F. Lin, H. C. Horng, Y. H. Hsiao, I. L. Shyu, and P. Chou, "The impact of gestational diabetes mellitus on postpartum urinary incontinence: a longitudinal cohort study on singleton pregnancies," *BJOG: An International Journal of Obstetrics and Gynaecology*, vol. 119, no. 11, pp. 1334–1343, 2012.

[68] S. Park, M. Y. Kim, S. H. Baik et al., "Gestational diabetes is associated with high energy and saturated fat intakes and with low plasma visfatin and adiponectin levels independent of prepregnancy BMI," *European Journal of Clinical Nutrition*, vol. 67, no. 2, pp. 196–201, 2013.

[69] P. Wang, M. C. Lu, C. W. Yu, L. C. Wang, and Y. H. Yan, "Influence of food intake on the predictive value of the gestational diabetes mellitus screening test," *Obstetrics & Gynecology*, vol. 121, no. 4, pp. 750–758, 2013.

[70] S. J. Yang, T. N. Kim, S. H. Baik et al., "Insulin secretion and insulin resistance in Korean women with gestational diabetes mellitus and impaired glucose tolerance," *The Korean Journal of Internal Medicine*, vol. 28, no. 3, pp. 306–313, 2013.

[71] G. J. Cho, L. Y. Kim, Y. N. Sung et al., "Secular trends of gestational diabetes mellitus and changes in its risk factors," *PLoS One*, vol. 10, no. 8, article e0136017, 2015.

[72] J. M. Heo, T. H. Kim, M. H. Hahn et al., "Comparison of the effects of gestational weight gain on pregnancy outcomes between non-diabetic and diabetic women," *Obstetrics & Gynecology Science*, vol. 58, no. 6, pp. 461–467, 2015.

[73] Y. Iimura, M. Matsuura, Z. Yao et al., "Lack of predictive power of plasma lipids or lipoproteins for gestational diabetes mellitus in Japanese women," *Journal of Diabetes Investigation*, vol. 6, no. 6, pp. 640–646, 2015.

[74] Y. J. Jung, J. Y. Kwon, H. Y. Cho, Y. W. Park, and Y. H. Kim, "Comparison of the performance of screening test for gestational diabetes in singleton versus twin pregnancies," *Obstetrics & Gynecology Science*, vol. 58, no. 6, pp. 439–445, 2015.

[75] B. K. Koo, J. H. Lee, J. Kim, E. J. Jang, and C.-H. Lee, "Prevalence of gestational diabetes mellitus in Korea: a national health insurance database study," *PLoS One*, vol. 11, no. 4, article e0153107, 2016.

[76] R. Ohara, M. Obata-Yasuoka, K. Abe, H. Yagi, H. Hamada, and H. Yoshikawa, "Effect of hyperemesis gravidarum on gestational diabetes mellitus screening," *International Journal of Gynecology & Obstetrics*, vol. 132, no. 2, pp. 156–158, 2016.

[77] J. S. Park, D. W. Kim, J. Y. Kwon, Y. W. Park, Y. H. Kim, and H. Y. Cho, "Development of a screening tool for predicting adverse outcomes of gestational diabetes mellitus: a retrospective cohort study," *Medicine*, vol. 95, no. 1, article e2204, 2016.

[78] M. Shimodaira, T. Yamasaki, and T. Nakayama, "The association of maternal ABO blood group with gestational diabetes mellitus in Japanese pregnant women," *Diabetes & Metabolic Syndrome: Clinical Research & Reviews*, vol. 10, no. 2, pp. S102–S105, 2016.

[79] D. Boriboonhirunsarn, P. Sunsaneevithayakul, and M. Nuchangrid, "Incidence of gestational diabetes mellitus diagnosed before 20 weeks of gestation," *Journal of the Medical Association of Thailand*, vol. 87, no. 9, pp. 1017–1021, 2004.

[80] C. Punthumapol and P. Tekasakul, "50 grams glucose challenge test for screening of gestational diabetes mellitus in each trimester in potential diabetic pregnancy," *Journal of the Medical Association of Thailand*, vol. 91, no. 6, pp. 787–793, 2008.

[81] P. Ruangvutilert, P. Chaemsaithong, K. Ruangrongmorakot, S. Kanokpongsakdi, and P. Sunsaneevithayakul, "Development of a modified 100-gram oral glucose tolerance test for diagnosis of gestational diabetes mellitus and its diagnostic accuracy," *Journal of the Medical Association of Thailand*, vol. 93, no. 10, pp. 1121–1127, 2010.

[82] P. C. Tan, J. N. Chai, L. P. Ling, and S. Z. Omar, "Maternal hemoglobin level and red cell indices as predictors of gestational diabetes in a multi-ethnic Asian population," *Clinical*

and *Experimental Obstetrics & Gynecology*, vol. 38, no. 2, pp. 150–154, 2011.

[83] S. Srichumchit, S. Luewan, and T. Tongsong, "Outcomes of pregnancy with gestational diabetes mellitus," *International Journal of Gynecology & Obstetrics*, vol. 131, no. 3, pp. 251–254, 2015.

[84] C. L. DeSisto, S. Y. Kim, and A. J. Sharma, "Prevalence estimates of gestational diabetes mellitus in the United States, pregnancy risk assessment monitoring system (PRAMS), 2007–2010," *Preventing Chronic Disease*, vol. 11, article E104, 2014.

[85] C. Chamberlain, G. Joshy, H. Li, J. Oats, S. Eades, and E. Banks, "The prevalence of gestational diabetes mellitus among aboriginal and Torres Strait Islander women in Australia: a systematic review and meta-analysis," *Diabetes/Metabolism Research and Reviews*, vol. 31, no. 3, pp. 234–247, 2015.

[86] C. E. Eades, D. M. Cameron, and J. M. M. Evans, "Prevalence of gestational diabetes mellitus in Europe: a meta-analysis," *Diabetes Research and Clinical Practice*, vol. 129, pp. 173–181, 2017.

[87] L. Yuen and V. W. Wong, "Gestational diabetes mellitus: challenges for different ethnic groups," *World Journal of Diabetes*, vol. 6, no. 8, pp. 1024–1032, 2015.

[88] D. J. P. Barker, "The origins of the developmental origins theory," *Journal of Internal Medicine*, vol. 261, no. 5, pp. 412–417, 2007.

[89] National Diabetes Data Group, "Classification and diagnosis of diabetes mellitus and other categories of glucose intolerance," *Diabetes*, vol. 28, no. 12, pp. 1039–1057, 1979.

[90] M. W. Carpenter and D. R. Coustan, "Criteria for screening tests for gestational diabetes," *American Journal of Obstetrics and Gynecology*, vol. 144, no. 7, pp. 768–773, 1982.

[91] American Diabetes Association, "Gestational diabetes mellitus," *Diabetes Care*, vol. 23, Supplement 1, pp. S77–S90, 2004.

[92] World Health Organization, *Definition, Diagnosis and Classification of Diabetes Mellitus and its Complications. Part 1: Diagnosis and Classification of Diabetes Mellitus*, Geneva, 1999.

[93] International Association of Diabetes and Pregnancy Study Groups Consensus Panel, B. E. Metzger, S. G. Gabbe et al., "International association of diabetes and pregnancy study groups recommendations on the diagnosis and classification of hyperglycemia in pregnancy," *Diabetes Care*, vol. 33, no. 3, pp. 676–682, 2010.

[94] J. Trujillo, A. Vigo, B. B. Duncan et al., "Impact of the International Association of Diabetes and Pregnancy Study Groups criteria for gestational diabetes," *Diabetes Research and Clinical Practice*, vol. 108, no. 2, pp. 288–295, 2015.

[95] L. Hartling, D. M. Dryden, A. Guthrie, M. Muise, B. Vandermeer, and L. Donovan, "Diagnostic thresholds for gestational diabetes and their impact on pregnancy outcomes: a systematic review," *Diabetic Medicine*, vol. 31, no. 3, pp. 319–331, 2014.

[96] International Association of Diabetes & Pregnancy Study Groups (IADPSG) Consensus Panel Writing Group and the Hyperglycemia & Adverse Pregnancy Outcome (HAPO) Study Steering Committee, B. E. Metzger, S. G. Gabbe et al., "The diagnosis of gestational diabetes mellitus: new paradigms or status quo?," *The Journal of Maternal-Fetal & Neonatal Medicine*, vol. 25, no. 12, pp. 2564–2569, 2012.

[97] G. T. C. Ko, J. C. N. Chan, V. T. F. Yeung, C.-C. Chow, L. W. W. Tsang, and C. S. Cockram, "A low socio-economic status is an additional risk factor for glucose intolerance in high risk Hong Kong Chinese," *European Journal of Epidemiology*, vol. 17, no. 3, pp. 289–295, 2001.

[98] S. Bo, G. Menato, C. Bardelli et al., "Low socioeconomic status as a risk factor for gestational diabetes," *Diabetes & Metabolism*, vol. 28, no. 2, pp. 139-140, 2002.

[99] Y. Zhu and C. Zhang, "Prevalence of gestational diabetes and risk of progression to type 2 diabetes: a global perspective," *Current Diabetes Reports*, vol. 16, no. 1, p. 7, 2016.

18

Early Subclinical Atherosclerosis in Gestational Diabetes: The Predictive Role of Routine Biomarkers and Nutrigenetic Variants

Marica Franzago,[1] Federica Fraticelli,[1] Marta Di Nicola,[2] Francesco Bianco,[3] Daniela Marchetti,[4] Claudio Celentano,[1] Marco Liberati,[1] Raffaele De Caterina,[3] Liborio Stuppia,[4] and Ester Vitacolonna[1]

[1]*Department of Medicine and Aging, School of Medicine and Health Sciences, "G. d'Annunzio" University, Chieti-Pescara, Chieti, Italy*
[2]*Laboratory of Biostatistics, Department of Medical, Oral and Biotechnological Sciences, "G. d'Annunzio" University, Chieti-Pescara, Chieti, Italy*
[3]*Institute of Cardiology, School of Medicine and Health Sciences, "G. d'Annunzio" University, Chieti-Pescara, Chieti, Italy*
[4]*Department of Psychological, Health and Territorial Sciences, School of Medicine and Health Sciences, "G. d'Annunzio" University, Chieti-Pescara, Chieti, Italy*

Correspondence should be addressed to Ester Vitacolonna; e.vitacolonna@unich.it

Academic Editor: Claudio De Lucia

Gestational diabetes mellitus (GDM) can be considered a silent risk for out-of-pregnancy diabetes mellitus (DM) and cardiovascular disease (CVD) later in life. We aimed to assess the predictive role of 3rd trimester lipid profile during pregnancy for the susceptibility to markers of subclinical atherosclerosis (CVD susceptibility) at 3 years in a cohort of women with history of GDM. A secondary aim is to evaluate the usefulness of novel nutrigenetic markers, in addition to traditional parameters, for predicting early subclinical atherosclerosis in such women in order to plan adequate early prevention interventions. We assessed 28 consecutive GDM women in whom we collected socio-demographic characteristics and clinical and anthropometric parameters at the 3rd trimester of pregnancy. In a single blood sample, from each patient, we assessed 9 single nucleotide polymorphisms (SNPs) from 9 genes related to nutrients and metabolism, which were genotyped by High Resolution Melting analysis. All women then attended a 3-year-postpartum follow-up and on that occasion performed an oral glucose tolerance test (OGTT, with 75 g oral glucose), the measurement of carotid artery intima-media thickness (cIMT), and analyses of metabolic parameters. In addition, we evaluated the physical activity level and the adherence to Mediterranean diet (MedDiet) using the International Physical Activity Questionnaire (IPAQ-*short version*) and PREDIMED questionnaires. We found an association between 3rd trimester triglycerides and cIMT ($p = 0.014$). We also found significant associations between the APOA5 CC genotype and cIMT after adjustments for age and body mass index ($p = 0.045$) and between the interaction CC APOA5/CC LDLR and cIMT ($p = 0.010$). At the follow-up, the cohort also featured a mean BMI in the overweight range and a high mean waist circumference. We found no difference in the MedDiet adherence, physical activity, and smoking but an inverse correlation between the PREDIMED and the IPAQ scores with the IMT. In conclusion, this preliminary study provides insight into the predictive role of lipid profile during pregnancy and of some genetic variants on cIMT taken as a parameter of subclinical CVD susceptibility in GDM.

1. Introduction

Gestational diabetes mellitus (GDM) is defined as "diabetes diagnosed in the 2nd or 3rd trimester of pregnancy, with or without remission after end of pregnancy" [1]. GDM prevalence has been reported to vary between 1% and 28% [2] and is increasing, especially in developed countries [3]. GDM may have clinical implications for both maternal and fetal adverse outcomes and for the later development of type 2 diabetes in the years following pregnancy. In addition to type 2 diabetes, women with GDM are also at greater risk of overt cardiovascular disease (CVD) later in life. Several modifiable and unmodifiable risk factors are involved in the connection between GDM and subsequent CVD: these include hyperglycemia and impaired glucose tolerance, atherogenic lipid profiles, higher age, and elevated high-sensitivity C-reactive protein (CRP) [4]. Particularly, the development of diabetes purports an increased risk of developing later CVD [5, 6]. Nevertheless, mechanisms linking GDM and CVD are still unclear [6–11]. Metabolic impairments, including dyslipidemia and vascular dysfunction, are common later in life in women with previous GDM (pGDM) [12, 13]. In these women, elevated markers of inflammation, decreased levels of adiponectin, increased peripheral resistance, and decreased cardiac output have been detected [11]. Women with pGDM also have higher total cholesterol (TC), low-density lipoprotein cholesterol (LDL-C), and triglycerides (TG), as well as lower high-density lipoprotein cholesterol (HDL-C), compared with healthy women of the same age, suggesting that pGDM women have a greater susceptibility to be exposed to "an atherogenic insult" [14, 15]. Here, an obesogenic lifestyle (unhealthy diet and physical inactivity) and a genetic predisposition [16] likely explains the later development of CVD in most such women.

Carotid artery intima-media thickness (cIMT) is a subclinical measure of early atherosclerosis that strongly predicts heart disease and stroke, particularly in women [17, 18], and also predicts the development of CVD from GDM [4, 19].

Several studies recently carried out in women with pGDM have shown higher values of endothelial dysfunction markers and of cIMT in such women compared with controls, despite the absence of evident metabolic abnormalities [10, 19–21]. Previous studies of ours [22, 23] also showed a relationship between several nutrigenetic variants and cardiometabolic risk factors in women with or without GDM, suggesting the need to consider such factors in association with routinely assessed markers (such as lipid profile during pregnancy) for their role in the development of post-GDM CVD.

In this context, in the present study, we aimed to assess the joint predictive role of lipid profile during pregnancy and of some genetic variants on cIMT taken as a parameter of subclinical atherosclerosis and indicating an early susceptibility to CVD in a cohort of women with GDM history. If proven predictive, such prediction models would allow the planning of adequate primary cardiometabolic disease (CMD) prevention interventions in post-GDM women.

2. Materials and Methods

2.1. Study Design and Participants. Twenty-eight consecutive pGDM women attending the Diabetes and Metabolism Unit and the Obstetrics and Gynaecology Clinic, School of Medicine and Health Sciences, "G. d'Annunzio" University of Chieti-Hospital "SS Annunziata" of Chieti, were recruited. Socio-demographic characteristics and clinical parameters, such as blood glucose, TC, HDL-C, LDL-C, TG, and blood pressure, were collected. BMI was measured at the beginning (BMI 1) and at the end of pregnancy (BMI 2). A blood sample was obtained from each patient and nine single nucleotide polymorphisms (SNPs) from 9 genes related to nutrients and metabolism were included in the analysis.

All 28 women attended a 3-year-postpartum follow-up. Postpartum glucose tolerance (75 g oral glucose tolerance test (OGTT)) was assessed. Clinical parameters were collected in all subjects. Cardiovascular and metabolic markers were analyzed, including total, HDL, and LDL cholesterol levels; TG; homocysteine; and carotid artery IMT. In addition, HbA1C and fasting blood glucose were measured.

Adherence to the Mediterranean diet (MedDiet) was evaluated through a validated 14-item questionnaire (PREDIMED), which generates a range of possible scores namely (i) no adherence (score ≤ 5), (ii) medium adherence ($6 \leq$ score ≤ 9), and (iii) maximum adherence (score ≥ 10) [24]. In addition, physical activity (PA) was assessed using a *short version* of the International Physical Activity Questionnaire (IPAQ), comprising 7 items concerning PA, 4 relating to demographic information, and the remaining 6 about the comprehension of the questionnaire [25]. IPAQ registers three different levels of intensity (low, moderate, and high PA).

All participants gave their written informed consent prior to their inclusion in the study. The study was approved by the Ethics Committee of the "G. d'Annunzio" University, Chieti-Pescara, Italy.

2.2. Inclusion and Exclusion Criteria. The inclusion criteria admitted women with ≥18 years of age with pGDM. The GDM diagnosis was confirmed when established both at the 16–18th and the 24–28th weeks of gestation, according to the International Association of Diabetes and Pregnancy Study Groups (IADPSG) criteria [26].

The exclusion criteria were women with type 1 or 2 prepregnancy diabetes, overt diabetes, or monogenic diabetes, specifically GCK diabetes.

2.3. Gene and SNP Selection. The genetic analysis was conducted at the Laboratory of Molecular Genetics, School of Medicine and Health Sciences, "G. d'Annunzio" University of Chieti. A total of 9 SNPs previously associated in literature with obesity, lipid, and glucose metabolism were selected. These SNPs, on different loci, have been associated with cardiovascular disease in previous studies, under the assumption that these variants may also contribute to cardiovascular risk assessment [22, 23].

In particular, three of these variants, namely, rs7903146 (*C* > *T*) in *TCF7L2*, rs1801282 (*C* > *G*) in *PPARG2*, and rs8192678 (*C* > *T*) in *PPARGC1A* are involved in carbohydrate metabolism; other three, namely, rs662799 (*T* > *C*) in *APOA5*, rs2228671 (*C* > *T*) in *LDLR*, and rs1260326 (*C* > *T*) in *GCKR* are involved in fat metabolism. In addition, two other SNPs, rs9939609 (*T* > *A*) in *FTO* and rs17782313 (*T* > C) near *MC4R*, associated with hunger control, were also selected. Finally, rs1801133 (*C* > *T*) in *MTHFR*, involved in folate metabolism, was also genotyped. It is of great relevance that all the selected gene variants make up a panel of CVD

Table 1: Characteristics of patients during pregnancy.

Variable	$N = 28$
Age (yr), *mean* ± *SD*	35.3 ± 3.8
School education, *n(%)*	
Low school	2 (7.1)
High school	14 (50.0)
University degree	12 (42.9)
Marital status, *n(%)*	
Single	5 (17.9)
Married	23 (82.1)
Employment, *n(%)*	
Employed	18 (64.3)
Unemployed	10 (35.7)
Prepregnancy BMI (kg/m^2), *mean* ± *SD*	27.4 ± 7.1
BMI at OGTT (kg/m^2), *mean* ± *SD*	30.8 ± 6.9
BMI at the end of pregnancy (kg/m^2), *mean* ± *SD*	31.6 ± 5.8
Weight variation, *mean* ± *SD*	
OGTT vs prepregnancy (kg)	6.2 ± 4.7
Delivery vs prepregnancy (kg)	6.3 ± 5.9
Systolic blood pressure (mmHg), *mean* ± *SD*	113.0 ± 16.8
Diastolic blood pressure (mmHg), *mean* ± *SD*	72.2 ± 10.9
3rd LDL-C (mg/dl), *mean* ± *SD*	150.5 ± 56.4
3rd HDL-C (mg/dl), *mean* ± *SD*	68.8 ± 13.5
3rd TC (mg/dl), *mean* ± *SD*	273.4 ± 51.0
3rd TG (mg/dl), *mean* ± *SD*	242.7 ± 75.8
Smoking habit, *n(%)*	
No	20 (71.4)
Yes	2 (7.1)
Ex	6 (21.4)
OGTT, *mean* ± *SD*	
T0	94.5 ± 6.3
T60	161.8 ± 27.1
T120	134.6 ± 34.5
Fasting blood glucose (mg/dl), *mean* ± *SD*	83.0 ± 8.0
Family history of DM (1st degree), *n(%)*	12 (42.9)
Previous GDM, *n(%)*	5 (17.9)

markers, which could provide a unique opportunity to use genetic information in clinical practice to predict early CVD in pGDM women [22, 23].

All SNPs were genotyped by High Resolution Melting (HRM) analysis. HRM was performed on 96-well PikoReal Real-Time PCR System (Thermo Scientific™) using the Luminaris Color HRM Master Mix (Thermo Scientific™) according to the manufacturer's instructions, as previously described [22].

2.4. Carotid Intima-Media Thickness Assessment. Carotid intima-media thickness (cIMT) was assessed in the Institute of Cardiology, School of Medicine and Health Sciences, "G. d'Annunzio" University of Chieti.

Left and right intima-media thickness (IMT) was measured on common carotid posterior wall, 1 centimeter from bulb bifurcation on each side, according to the latest European Society of Cardiology (ESC) and European Society of Hypertension (ESH) guidelines [27].

All the exams were performed with a dedicated Esaote MyLab 30 Gold portable ultrasound, with a standard 7.5 MHz linear probe, provided with Quality Intima Media Thickness (QIMT™) software. The software uses radio frequency data processing signal in real time and ensures high accuracy and low intra- and interobserver variability [28]. One expert operator (FB) performed all the exams in a blinded fashion from genetics; before the automatic measurement of QIMT, a manual image acquisition of carotid vessels was obtained with each participant lying supine, with the neck hyperextended. At each patient was attributed the mean value between three measurements for QIMT. Concordance correlation coefficient between the three measurements was 0.99 (95% CI: 0.98-0.99).

2.5. Statistical Analysis. We estimated the minimum required sample size for the correlation analysis on the basis of previously observed data or published results. The minimum sample size ($n = 28$) was determined in order to obtain an expected correlation coefficient ($r = 0.5$) [20] between cIMT and lipid profile parameters with at least 80% of desired statistical power level and an alpha error rate of 5%.

The quantitative variables were summarized as mean and standard deviation (SD) or median and interquartile range (IQR), according to their distribution. Qualitative variables were summarized as frequency and percentage. Shapiro-Wilk's test was performed to evaluate the departures from normality distribution for each variable.

Lin's concordance correlation coefficient (CCC) was calculated along with the 95% confidence intervals of assessing the intraobserver reproducibility of measurements.

Nonparametric Kruskal-Wallis test was performed to test the effect of different APOA5 genotypes on levels of cIMT and on levels of TC, HDL-C, LDL-C, and TG.

The relationship between cIMT and TC, HDL-C, LDL-C, and TG at the 3rd trimester was explored by linear multiple regression analysis adjusted for age and BMI. The univariate regressions between cIMT and lipid profile at the 3rd trimester of pregnancy were reported graphically as a scattergram.

Hardy-Weinberg equilibrium (HWE) deviations in the genotype frequency distributions were calculated using the chi-square analysis.

The level of statistical significance was set at $p < 0.05$. Statistical analysis was performed using the Statistical Package for Social Science (SPSS) software for Windows (SPSS, Chicago, IL, USA) and Stata v14.1 (StataCorp, College Station, TX).

3. Results

The demographic and clinical characteristics of the cohort of women, both during pregnancy and at follow-up, are reported in Tables 1 and 2, respectively. A total of 28 women were included in the study. No difference has been

Table 2: Characteristics of patients at follow-up.

Variable	*N* = 28
Age (yr), *mean* ± *SD*	37.9 ± 4.2
Height (m), *mean* ± *SD*	1.60 ± 0.06
Weight (kg), *mean* ± *SD*	71.4 ± 20.7
BMI (kg/m^2), *mean* ± *SD*	26.7 ± 9.2
Waist circumference (cm), *mean* ± *SD*	86.2 ± 16.1
Systolic blood pressure (mmHg), *mean* ± *SD*	118.5 ± 14.4
Diastolic blood pressure (mmHg), *mean* ± *SD*	74.8 ± 8.9
LDL-C (mg/dl), *mean* ± *SD*	110.1 ± 30.4
HDL-C (mg/dl), *mean* ± *SD*	54.2 ± 12.7
TC (mg/dl), *mean* ± *SD*	186.5 ± 33.2
TG (mg/dl), *mean* ± *SD*	110.8 ± 72.1
Fasting blood glucose (mg/dl), *mean* ± *SD*	91.4 ± 9.5
OGTT (mg/dl), *mean* ± *SD*	
T0	95.6 ± 9.4
T60	133.9 ± 35.7
T120	106.7 ± 24.4
HbA1C (mmol/mol), *mean* ± *SD*	35.4 ± 4.1
IPAQ, *n(%)*	
Low	14 (50.0)
Moderate	9 (32.1)
High	5 (17.9)
PREDIMED, *median* (Q_1-Q_3)	7.5 (6.0–9.0)
cIMT (mm), *mean* ± *SD*	0.51 ± 0.09
Homocisteina, *mean* ± *SD*	9.6 ± 3.1

found in the adherence to the MedDiet, PA, and smoking among the sample.

Although not statistically significant, an inverse correlation between the PREDIMED and the IPAQ scores with the cIMT values was found (Rho = −0.060, $p = 0.768$ and Rho = −0.276, $p = 0.163$, respectively). In addition, our results showed a connection between the women's waist circumference and cIMT values (Rho = 0.378, $p = 0.057$) at the follow-up, which, however, does not reach a statistical significance.

Furthermore, a significant positive relation between the 3rd trimester TG and cIMT (Rho = 0.468; $p = 0.014$) was found (Figure 1). The genotype distribution of investigated SNPs in patients is reported in Table 3. All the investigated genotype frequencies were within the Hardy-Weinberg ?equilibrium range (χ^2 test p value > 0.05). Also, a significant association was found in the codominant model (TT vs. TC vs. CC) between APOA5 CC genotype and cIMT after adjustments for age and BMI (0.50 ± 0.07 vs 0.48 ± 0.08 vs 0.65 ± 0.08; $p = 0.045$) (Figure 2). Finally, a significant association between the interaction CC APOA5/CC LDLR and cIMT ($p = 0.010$) has been observed.

No statistically significant differences were found among the 3rd trimester lipid profile, PREDIMED, and IPAQ scores in different APOA5 genotypes.

No other significant differences were detected with respect to other genes.

4. Discussion

The main aim of the present study was to assess the joint predictive role of lipid profile during pregnancy and of some genetic variants, cIMT taken as a parameter of subclinical atherosclerosis, and indicating an early susceptibility to CVD in a cohort of women with GDM history. Another aim was to examine new nutrigenetic markers as well as traditional parameters to predict early subclinical atherosclerosis in pGDM and to plan adequate early prevention interventions.

Several routine parameters and biochemical markers are currently available to quantify the risk in pGDM women to develop diabetes after pregnancy [3]. Although the incidence of CVD events in young women is low, an early identification of possible CMD risk may provide an irreplaceable opportunity for well-timed intervention and timely prevention. In order to reduce not only the occurrence of diabetes but also its subsequent cardiovascular complications, it is necessary to improve the provision of postpartum follow-ups. In fact, many authors have highlighted the close relationship between common CVD risk factors and a GDM history. In addition to traditional parameters, cIMT and arterial stiffness (RFQAS) values can be significant in assessing the risk for heart disease and strokes [18]. Bo et al. [20] measured cIMT in 82 women with a history of GDM and 113 without one, 6.5 years after delivery: their study showed that women with pGDM, regardless of their BMI and the presence of metabolic abnormalities, displayed remarkably higher E-selectin, ICAM-1, and IMT values than controls. IMT proved to be significantly associated with pGDM in a regression model, after adjustments for BMI, waist circumference, blood pressure, and glucose values. Volpe et al. [21] measured cIMT in 28 women with and 24 without a history of GDM 2 years after delivery, finding that young women with pGDM presented early signs of vessel involvement, albeit within upper normal levels. GDM and control groups differed in terms of their main metabolic syndrome components, such as waist circumference, blood pressure, fasting plasma glucose, and TG, all significantly higher in GDM women than in the control group.

Kaul et al. [29] observed that GDM was associated with 1.4 times higher rates of CVD. Then, Retnakaran and Shah [11] confirmed similar results, noting that women with GDM have an elevated risk of bad cardiovascular outcomes, even in the absence of type 2 diabetes.

Hypertriglyceridemia and low HDL-C are known to be characteristic traits of type 2 diabetes. It may not be surprising that in our previous studies their presence was detected in women with pGDM. Although the CV risk implications of hypertriglyceridemia and low HDL-C remain controversial, the CV significance of LDL-C and its main lipoprotein (apolipoprotein B (apoB)) is well established [30]. In our previous studies, GDM women showed significantly higher serum concentrations of TC and LDL-C during the 3rd trimester than the control group, and a significant correlation was

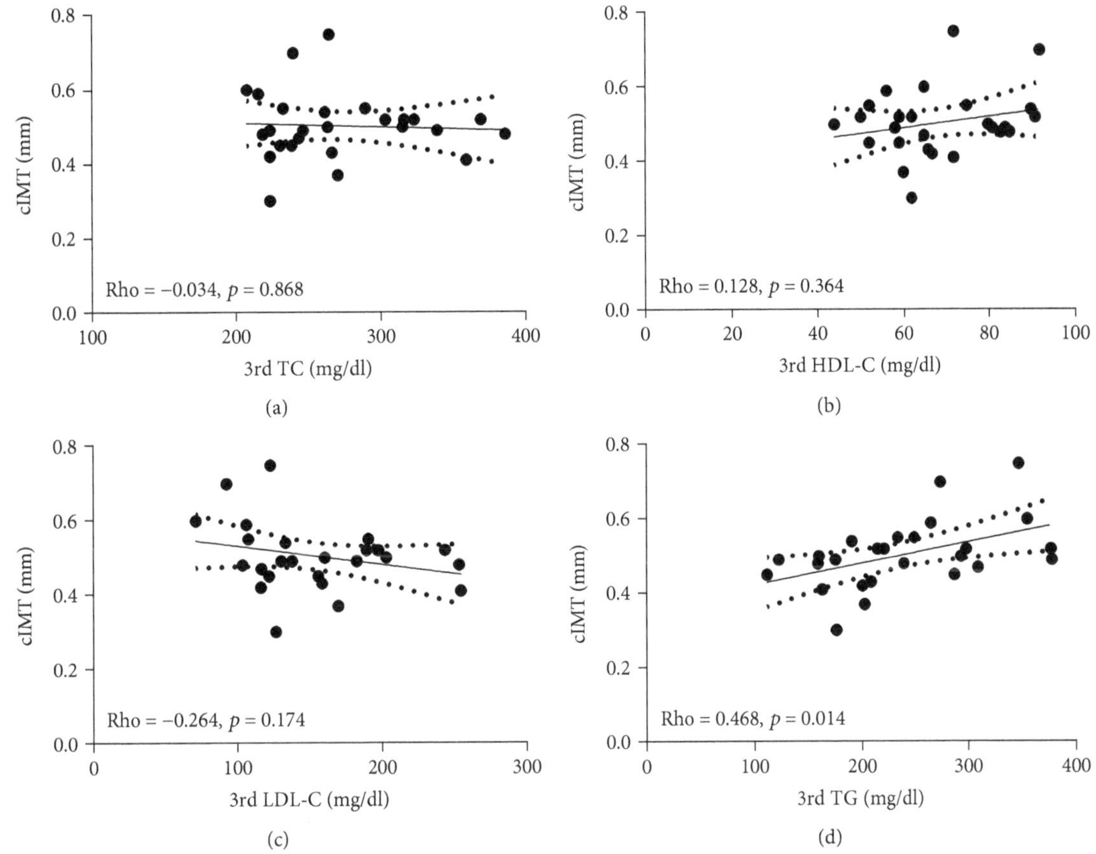

FIGURE 1: Nonparametric correlation analysis between cIMT and lipid profile during 3rd trimester of pregnancy.

TABLE 3: Genotypes distribution.

Genotype n (%)				No carrier	Carrier	HWE (p value)
TCF7L2	CC	CT	TT	CC	CT + TT	
rs7903146 (C > T)	8 (28.6)	10 (35.7)	10 (35.7)	8 (28.6)	20 (71.4)	*0.095*
PPARG2	CC	CG	GG	CC	CG + GG	
rs1801282 (C > G)	21 (75.0)	7 (25.0)	—	21 (75.0)	7 (25.0)	*0.389*
PPARGC1A	CC	CT	TT	CC	CT + TT	
rs8192678 (C > T)	9 (32.1)	16 (57.1)	3 (10.7)	9 (32.1)	19 (87.8)	*0.460*
APOA5	TT	CT	CC	TT	CT + CC	
rs662799 (T > C)	13 (46.4)	12 (42.9)	3 (10.7)	13 (46.4)	15 (53.6)	*0.857*
MC4R	TT	CT	CC	TT	CT + CC	
rs17782313 (T > C)	19 (67.9)	6 (21.4)	3 (10.7)	19 (67.9)	9 (32.1)	*0.099*
LDLR	CC	CT	TT	CC	CT + TT	
rs2228671 (C > T)	22 (78.6)	6 (21.4)	—	22 (78.6)	6 (21.4)	*0.460*
GCKR	CC	CT	TT	CC	CT + TT	
rs1260326 (C > T)	4 (14.3)	16 (57.1)	8 (28.6)	4 (14.3)	24 (85.7)	*0.293*
FTO	TT	TA	AA	TT	TA + AA	
rs9939609 (T > A)	8 (28.6)	10 (35.7)	10 (35.7)	8 (28.6)	20 (71.4)	*0.509*
MTHFR	CC	CT	TT	CC	CT + TT	
rs1801133 (C > T)	5 (17.9)	18 (64.3)	5 (17.9)	5 (17.9)	23 (82.1)	*0.190*

HWE − Hardy-Weinberg equilibrium.

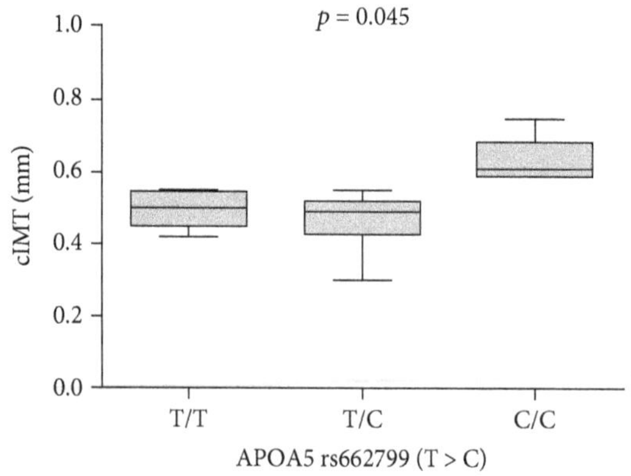

FIGURE 2: Box-whisker graphs of cIMT values with respect to APOA5 genotypes. Box-whisker plots show the 25th and 75th percentile range (box) with Tukey 95% confidence intervals (whiskers) and median values (transverse lines in the box). p value in figure is relative to Kruskal-Wallis test.

observed between lipid parameters and some polymorphisms in genes APOA5 and LDLR; also, TG were higher in GDM women than controls, although not reaching statistical significance [23]. Interestingly, in our present study, an association between 3rd trimester TG and cIMT has been found ($p = 0.014$).

These remarkable results echo those of Di Cianni et al. [31], who reported that TC, TG, LDL-C, glucose, and systolic blood pressure were all significantly higher among the GDM cohort, suggesting a condition similar to the metabolic syndrome occurring in these women. These peculiar changes in lipoprotein profile may favour endothelial damage in pregnancy [32, 33]. The GDM lipid profile is very similar to the one accompanying the insulin resistance in the metabolic syndrome. More recently, Gongora and Wenger [34] showed that women with GDM have a more atherogenic lipid profile by three months postpartum, characterized by an increase of cIMT compared to controls and that the risk of developing metabolic syndrome increased by up to 10% in those with pGDM.

It is known that pregnancy is a stress test, as hyperglycemia seems to have a significant impact on the CV system during this limited period [35]; we could hypothesize that lipid pattern modifications during pregnancy with GDM are an injury which results in a possible susceptibility to future CVD risk. Unfortunately, the mechanisms involved in an increased risk of CVD in pGDM need to be further investigated. GDM women's lipid profile displays a preponderance of small dense LDL particles; also, they present an increased susceptibility of LDL oxidation during pregnancy [30].

These data reveal the necessity of monitoring women with GDM adequately and long term, to prevent both CVD and diabetes risks. Unfortunately, several studies showed low rates of postdelivery glucose testing [36, 37]. It should be emphasised that, to date, the postpartum screening of women with pGDM is still suboptimal [3]; therefore, this issue also prompts the need to identify a practical and feasible tool which ideally should include panel genes and routine clinical and metabolic parameters, to identify GDM women at high risk of diabetes and CVD [23] and summon them for follow-ups. Previous investigations highlighted that women with pGDM have an increased risk of CVD later in life as a result of a combination of genetic factors and gene-diet interaction.

Furthermore, it is essential to define the characteristics of the studied gene variants. Interestingly, a previous Italian study showed that APOA5-1131T > C may affect the risk of early-onset myocardial infarction (MI), with an odds ratio of 1.44 (CI: 1.23–1.69) per C allele [38]. Apolipoprotein A-V gene, as described for the first time in 2001, is located proximal to the APOAI, APOCIII, and APOA-IV gene cluster on human 11q23 [39]. APOA5 encodes apolipoprotein (apo) AV, which is expressed in the liver and circulates on chylomicrons (CM), very low density lipoproteins (VLDL), and HDL. Common genetic variants of the apolipoprotein gene family members are related to variations in serum lipid levels.

Recently, a meta-analysis [40] showed that the APOA5 rs662799 C allele is associated with elevated circulating TG levels, regardless of ethnicity, indicating a possible mediating role for circulating TG in the association between the risk variant at APOA5 and the atherosclerotic process [41, 42]. This variant was correlated with not only higher plasma TG but also with lower HDL-C levels by our [22, 23] and other groups [38, 43]. Emerging data about APOA5-1131T > C suggested that APOA5 gene may have a direct effect above and beyond its effect on TG but, until now, needs to be confirmed by further studies [38]. In the Framingham Heart Study, an almost 2-fold increased risk of CVD was observed in females carrying the C allele of the −1131T > C [44]. Moreover, the relationship with IMT was observed for the rare allele of the −1131T > C SNP in overweight and obese subjects [45, 46].

Qiao et al. [47] observed that in type 2 diabetes patients, TG levels and the TG/HDL-C ratio were greater in those with TC and CC genotypes than in those with TT genotype subjects ($p < 0.05$). In addition, diabetic patients with CC genotype had greater carotid IMT than those with TT genotype ($p = 0.080$), although these data do not reach statistical significance.

We found a significant association between APOA5 CC genotype and cIMT ($p = 0.045$). Current evidence indicates that the increased risk of CVD is influenced by a merging of modifiable risk factors, ages, and/or genetics; however, the proportion of the contribution of these factors in modulating is still debated. Our findings suggest that even though the age of our study cohort was very young, women with C genotype probably experience the disadvantage of such genetic factor leading to CVD susceptibility in the form of a cIMT increase.

LDLR gene can regulate cholesterol metabolism. Among the several genetic variants identified at LDLR locus, the rs2228671 has been intensively studied and it has shown the strongest association with total and LDL-C levels across multiple populations [48–50] with the T allele being associated consistently, to a decreased risk of CAD [48]. Our previous findings are consistent with the previous literature; in fact, we showed that carriers of the rs2228671 T allele were significantly associated with the 3rd trimester LDL-C levels in GDM women [22, 23].

Furthermore, we observed a significant association between CC APOA5/CC LDLR interaction and cIMT ($p = 0.010$). Surprisingly, women with CC genotype in APOA5 rs662799 in the absence of the T protective allele of LDLR rs2228671 present a cIMT increase. It would be interesting to further investigate the causal molecular mechanism underlying this interaction. We could hypothesize that the interaction effect of LDLR rs2228671 and APOA5 rs662799 implies a probable mitigation on cIMT values.

As expressed by Mecacci et al. [35], GDM can be considered as a "window into future health" in which it is advisable to adopt a healthy lifestyle to prevent or delay diabetes and/or CVD development postpartum.

In our previous study [23], we found that women with GDM had a greater BMI than the control group both in pre-pregnancy and at the end of pregnancy. In the present study, we analyzed women's lifestyle at follow-up: the pGDM women had a mean BMI that falls within the overweight range, as well as a high mean waist circumference (86.2 ± 16.1 cm). Moreover, no difference of adherence to the MedDiet, PA, and smoking was observed, although an inverse correlation between both the PREDIMED and the IPAQ scores with the cIMT values was found. This is an interesting feature supporting the potential role of preventive intervention. In fact, we noted that our cohort had a median MedDiet score of 7.5 (medium adherence), suggesting a poor adherence to healthy nutritional habits; also, a high percentage of them reported lower levels of PA. These modifiable risk factors can be easily acted upon to allow for early cardiovascular prevention.

In this view, tailored nutrition and lifestyle prescription represent a promising strategy for the prevention and management of metabolic syndrome [51]. In this regard, the main goals are a correct identification and stratification of GDM women at risk for CVD and an evaluation of the preventive strategies, as well as the improvement of postpartum screening.

Longer-term studies are indicated to define a potential role of lifestyle intervention [4]. Follow-up after GDM could be enhanced by similar quality and accountability measures requiring that patients and clinicians discuss future risks and referral to primary care as a standard of practice [36].

To our knowledge, this is the first study using multisectoral innovative biomarkers to evaluate the cardiometabolic risk in pGDM. Therefore, women with pGDM could be enrolled in follow-up programs designed to ensure continuous monitoring, thus providing effective prevention of both type 2 diabetes and CVD [7, 15].

It would be clinically valuable to have a risk marker during pregnancy so that long-term follow-ups and appropriate strategies of interventions can be focused on the women at greatest risk in a timely manner [52].

This study has some limitations. First of all, the sample size: this may have limited the statistical significance of metabolic and vascular function data. Second, non-pGDM women have not been involved. The present research is a preliminary small-scale study to evaluate the joint predictive role of lipid profile during pregnancy and of some genetic variants on cIMT taken as a parameter of subclinical atherosclerosis in a cohort of women with GDM history. Results obtained about the potential role of routine biomarkers and nutrigenetic variants in our small sample could be validated in a larger study.

However, our study provides a remarkable insight into the potential predictive role of both genetic factors and 3rd trimester lipid profile for CVD susceptibility in pGDM. It will be crucial to replicate and expand our findings and further studies are warranted for better understanding of the potential gene-gene and gene-environment interactions, thus attributing a significant prognostic role to new and old biomarkers during pregnancy.

Conflicts of Interest

The authors declare that there is no conflict of interests associated with this manuscript.

Authors' Contributions

The study was designed by EV, LS, RDC, and MF. CC and ML contributed to clinical evaluation and support to the recruitment of patients. MF, FF, MDN, and EV contributed to data acquisition, analysis, and interpretation. The experiments were performed by MF. Nutritional status was assessed by FF. Carotid intima-media thickness was assessed by FB. The manuscript was drafted by MF, FF, and EV. DM contributed to data analysis. MDN was the statistician that performed the statistical analyses; she also helped in the drafting and editing of the manuscript. All authors were involved in critical revision and approved the final version of the manuscript before submission. EV, LS, and MDN are the guarantors of this work and, as such, had full access to all the data in the study and take responsibility for the integrity of the data and the accuracy of the data analysis. Marica Franzago and Federica Fraticelli contributed equally to this work.

References

[1] American Diabetes Association (ADA), "Standards of medical care in diabetes—2018," *Diabetes Care*, vol. 41, Supplement 1, pp. S13–S27, 2018.

[2] M. Hod, A. Kapur, D. A. Sacks et al., "The International Federation of Gynecology and Obstetrics (FIGO) initiative on gestational diabetes mellitus: a pragmatic guide for diagnosis, management, and care," *International Journal of Gynecology & Obstetrics*, vol. 131, Supplement 3, pp. S173–S211, 2015.

[3] S. Burlina, M. G. Dalfrà, and A. Lapolla, "Clinical and biochemical approach to predicting post-pregnancy metabolic decompensation," *Diabetes Research and Clinical Practice*, 2018.

[4] J. Harreiter, G. Dovjak, and A. Kautzky-Willer, "Gestational diabetes mellitus and cardiovascular risk after pregnancy," *Womens Health*, vol. 10, no. 1, pp. 91–108, 2014.

[5] M. J. Legato, A. Gelzer, R. Goland et al., "Gender-specific care of the patient with diabetes: review and recommendations," *Gender Medicine*, vol. 3, no. 2, pp. 131–158, 2006.

[6] D. K. Tobias, J. J. Stuart, S. Li et al., "Association of history of gestational diabetes with long-term cardiovascular disease risk in a large prospective cohort of US women," *JAMA Internal Medicine*, vol. 177, no. 12, pp. 1735–1742, 2017.

[7] B. Daly, K. A. Toulis, N. Thomas et al., "Increased risk of ischemic heart disease, hypertension, and type 2 diabetes in women with previous gestational diabetes mellitus, a target group in general practice for preventive interventions: a population-based cohort study," *PLoS Medicine*, vol. 15, no. 1, article e1002488, 2018.

[8] D. B. Carr, K. M. Utzschneider, R. L. Hull et al., "Gestational diabetes mellitus increases the risk of cardiovascular disease in women with a family history of type 2 diabetes," *Diabetes Care*, vol. 29, no. 9, pp. 2078–2083, 2006.

[9] B. R. Shah, R. Retnakaran, and G. L. Booth, "Increased risk of cardiovascular disease in young women following gestational diabetes mellitus," *Diabetes Care*, vol. 31, no. 8, pp. 1668-1669, 2008.

[10] E. P. Gunderson, V. Chiang, M. J. Pletcher et al., "History of gestational diabetes mellitus and future risk of atherosclerosis in mid-life: the Coronary Artery Risk Development in Young Adults study," *Journal of the American Heart Association*, vol. 3, no. 2, article e000490, 2014.

[11] R. Retnakaran and B. R. Shah, "Role of type 2 diabetes in determining retinal, renal and cardiovascular outcomes in women with previous gestational diabetes mellitus," *Diabetes Care*, vol. 40, no. 1, pp. 101–108, 2017.

[12] S. M. Heitritter, C. G. Solomon, G. F. Mitchell, N. Skali-Ounis, and E. W. Seely, "Subclinical inflammation and vascular dysfunction in women with previous gestational diabetes mellitus," *The Journal of Clinical Endocrinology and Metabolism*, vol. 90, no. 7, pp. 3983–3988, 2005.

[13] M. Edwards, S. Meltzer, E. Rahme, and K. Dasgupta, "Predictors of postpartum lipid abnormalities in women with gestational diabetes," *Canadian Journal of Diabetes*, vol. 36, no. 6, pp. 305–309, 2012.

[14] A. C. O'Higgins, V. O'Dwyer, C. O'Connor, S. F. Daly, B. T. Kinsley, and M. J. Turner, "Postpartum dyslipidaemia in women diagnosed with gestational diabetes mellitus," *Irish Journal of Medical Science*, vol. 186, no. 2, pp. 403–407, 2017.

[15] G. Di Cianni, E. Lacaria, C. Lencioni, and V. Resi, "Preventing type 2 diabetes and cardiovascular disease in women with gestational diabetes - the evidence and potential strategies," *Diabetes Research and Clinical Practice*, 2018.

[16] K. Goueslard, J. Cottenet, A. S. Mariet et al., "Early cardiovascular events in women with a history of gestational diabetes mellitus," *Cardiovascular Diabetology*, vol. 15, no. 1, p. 15, 2016.

[17] E. B. Mathiesen, S. H. Johnsen, T. Wilsgaard, K. H. Bønaa, M. L. Løchen, and I. Njølstad, "Carotid plaque area and intima-media thickness in prediction of first-ever ischemic stroke: a 10-year follow-up of 6584 men and women: the Tromsø study," *Stroke*, vol. 42, no. 4, pp. 972–978, 2011.

[18] S. H. Johnsen, E. B. Mathiesen, O. Joakimsen et al., "Carotid atherosclerosis is a stronger predictor of myocardial infarction in women than in men: a 6-year follow-up study of 6226 persons: the Tromsø study," *Stroke*, vol. 38, no. 11, pp. 2873–2880, 2007.

[19] J. W. Li, S. Y. He, P. Liu, L. Luo, L. Zhao, and Y. B. Xiao, "Association of gestational diabetes mellitus (GDM) with subclinical atherosclerosis: a systemic review and meta-analysis," *BMC Cardiovascular Disorders*, vol. 14, no. 1, 2014.

[20] S. Bo, S. Valpreda, G. Menato et al., "Should we consider gestational diabetes a vascular risk factor?," *Atherosclerosis*, vol. 194, no. 2, pp. e72–e79, 2007.

[21] L. Volpe, I. Cuccuru, C. Lencioni et al., "Early subclinical atherosclerosis in women with previous gestational diabetes mellitus," *Diabetes Care*, vol. 31, no. 5, article e32, 2008.

[22] M. Franzago, F. Fraticelli, A. Nicolucci et al., "Molecular analysis of a genetic variants panel related to nutrients and metabolism: association with susceptibility to gestational diabetes and cardiometabolic risk in affected women," *Journal Diabetes Research*, vol. 2017, article 4612623, 7 pages, 2017.

[23] M. Franzago, F. Fraticelli, D. Marchetti et al., "Nutrigenetic variants and cardio-metabolic risk in women with or without gestational diabetes," *Diabetes Research and Clinical Practice*, vol. 137, pp. 64–71, 2018.

[24] M. A. Martínez-González, A. García-Arellano, E. Toledo et al., "A 14-item Mediterranean diet assessment tool and obesity indexes among high risk subjects: the PREDIMED trial," *PLoS One*, vol. 7, no. 8, article e43134, 2012.

[25] A. Mannocci, D. Di Thiene, A. Del Cimmuto et al., "International physical activity questionnaire: validation and assessment in an Italian sample," *Italian Journal of Public Health*, vol. 7, no. 4, pp. 369–376, 2010.

[26] International Association of Diabetes and Pregnancy Study Groups Consensus Panel, "International association of diabetes and pregnancy study groups recommendations on the diagnosis and classification of hyperglycemia in pregnancy," *Diabetes Care*, vol. 33, no. 3, pp. 676–682, 2010.

[27] G. Mancia, R. Fagard, K. Narkiewicz et al., "2013 ESH/ESC practice guidelines for the management of arterial hypertension," *Blood Pressure*, vol. 23, no. 1, pp. 3–16, 2014.

[28] L. Di Geso, E. M. Zardi, A. Afeltra et al., "Comparison between conventional and automated software-guided ultrasound assessment of bilateral common carotids intima-media thickness in patients with rheumatic diseases," *Clinical Rheumatology*, vol. 31, no. 5, pp. 881–884, 2012.

[29] P. Kaul, A. Savu, K. A. Nerenberg et al., "Impact of gestational diabetes mellitus and high maternal weight on the development of diabetes, hypertension and cardiovascular disease: a population level analysis," *Diabetic Medicine*, vol. 32, no. 2, pp. 164–173, 2015.

[30] R. Retnakaran, "Hyperglycemia in pregnancy and its implications for a woman's future risk of cardiovascular disease," *Diabetes Research and Clinical Practice*, 2018.

[31] G. Di Cianni, R. Miccoli, L. Volpe, C. Lencioni, and S. Del Prato, "Intermediate metabolism in normal pregnancy and in gestational diabetes," *Diabetes/Metabolism Research and Reviews*, vol. 19, no. 4, pp. 259–270, 2003.

[32] N. Sattar, A. Bendomir, C. Berry, J. Shepherd, I. A. Greer, and C. J. Packard, "Lipoprotein subfraction concentrations in preeclampsia: pathogenic parallels to atherosclerosis," *Obstetrics & Gynecology*, vol. 89, no. 3, pp. 403–408, 1997.

[33] G. León-Reyes, R. F. Maida-Claros, A. X. Urrutia-Medina et al., "Oxidative profiles of LDL and HDL isolated from

women with preeclampsia," *Lipids in Health and Disease*, vol. 16, no. 1, p. 90, 2017.

[34] M. C. Gongora and N. K. Wenger, "Cardiovascular complications of pregnancy," *International Journal of Molecular Sciences*, vol. 16, no. 10, pp. 23905–23928, 2015.

[35] F. Mecacci, S. Ottanelli, and F. Petraglia, "Mothers with HIP - the short term and long-term impact, what is new?," *Diabetes Research and Clinical Practice*, vol. 18, article 30532-1, 2018.

[36] J. A. Bernstein, E. Quinn, O. Ameli et al., "Follow-up after gestational diabetes: a fixable gap in women's preventive healthcare," *BMJ Open Diabetes Research & Care*, vol. 5, no. 1, article e000445, 2017.

[37] S. Poola-Kella, R. A. Steinman, B. Mesmar, and R. Malek, "Gestational diabetes mellitus: post-partum risk and follow up," *Reviews on Recent Clinical Trials*, vol. 13, no. 1, pp. 5–14, 2018.

[38] R. De Caterina, P. J. Talmud, P. A. Merlini et al., "Strong association of the *APOA5*-1131T>C gene variant and earlyonset acute myocardial infarction," *Atherosclerosis*, vol. 214, no. 2, pp. 397–403, 2011.

[39] L. A. Pennacchio, M. Olivier, J. A. Hubacek et al., "An apolipoprotein influencing triglycerides in humans and mice revealed by comparative sequencing," *Science*, vol. 294, no. 5540, pp. 169–173, 2001.

[40] Y. Pi, L. Zhang, Q. Yang et al., "Apolipoprotein A5 gene promoter region-1131T/C polymorphism is associated with risk of ischemic stroke and elevated triglyceride levels: a meta-analysis," *Cerebrovascular Diseases*, vol. 33, no. 6, pp. 558–565, 2012.

[41] Z. Zhang, B. Peng, R. Gong et al., "Apolipoprotein A5 polymorphisms and risk of coronary artery disease: a meta-analysis," *Bioscience Trends*, vol. 5, no. 4, pp. 165–172, 2011.

[42] A. Au, L. R. Griffiths, L. Irene, C. W. Kooi, and L. K. Wei, "The impact of APOA5, APOB, APOC3 and ABCA1 gene polymorphisms on ischemic stroke: evidence from a meta-analysis," *Atherosclerosis*, vol. 265, pp. 60–70, 2017.

[43] Y. W. Yin, Q. Q. Sun, P. J. Wang et al., "Genetic polymorphism of apolipoprotein A5 gene and susceptibility to type 2 diabetes mellitus: a meta-analysis of 15,137 subjects," *PLoS One*, vol. 9, no. 2, article e89167, 2014.

[44] C. Q. Lai, S. Demissie, L. A. Cupples et al., "Influence of the APOA5 locus on plasma triglyceride, lipoprotein subclasses, and CVD risk in the Framingham Heart Study," *Journal of Lipid Research*, vol. 45, no. 11, pp. 2096–2105, 2004.

[45] R. Elosua, J. M. Ordovas, L. A. Cupples et al., "Variability at the *APOA5* locus is associated with carotid atherosclerosis with a modifying effect of obesity: the Framingham Heart Study," *Journal of Lipid Research*, vol. 47, no. 5, pp. 990–996, 2006.

[46] M. Guardiola, M. Cofán, I. de Castro-Oros et al., "APOA5 variants predispose hyperlipidemic patients to atherogenic dyslipidemia and subclinical atherosclerosis," *Atherosclerosis*, vol. 240, no. 1, pp. 98–104, 2015.

[47] Y. Qiao, R. Liu, H. M. Tian, Y. Liu, O. Qiang, and B. W. Liu, "Association of apolipoprotein A5 gene -1131T/C polymorphism with serum lipids and carotid intima-media thickness in patients with type 2 diabetes mellitus," *Sichuan Da Xue Xue Bao Yi Xue Ban*, vol. 39, no. 6, pp. 965–8, 999, 2008.

[48] P. Linsel-Nitschke, A. Götz, J. Erdmann et al., "Lifelong reduction of LDL-cholesterol related to a common variant in the LDL-receptor gene decreases the risk of coronary artery disease—a Mendelian randomisation study," *PLoS One*, vol. 3, no. 8, article e2986, 2008.

[49] N. Martinelli, D. Girelli, B. Lunghi et al., "Polymorphisms at LDLR locus may be associated with coronary artery disease through modulation of coagulation factor VIII activity and independently from lipid profile," *Blood*, vol. 116, no. 25, pp. 5688–5697, 2010.

[50] H. Ye, Q. Zhao, Y. Huang et al., "Meta-analysis of low density lipoprotein receptor (LDLR) rs2228671 polymorphism and coronary heart disease," *BioMed Research International*, vol. 2014, Article ID 564940, 6 pages, 2014.

[51] J. de Toro-Martín, B. Arsenault, J.-P. Després, and M.-C. Vohl, "Precision nutrition: a review of personalized nutritional approaches for the prevention and management of metabolic syndrome," *Nutrients*, vol. 9, no. 8, 2017.

[52] H. Fadl, A. Magnuson, I. Östlund, S. Montgomery, U. Hanson, and E. Schwarcz, "Gestational diabetes mellitus and later cardiovascular disease: a Swedish population based case-control study," *BJOG*, vol. 121, no. 12, pp. 1530–1536, 2014.

19

Depressive Symptoms in Women with Gestational Diabetes Mellitus: The LINDA-Brazil Study

Patrícia Damé,[1] Kadhija Cherubini,[1] Pâmella Goveia,[1] Geórgia Pena,[1] Leony Galliano,[2] Cristina Façanha,[3,4] and Maria Angélica Nunes[1]

[1]*Postgraduate Program in Epidemiology, School of Medicine, Federal University of Rio Grande do Sul, Porto Alegre, RS, Brazil*
[2]*Postgraduate Program in Physical Education, Superior School of Physical Education, Federal University of Pelotas, Pelotas, RS, Brazil*
[3]*Integrated Center for Diabetes and Hypertension, Ceará State Health Department, Fortaleza, CE, Brazil*
[4]*School of Medicine, Unichristus University Center, Fortaleza, CE, Brazil*

Correspondence should be addressed to Maria Angélica Nunes; maanunes@gmail.com

Academic Editor: Basilio Pintaudi

This study aimed to assess the frequency and severity of depressive symptoms and their relationship with sociodemographic characteristics in women with gestational diabetes mellitus (GDM) who participated in the LINDA-Brazil study. We conducted cross-sectional analyses of 820 women with GDM who were receiving prenatal care in the public health system. We conducted structured interviews to obtain clinical and sociodemographic information and applied the Edinburgh Postnatal Depression Scale (EPDS) to assess depressive symptoms. We classified the presence and severity of depressive symptoms using scores of ≥12 and ≥18, respectively. We used Poisson regression to estimate prevalence ratios (PR). Most of the women lived with a partner (88%), 50% were between 30 and 39 years old, 39% had finished high school, 39% had a family income of 1-2 minimum wages, and 47% were obese before their pregnancies. The presence of depressive symptoms was observed in 31% of the women, and severe depressive symptoms were observed in 10%; 8.3% reported self-harm intent. Lower parity and higher educational levels were associated with lower EPDS score. Depressive symptoms were common and frequently severe among women with GDM, indicating the need to consider this situation when treating such women, especially those who are more socially vulnerable. This trial is registered with NCT02327286, registered on 23 December 2014.

1. Introduction

Pregnancy is one of life's most important events, involving social, psychological, and hormonal changes [1]. It is also a time of great vulnerability to the development of mental disorders, especially depressive disorders [2]. Maternal depression has been linked to negative health-related behaviors and associated with morbidity and mortality [2]. This disorder is a major health problem for women of all nationalities. In a review of depression in pregnant women, prevalence rates were found to be 7.4%, 12.8%, and 12.0% in the first, second, and third trimesters, respectively [1]. It is estimated that 25% to 35% of women have depressive symptoms during pregnancy, and up to 20% of them may meet the criteria for major depression in low- and middle-income countries [3]. In a systematic review of 51 studies (with 48,904 participants), 20 of which were conducted in low- and middle-income countries, depression ranged from 17.3% to 57% [2]. Studies in Brazil showed prevalence ranging from 17.3% to 37.9% [2].

Studies that have aimed to assess depression in women with gestational diabetes are rare in the literature. Gestational diabetes mellitus (GDM), a hyperglycemic state detected during pregnancy, is an established risk factor for diabetes [4]. Diabetes is a major cause of morbidity and mortality and is one of the four main chronic diseases identified by the World Health Organization as a focus for prevention and control [5]. GDM also causes adverse outcomes and is related to depressive symptoms, which may affect adherence to treatment and compound pregnancy outcomes. Since GDM and depressive symptoms may have adverse effects on mothers and their children, it is important to investigate the factors related to the presence of depressive symptoms among women with gestational diabetes.

Thus, this study aimed to assess the frequency and severity of depressive symptoms according to the Edinburgh Postnatal Depression Scale (EPDS) and their relationship to clinical and sociodemographic characteristics in the women with GDM who participated in the LINDA-Brazil study.

2. Methods

2.1. Setting and Sample. We studied 820 women with GDM who were receiving care at tertiary prenatal care facilities within the Brazilian National Health System in 2014 and 2015 in three cities: Porto Alegre, Fortaleza, and Pelotas. This was a cross-sectional study developed during the recruitment for a large clinical trial called LINDA-Brazil, a multicenter-randomized clinical trial that aimed to evaluate the effectiveness of a lifestyle intervention program in preventing type 2 diabetes after pregnancies complicated by GDM in women identified as being at higher risk. The design of the LINDA-Brazil study has been described elsewhere [4].

Eligibility criteria included being 18 years or older, having been diagnosed with GDM, and living within an easily accessible distance to the trial sites, which were located in urban and rural areas of Fortaleza, Pelotas, and Porto Alegre and their metropolitan areas. During the first contact, the study's protocol was explained and an initial signed consent form was obtained.

2.2. Measurements. Data on sociodemographic and anthropometric characteristics as well as gestational age, obstetric history (abortion and parity), and GDM diagnosis and treatment were obtained through interviews at the prenatal clinics and reviews of medical records. Socioeconomic status was determined using two indicators: educational level and household income. We used multiples of the minimum wage to measure household income. The minimum wage is the lowest amount an employer can legally pay employees per month. In Brazil, one minimum wage is equivalent to 300 U.S. dollars.

Depressive symptoms during the previous seven days were assessed using the Edinburgh Postnatal Depression Scale (EPDS) and were rated on a scale of 0–30. The EPDS is one of the most widely used screening questionnaires for pregnant and postpartum women and has been validated to Brazilian Portuguese [6].

We conducted interviews during gestation at referral centers for women with high-risk pregnancies before or after their doctor appointments. Structured questionnaires were applied face-to-face by trained interviewers. The questionnaires took approximately 20 minutes to complete, and it took about five minutes to apply the EPDS, which consists of a ten-question questionnaire and is supported by a card with multiple-choice answers to avoid constraints.

A diagnosis of gestational diabetes was made according to the diagnostic criteria used at each center. The criteria were frequently based on a two-step approach (a fasting plasma glucose test followed by an oral glucose test). Initially, diagnoses were often made using a single elevated two-hour plasma glucose test. However, more recently, the criteria developed by the International Association of Diabetes and Pregnancy Study Group have become more commonly used.

2.3. Outcome. A score ≥ 12 was used to classify the presence of clinically relevant symptoms. A score ≥ 18 indicated severity of the symptoms. The EPDS included a specific question to assess self-harm intent.

2.4. Data Management and Analysis. Poisson regression with robust variance [7] was performed to estimate prevalence ratios (PR). Adjusted prevalence ratios included remaining variables. We defined the presence and severity of symptoms as dependent variables. SAS 9.4 was used for all statistical analyses, using 95% confidence intervals (95% CI).

2.5. Ethical Aspects. All participants were informed of the research protocol and signed informed consent forms. The study was approved by the Ethics in Research Committee of the Hospital de Clínicas de Porto Alegre (Project 120097, May 4, 2012).

3. Results

Half of the women (50%) were 30 to 39 years old and most of them lived with a partner (88%) and were of low socioeconomic status. The average gestational age was 31 weeks. Only 39% had finished high school and 39% had a family income of 1-2 minimum wages. Many women were obese before their pregnancies (47%). At the time of the interview, 12% were using insulin to treat their GDM, 53% had had one or two prior C-sections and normal delivery, and 71% had no history of abortion. Thirty-one percent of women evaluated showed depressive symptoms, and approximately 10% showed severe symptoms. Furthermore, 8.3% had thought about harming themselves during the previous seven days. Table 1 shows the frequencies found of the presence and severity of depressive symptoms and self-harm intent.

Adjusted prevalence ratios showed that higher educational and lower parity levels were inversely associated with frequency of depressive symptoms. After adjustment, household income, age, living with a partner, prepregnancy body mass index, abortion, and insulin use during pregnancy were not associated with depressive symptoms in any level (Table 2).

4. Discussion

Our study highlights the prevalence of depressive symptoms (31%), their severity (10%), and the frequency of self-harm intent (8.3%) in women with GDM who received tertiary prenatal care. Most of the women were of low socioeconomic status, and many of them were obese before their pregnancies, which show that this population is at greater risk for type 2 diabetes and other chronic diseases. Higher educational and lower parity levels were associated with lower frequency of depressive symptoms in this population.

Studies of depression in women with GDM are scarce in the literature, and most of them have evaluated prepregnancy

Table 1: Frequency of depressive symptom scores obtained using the Edinburgh Postnatal Depression Scale, according to sociodemographic characteristics ($n = 820$).

Variables	Score <12 n (%)	≥12 n (%)	≥18 n (%)	Self-harm intent n (%)
Total	563 (69)	257 (31)	81 (9.9)	68 (8.3)
Age (years)				
18 to 29	223 (70)	97 (30)	31 (10)	26 (8)
30 to 39	279 (68)	132 (32)	39 (9)	34 (8)
≥40	60 (69)	27 (31)	11 (13)	8 (9.2)
Living with a partner				
Yes	511 (71)	214 (29)	67 (9)	57 (8)
No	52 (55)	43 (45)	14 (15)	11 (12)
Education				
Complete/incomplete university degree	73 (84)	14 (16)	6 (7)	3 (4)
Complete high school	230 (73)	86 (27)	22 (7)	18 (6)
Incomplete high school	140 (63)	81 (37)	30 (14)	29 (13)
Incomplete elementary school	120 (61)	76 (39)	23 (12)	18 (9)
Household income (minimum wages)				
≥3	92 (77)	27 (23)	4 (3)	2 (2)
2 to <3	133 (76)	42 (24)	10 (6)	7 (4)
1 to <2	210 (66)	107 (34)	43 (14)	28 (9)
<1	120 (61)	77 (39)	23 (12)	28 (14)
Prepregnancy body mass index				
<25 kg/m^2	126 (70)	55 (30)	17 (9)	14 (8)
Overweight	167 (69)	74 (31)	22 (9)	20 (8)
Obese class I	145 (66)	74 (34)	23 (11)	17 (8)
Obese class II/III	106 (69)	47 (31)	16 (11)	15 (10)
Insulin use during pregnancy				
No	500 (69)	224 (31)	74 (10)	64 (9)
Yes	63 (66)	33 (34)	7 (7)	4 (4)
Parity				
0	140 (76)	44 (24)	10 (5)	11 (6)
1 to 2	260 (69)	117 (31)	40 (11)	30 (8)
≥3	87 (58)	64 (42)	18 (12)	20 (13)
Abortions				
0	355 (70)	150 (30)	43 (9)	42 (8)
1 to 3	128 (64)	73 (36)	25 (12)	19 (9)
≥4	4 (57)	3 (43)	1 (14)	0 (0)

diabetes or postpartum depression [8, 9] in contrast to the present study, which deals with data from the gestational period. Also, it bears highlighting that different instruments and cut-off scores are used in literature to evaluate depressive symptoms. This may explain the differences found in prevalence and may hinder comparisons of the findings.

Still, the gestational trimester during which the data collection occurred should be observed. A longitudinal study using the Center for Epidemiologic Studies-Depression (CES-D) score pointed out that there are differences in the prevalence of depressive symptoms according to gestational trimester [10]. The data show a slight decrease in the prevalence of depressive symptoms from the first (15%) to the second trimester (14%) but a relevant increase from the second to the third trimester (30%) [10]. In the LINDA-Brazil study, the mean gestational age in the data collection corresponded to the third trimester (31 weeks), which may explain the higher prevalence of depressive symptoms that was found. In contrast, an evaluation of 137 pregnant women with prediabetes that used the Hospital Anxiety and Depression Scale (HADS) indicated that there was no difference in depressive symptoms between the first and last gestational trimesters [8].

It has been estimated that the prevalence of depression in women with GDM ranges from 4.1% to 80.0%, according to a recent systematic review that included 16 studies. The high

TABLE 2: Association between sociodemographic characteristics and the Edinburgh Postnatal Depression Scale ($n = 820$).

Variables	EPDS ≥ 12 PR (95% CI)*	p	EPDS ≥ 18 PR (95% CI)*	p
Age (years)				
18 to 29	1.0	—	1.0	—
30 to 39	1.0 (0.8–1.3)	0.913	0.8 (0.5–1.3)	0.375
≥40	0.9 (0.6–1.3)	0.497	1.0 (0.5–2.2)	0.931
Living with a partner				
Yes	1.0	—	1.0	—
No	1.3 (0.9–1.7)	0.099	1.5 (0.8–3.0)	0.232
Education				
Complete/incomplete university degree	1.0	—	1.0	—
Complete high school	1.5 (0.8–2.7)	0.156	0.7 (0.3–1.7)	0.404
Incomplete high school	1.9 (1.0–3.4)	<0.05	1.3 (0.5–3.3)	0.647
Incomplete elementary school	1.9 (1.0–3.5)	<0.05	0.9 (0.3–2.5)	0.768
Household income (minimum wages)				
≥3	1.0	—	1.0	—
2 to <3	1.3 (0.8–2.1)	0.343	2.9 (0.7–12.8)	0.151
1 to <2	1.6 (1.0–2.5)	0.058	5.7 (1.4–23.3)	<0.05
<1	1.5 (0.9–2.5)	0.082	3.7 (0.8–16.4)	0.086
Prepregnancy body mass index				
<25 kg/m^2	1.0	—	1.0	
Overweight	1.1 (0.8–1.4)	0.757	1.0 (0.5–1.9)	0.971
Obese class I	1.1 (0.8–1.5)	0.701	1.1 (0.6–2.2)	0.720
Obese class II/III	0.9 (0.7–1.3)	0.713	0.9 (0.4–1.9)	0.820
Parity				
0	1.0	—	1.0	—
1 to 2	1.3 (0.9–1.8)	0.150	2.1 (1.0–4.5)	0.065
≥3	1.6 (1.1-2.3)	<0.05	2.1 (0.8–5.3)	0.130
Abortions				
0	1.0	—	1.0	—
1 to 2	1.2 (0.9–1.5)	0.205	1.4 (0.8–2.3)	0.226
≥3	1.3 (0.8–2.2)	0.324	1.5 (0.5–4.6)	0.516

*Adjusted prevalence ratios estimated using robust Poisson regression, including the table's remaining variables.

variability of the results is due to differences among populations and when the data were collected, in addition to the factors that were mentioned above [11]. Furthermore, no specific studies were found on GDM and depression in the Brazilian population.

Moreover, a systematic review [1] identified that studies using an EPDS score of ≥12 (as was used in our study) in the general population of pregnant women showed lower levels of depression (5% to 8.7%) [12, 13] compared to studies conducted with women of low socioeconomic status (29% to 51%), even considering higher EPDS cut-off points (scores of ≥13 and ≥14) [14, 15]. In low- and middle-income countries like Brazil, maternal depression remains underrecognized and undertreated and is related to negative health outcomes, increasing the risk of comorbidities [2] such as GDM [16, 17].

Some studies have evaluated or reviewed depression and sociodemographic aspects, as this study did [2, 18–20]. A review of these aspects showed that age, marital status, and income have an impact on depression [1], in contrast to what was observed in the LINDA-Brazil study, which identified only higher educational and lower parity levels as being inversely associated with depressive symptoms. Importantly, there are also indications that women with histories of depression are more likely to have GDM [20]. However, the present study did not consider this issue.

Low socioeconomic and educational status, inadequate social support, and a history of mental illness have been consistently identified as risk factors for antepartum and postpartum depression in low- and middle-income countries [2]. A recent systematic review of 104 studies on maternal depression showed frequencies ranging from 16.2% to 24.3% in Brazilian studies and those that used the EPDS to evaluate depressive symptoms. These findings support the hypothesis that differences in depression rates may reflect demographic differences and the different instruments used to estimate or classify depression [21].

Regarding self-harm intent, many studies have related it to suicidal ideation. In this context, frequencies ranged from

2.6% to 27.8% [2]. However, this study used one specific question in the EPDS questionnaire to assess self-harm intent in the previous week, illustrating that the ability to compare these data with those of other studies is limited.

One of the limitations of this study is that we collected data only in the third trimester (at a mean of 31 weeks) and not in other gestational trimesters or before delivery. Neither did we investigate the women's social support systems or whether they had histories of depression. It was not possible to make comparisons with pregnant women without diabetes since all of the women studied had GDM. Finally, the EPDS only evaluates depressive symptoms and does not diagnose depression. Thus, it tends to overestimate depression prevalence [18]. Furthermore, differences in cultural and economic factors may be related to under- or overreporting depressive symptoms. Another issue that merits discussion is the different diagnostic criteria used for the study population. Some of the patients were diagnosed using fasting glycaemia while others underwent a complex procedure that included one or two glucose tolerance tests according to a two-step diagnostic procedure. This study was not able to evaluate whether this difference affected the prevalence of depressive symptoms found in the study population.

Screening for depression (especially during early pregnancy) may be important at different times. Further research on women with GDM would be useful to determine whether depression is a substantial risk factor for GDM and to explore other negative outcomes. Such studies could potentially decrease the costs of maternal and neonatal care and reduce short- and long-term morbidity.

5. Conclusion

This study found a high proportion of pregnant women with GDM who presented depressive symptoms. Such a frequency is worrisome, given its known negative impact on pregnancy outcomes. Our results suggest the need to consider depressive symptoms in the treatment of women whose pregnancies are complicated by gestational diabetes, especially in more vulnerable populations.

Disclosure

The views expressed in this manuscript are those of the authors and do not reflect the opinion of the study's sponsors, who had no role in study's design, data collection, analysis or interpretation, or writing the manuscript.

Conflicts of Interest

The authors declare that there is no conflict of interest regarding the publication of this paper.

Acknowledgments

This study received funding from the Brazilian National Council of Technological and Scientific Development (Grant no. 563942/2010-0) and the Eli Lilly Non-Communicable Diseases Partners (Grant no. 2012/2016).

References

[1] H. A. Bennett, A. Einarson, A. Taddio, G. Koren, and T. R. Einarson, "Prevalence of depression during pregnancy: systematic review," *Obstetrics and Gynecology*, vol. 103, no. 4, pp. 698–709, 2004.

[2] B. Gelaye, M. B. Rondon, R. Araya, and M. A. Williams, "Epidemiology of maternal depression, risk factors, and child outcomes in low-income and middle-income countries," *Lancet Psychiatry*, vol. 3, no. 10, pp. 973–982, 2016.

[3] A. Rahman, Z. Iqbal, and R. Harrington, "Life events, social support and depression in childbirth: perspectives from a rural community in the developing world," *Psychological Medicine*, vol. 33, no. 7, pp. 1161–1167, 2003.

[4] M. I. Schmidt, B. B. Duncan, C. Castilhos et al., "Lifestyle INtervention for Diabetes prevention After pregnancy (LINDA-Brasil): study protocol for a multicenter randomized controlled trial," *BMC Pregnancy and Childbirth*, vol. 16, p. 68, 2016.

[5] World Health Organization and Public Health Agency of Canada, *Preventing Chronic Diseases: A Vital Investment*, World Health Organization; Public Health Agency of Canada, Geneva, Ottawa, 2005.

[6] I. S. Santos, A. Matijasevich, B. F. Tavares et al., "Validation of the Edinburgh Postnatal Depression Scale (EPDS) in a sample of mothers from the 2004 Pelotas birth cohort study," *Cadernos de Saúde Pública*, vol. 23, no. 11, pp. 2577–2588, 2007.

[7] A. J. D. Barros and V. N. Hirakata, "Alternatives for logistic regression in cross-sectional studies: an empirical comparison of models that directly estimate the prevalence ratio," *BMC Medical Research Methodology*, vol. 3, p. 21, 2003.

[8] N. C. Do, A. L. Secher, P. Cramon et al., "Quality of life, anxiety and depression symptoms in early and late pregnancy in women with pregestational diabetes," *Acta Obstetricia et Gynecologica Scandinavica*, vol. 96, 2016.

[9] J. M. Nicklas, L. J. Miller, C. A. Zera, R. B. Davis, S. E. Levkoff, and E. W. Seely, "Factors associated with depressive symptoms in the early postpartum period among women with recent gestational diabetes mellitus," *Maternal and Child Health Journal*, vol. 17, no. 9, pp. 1665–1672, 2013.

[10] R. Setse, R. Grogan, L. Pham et al., "Longitudinal study of depressive symptoms and health-related quality of life during pregnancy and after delivery: the health status in pregnancy (HIP) study," *Maternal and Child Health Journal*, vol. 13, no. 5, pp. 577–587, 2009.

[11] G. P. Ross, H. Falhammar, R. Chen, H. Barraclough, O. Kleivenes, and I. Gallen, "Relationship between depression and diabetes in pregnancy: a systematic review," *World Journal of Diabetes*, vol. 7, no. 19, p. 554, 2016.

[12] H. Verdoux, A. L. Sutter, E. Glatigny-Dallay, and A. Minisini, "Obstetrical complications and the development of postpartum depressive symptoms: a prospective survey of the MATQUID cohort," *Acta Psychiatrica Scandinavica*, vol. 106, no. 3, pp. 212–219, 2002.

[13] M. Pajulo, E. Savonlahti, A. Sourander, H. Helenius, and J. Piha, "Antenatal depression, substance dependency and social support," *Journal of Affective Disorders*, vol. 65, no. 1, pp. 9–17, 2001.

[14] H. L. Bolton, P. M. Hughes, P. Turton, and P. Sedgwick, "Incidence and demographic correlates of depressive symptoms during pregnancy in an inner London population," *Journal*

of Psychosomatic Obstetrics and Gynaecology, vol. 19, no. 4, pp. 202–209, 1998.

[15] M. D. Mckee, M. Cunningham, K. R. Jankowski, and L. Zayas, "Health-related functional status in pregnancy: relationship to depression and social support in a multi-ethnic population," *Obstetrics and Gynecology*, vol. 97, no. 6, pp. 988–993, 2001.

[16] S. N. Hinkle, G. M. Buck Louis, S. Rawal, Y. Zhu, P. S. Albert, and C. Zhang, "A longitudinal study of depression and gestational diabetes in pregnancy and the postpartum period," *Diabetologia*, vol. 59, no. 12, pp. 2594–2602, 2016.

[17] J. G. Katon, J. Russo, A. R. Gavin, J. L. Melville, and W. J. Katon, "Diabetes and depression in pregnancy: is there an association?" *Journal of Womens Health*, vol. 20, no. 7, pp. 983–989, 2011.

[18] E. F. Melo, J. G. Cecatti, R. C. Pacagnella, D. F. B. Leite, D. E. Vulcani, and M. Y. Makuch, "The prevalence of perinatal depression and its associated factors in two different settings in Brazil," *Journal of Affective Disorders*, vol. 136, no. 3, pp. 1204–1208, 2012.

[19] C. Morrison, J. G. McCook, and B. A. Bailey, "First trimester depression scores predict development of gestational diabetes mellitus in pregnant rural Appalachian women," *Journal of Psychosomatic Obstetrics and Gynaecology*, vol. 37, no. 1, pp. 21–25, 2016.

[20] K. Natasha, A. Hussain, and A. K. A. Khan, "Prevalence of depression among subjects with and without gestational diabetes mellitus in Bangladesh: a hospital based study," *Journal of Diabetes and Metabolic Disorders*, vol. 14, p. 64, 2015.

[21] L. Chasan-Taber, R. T. Fortner, A. Gollenberg, J. Buonnaccorsi, N. Dole, and G. Markenson, "A prospective cohort study of modifiable risk factors for gestational diabetes among Hispanic women: design and baseline characteristics," *Journal of Womens Health*, vol. 19, no. 1, pp. 117–124, 2010.

20

Seasonal Pattern in the Diagnosis of Gestational Diabetes Mellitus in Southern Sweden

Anastasia Katsarou,[1,2] Rickard Claesson,[1,3] Claes Ignell,[1,4] Nael Shaat,[1,2] and Kerstin Berntorp[1,2]

[1] *Department of Clinical Sciences, Lund University, Malmö, Sweden*
[2] *Department of Endocrinology, Skåne University Hospital, Malmö, Sweden*
[3] *Department of Obstetrics and Gynaecology, Office for Healthcare "Kryh", Ystad, Sweden*
[4] *Department of Obstetrics and Gynaecology, Office for Healthcare "Sund", Helsingborg, Sweden*

Correspondence should be addressed to Anastasia Katsarou; anastasia.katsarou@med.lu.se

Academic Editor: Ulrike Rothe

Aim. The aim of this study was to examine seasonal patterns in glucose tolerance and in the diagnosis of gestational diabetes mellitus (GDM). *Methods.* Altogether, 11 538 women underwent a 75-g oral glucose tolerance test (OGTT) in the twenty-eighth week of pregnancy during the years 2003–2005 in southern Sweden. GDM was defined by the 2-h capillary glucose concentration in the OGTT (≥8.9 mmol/L). Chi-squared test, analysis of variance, and regression analyses were used for statistical evaluations. *Results.* The seasonal frequency of GDM ranged from 3.3% in spring to 5.5% in summer ($p < 0.0001$). Mean 2-h glucose concentrations followed the same seasonal trend, with a difference of 0.15 mmol/L between winter and summer ($p < 0.0001$). The 2-h glucose level increased by 0.009 mmol/L for every degree increase in temperature ($p < 0.0001$). In regression analysis, summer (June–August) was associated with increased 2-h glucose level ($p < 0.001$) and increased frequency of GDM compared to the other seasons (odds ratio 1.51, 95% confidence interval 1.24–1.83, and $p < 0.001$). *Conclusions.* Our findings suggest seasonal variation in the 2-h glucose concentration in the OGTT and in the proportion of women diagnosed with GDM, with a peak in the summer.

1. Introduction

While seasonality in the onset of type 1 diabetes is well documented [1], less is known about seasonality in the diagnosis of type 2 and gestational diabetes mellitus (GDM). Doró et al. (2006) reported an increased incidence of type 2 diabetes onset in winter [2]. A similar pattern in HbA1c and glucose levels has been reported in diabetes patients, possibly because of seasonal variations in environmental conditions, such as diet and exercise [3–6]. In contrast, Schmidt et al. (1994) reported a 4-fold increase in the frequency of GDM in the summer compared with the winter, which they related to increased 2-h glucose levels in the oral glucose tolerance test (OGTT) at higher ambient temperatures [7]. Similar results of temperature-induced differences in post-load venous glucose levels have previously been reported by Akanji et al. in subjects with and without diabetes [8, 9]. However, two other studies from Australia and the UK found no clinically significant evidence of any seasonal variation in the prevalence of GDM or the 2-h glucose levels in the OGTT [10, 11].

The prevalence of GDM in a given population depends on the screening approach and on the diagnostic criteria used [12]. In southern Sweden, universal screening for GDM with a 75-g OGTT has been performed at the antenatal clinics since 1995, with no major changes in the diagnostic procedure. The diagnosis of GDM is based on the 2-h capillary glucose concentration [13]. During the years 2003–2005, pregnant women, representing different glucose categories according to the OGTT, were invited to take part in a follow-up study postpartum, the Mamma Study. During the period of recruitment, a large number of test results were made available and they form the basis of the present study. The aim was to determine whether there were any differences in glucose tolerance by season and, consequently, if the frequency of GDM showed any seasonal variation. Such differences are important to elucidate, since they may affect the diagnostic procedure and interpretation of the results.

2. Materials and Methods

2.1. GDM Screening. The screening programme for GDM in southern Sweden has been described in detail elsewhere [13]. Briefly, a 75-g OGTT is offered to all women in the twenty-eighth week of gestation after overnight fasting and also in week 12 if there is a history of GDM in previous pregnancies or a first-degree relative with diabetes. The HemoCue blood glucose 201+ system (HemoCue AB, Ängelholm, Sweden) is used to perform immediate analysis of capillary glucose concentrations, which are reported as equivalent plasma glucose concentrations [14]. To ascertain the quality of the individual testing, double sampling is used, with acceptance of a divergence of ≤0.3 mmol/L. If this is not reached, a third sample is taken, and if the divergence between two of the samples is still not acceptable, the equipment is checked and the OGTT is not regarded as being valid.

The diagnostic criteria for GDM used in the present study are a slight modification of those recommended by the World Health Organization in 1999, defining GDM as a 2-h venous plasma glucose concentration of ≥7.8 mmol/L, corresponding to a capillary plasma glucose concentration of ≥8.9 mmol/L [15]. The diagnosis was based on the mean of the two measurements.

2.2. Study Population. Recruitment to the Mamma Study took place during the years 2003–2005 and involved four of the five delivery departments in the county of Skåne in southern Sweden [16]. During the recruitment period, OGTT results from the local antenatal clinics were sent to the study coordinator, enabling identification of the test results of women who consented to be enrolled; it also ensured correct sampling technique [13]. Initially, 11 976 OGTT results in total were reported. If a woman had more than one pregnancy during the study period, only the first one was included. Likewise, if a woman underwent more than one OGTT during the same pregnancy, only the one performed in pregnancy week 28 was included. This restricted data set (n = 11 538) formed the basis of the present evaluation. Mean monthly temperatures during the study period were obtained from the Swedish Meteorological and Hydrological Institute (http://opendata-download-metobs.smhi.se/explore/?parameter=3#).

The study was carried out in accordance with the Declaration of Helsinki. Written informed consent was obtained from all participants, and the study protocol was approved by the Ethics Committee of Lund University (LU 259-00).

2.3. Statistical Analysis. OGTT results from the 3-year study period were grouped together into months and seasons (winter: December–February; spring: March–May; summer: June–August; autumn: September–November). Chi-squared test was used to test for differences in frequencies between months and seasons, and one-way analysis of variance (ANOVA) was used to test for the corresponding differences in means. Multivariable logistic regression was used to examine whether month or season was associated with the diagnosis of GDM and multivariable linear regression was used to examine the corresponding associations with 2-h glucose levels. The relationship between mean monthly temperatures and mean monthly 2-h glucose concentrations was evaluated by simple linear regression.

IBM SPSS Statistics 22 for Windows (IBM Corporation, Armonk, NY) was used for analysis. Two-sided p values of less than 0.05 were considered to be statistically significant.

3. Results

Of the 11 538 women who underwent an OGTT during the study period, a total of 487 women (4.2%) were diagnosed with GDM.

Table 1 shows the study material, organized by month and season. The monthly frequency of GDM ranged from 2.9% in March to 5.8% in June, and the seasonal frequency of GDM ranged from 3.3% in spring to 5.5% in summer. The differences in frequencies were statistically significant, both for month ($p = 0.01$) and for season ($p < 0.0001$). The mean age of participating women was 29.9 (standard deviation 5.1) years, and the ages ranged from 15 to 49 years. The age of the women differed statistically significantly between months and seasons ($p < 0.001$). However, no significant differences in the monthly distributions of age were noted.

Mean monthly temperature ranged from −0.6°C in winter to 17.7°C in summer (Table 1). In a simple linear regression with 2-h plasma glucose as the dependent variable and mean monthly temperature as the predictor variable, the coefficient in the equation was 0.009, suggesting that the 2-h glucose level increased by 0.009 mmol/L for every degree increase in temperature ($p < 0.0001$).

Figure 1 illustrates the monthly mean 2-h glucose level during the OGTT (with 95% confidence interval (CI)) and the monthly percentage of women with GDM. Though numerically small, the differences in 2-h glucose levels were statistically significant ($p < 0.001$), with the lowest values observed from January to March and peak levels from June to August. A similar seasonal trend was seen for the percentage of women with 2-h glucose levels in the GDM range (2-h glucose level ≥ 8.9 mmol/L). There were no differences in the distribution of glucose concentrations between months or seasons.

In regression analysis, adjusting for age, the summer months (June to August) were found to be associated with increased 2-h glucose levels ($p < 0.001$) and increased frequency of GDM compared to all other months (OR = 1.51 (95% CI: 1.24–1.83); $p < 0.001$).

4. Discussion

In this observational study of 11 538 pregnancies, we found seasonal variations in the 2-h glucose level in the OGTT performed in the twenty-eighth week of gestation, giving

TABLE 1: Description of the study material, organized by month and season.

	OGTT *n*	GDM *n* (%)	2-h glucose, mmol/L Mean (SD)	Age, years, mean (SD)	Temperature, °C, mean
Month					
January	1 094	36 (3.3)	6.4 (1.3)	30.4 (5.0)	0
February	928	34 (3.7)	6.4 (1.3)	30.1 (5.3)	−0.6
March	1 082	31 (2.9)	6.4 (1.2)	30.1 (5.2)	2.4
April	1 027	34 (3.3)	6.5 (1.3)	30.1 (5.0)	7.5
May	1 057	41 (3.9)	6.5 (1.4)	30.4 (5.1)	12.1
June	1 009	59 (5.8)	6.6 (1.4)	29.8 (5.1)	15.2
July	974	50 (5.1)	6.6 (1.3)	30.0 (5.0)	17.7
August	928	52 (5.6)	6.6 (1.3)	29.6 (5.0)	17.6
September	781	33 (4.2)	6.5 (1.3)	29.5 (5.3)	14.4
October	835	42 (5.0)	6.6 (1.3)	29.6 (5.1)	8.4
November	897	38 (4.2)	6.6 (1.3)	29.6 (5.2)	5.3
December	926	37 (4.0)	6.5 (1.3)	29.8 (5.1)	2.9
Season					
Winter	2 948	107 (3.6)	6.4 (1.3)	30.1 (5.1)	0.7
Spring	3 166	106 (3.3)	6.5 (1.3)	30.2 (5.1)	7.3
Summer	2 911	161 (5.5)	6.6 (1.4)	29.8 (5.0)	16.8
Autumn	2 513	113 (4.5)	6.6 (1.3)	29.6 (5.2)	9.2

GDM, gestational diabetes mellitus; OGTT, oral glucose tolerance test; SD, standard deviation.

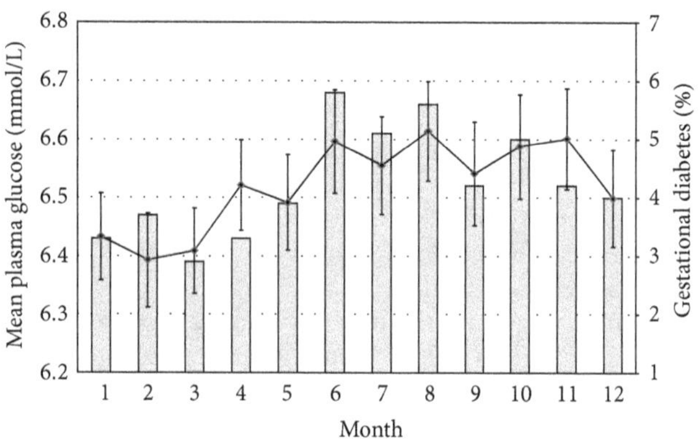

FIGURE 1: Monthly mean 2-h glucose levels and the monthly percentage of women with gestational diabetes mellitus.

seasonal variations in the percentage of women diagnosed with GDM—with a peak in the summer.

Until recently, there have only been three previous studies in the literature evaluating seasonality in GDM [7, 10, 11]. Using a 2-h venous plasma glucose concentration of ≥7.8 mmol/L to define GDM during a standardized 75-g OGTT in 1 113 consecutively tested women in Brazil, Schmidt et al. (1994) reported that the frequency of GDM varied in relation to the ambient temperature, from 4.8% in winter to 14.8% in summer [7]. For every degree increase in temperature, the mean 2-h glucose level increased by 0.07 mmol/L, while the fasting glucose levels were unaffected by temperature. Standardizing the results at 23°C indicated that women were overdiagnosed by 19% at higher temperatures and underdiagnosed by 45% at lower temperatures [7]. Similar results have been described in small-scale studies outside of pregnancy [8, 9]. Increased arterialisation of the venous blood at elevated temperatures has been suggested to be a plausible explanation [17]. Whether these variations in glucose levels result from an acute effect of temperature rather than a chronic one is not fully understood, although some experimental studies have indicated an acute effect [18, 19]. Interestingly, in a very recent study from the coastal area of Australia, Moses et al. reported significantly lower median 1-h and 2-h glucose levels in the OGTT in the winter compared with the overall 1-h and 2-h results, when evaluated in a cohort of 7 369 pregnant women prospectively followed up during a 3-year period [20]. Furthermore, in a population-based study from South Australia, Verburg et al. recently reported seasonal variation in the diagnosis of GDM based on the estimated date of conception [21].

Since the present study was based on capillary glucose measurements, previous findings cannot be directly extrapolated to results using our methodology. However, temperature-induced changes in peripheral blood flow may very well affect the composition of capillary blood as well, representing a mixture of arterial and venous blood. According to national statistics, the average temperature in the region varied between −0.6°C in winter and +17.7°C in summer during the study period. With respect to the simple linear regression analysis, indicating that for every one degree increase in temperature the glucose concentration increased by 0.009 mmol/L, this difference in temperature between summer and winter corresponds to a difference of 0.15 mmol/L in glucose concentration. It is important to note that OGTT as such has a rather low reproducibility, especially for 2-h glucose levels in the intermediate range [22–24]. This means that a difference of 0.15 mmol/L would have diagnostic implications in women with glucose concentrations close to the diagnostic limit, thereby increasing the frequency of GDM in the summer.

Though not regarded as a diagnostic standard [25], capillary finger-tip tests have been used in the screening programme for GDM in southern Sweden ever since they were first introduced in 1995 [13]. For practical reasons, this was regarded as a prerequisite when introducing the OGTT on a large scale. Glucose measurements based on capillary samples are generally believed to show greater variation than venous glucose measurements [26]. If the hand is cold there is a risk of squeezing and "milking" of the finger, increasing the proportion of extracellular fluid, resulting in a lower glucose concentration. However, since glucose measurements in the present study were based on measurements after two hours at room temperature in the antenatal clinic, such an explanation would seem less likely.

In contrast to our findings and those of Schmidt et al. [7], Janghorbany et al. (2006) could not prove any seasonality in glucose tolerance or in the incidence of GDM in 4 942 pregnancies in Plymouth, UK [11]. However, it is important to note that Plymouth has a very mild climate, with little seasonal variation. Furthermore, only 11% (n = 539) of the women underwent an OGTT during pregnancy and the incidence figures were based on those with an abnormal OGTT (n = 90), as opposed to all the others who either had a normal OGTT or initially screened negative by random plasma glucose testing or risk factors. In a study from Australia, Moses and Griffiths (1995) examined seasonal trends in 2 749 women consecutively tested with a 75-g OGTT [10]. Interestingly, after adjustments for various risk factors, multiple regression analysis revealed a significant association between the monthly temperature and the 2-h glucose level in the OGTT; the 2-h glucose level increased by 0.026 mmol/L for every degree increase in temperature [10]. However, Chi-squared analysis did not suggest any seasonal variation in the diagnosis of GDM, and it was concluded that the association between 2-h glucose and temperature was unlikely to be of any clinical importance in the temperate coastal area of Australia, with the mean monthly temperature during the study period ranging from 13.6°C in July to 22.3°C in January [10].

Our results do not agree with previous observations by Doró et al. from Hungary, of an increased incidence of type 2 diabetes in winter, although it should be noted that the incidence figures reported were based on the initiation of antidiabetic therapy in individuals with previously diagnosed diabetes, therefore not representing the "true" diabetes onset [2]. Likewise, worsening of metabolic control in subjects with type 2 diabetes in winter has been described in a number of studies [3–6]. Since diet and exercise are hallmarks of the treatment of type 2 diabetes, it is reasonable to assume that environmental factors, such as diet and exercise patterns, have an important role in the seasonal variation in glucose metabolism in patients with diabetes. Seasonal variation in the diagnosis of GDM possibly reflects seasonality of environmental influences early in gestation, during placental development, affecting placental metabolism and glucose homeostasis later on in pregnancy [21]. Many factors vary with season, including the nutritional quality of foods, temperature, the number of hours of sunshine, and vitamin D synthesis. Maternal vitamin D deficiency in early pregnancy has been associated with increased risk of GDM [27]. Moreover, seasonal variation in vitamin D status, quantified as the total number of hours of sunshine during the three months preceding the onset of diabetes, was suggested as an explanation for the seasonality of type 2 diabetes reported by Doró et al. [28].

The strength of the present study was the uniform diagnostic procedure for GDM, based on universal screening with a 75-g OGTT and enabling identification of a large cohort of women in one particular week of gestation. Unfortunately, we did not have access to individual data other than age, so the figures are crude and unadjusted for other potentially important risk factors, such as body mass index and ethnicity [29]. However, we have no reason to believe that this would have any major effect on the results, due to the size of the material and the exclusive use of OGTT. Another weakness of the study was that we only had information on mean monthly temperatures during the study period and not the mean temperature on specific days, which makes it difficult to draw any firm conclusions on the effect of temperature on our results.

We have previously shown that approximately 5-6% of women with GDM in our region have positive islet cell autoantibodies as a marker of autoimmune pathogenesis and therefore of type 1 diabetes [30, 31]. Of these, 50% had developed type 1 diabetes within ten years postpartum [30]. Seasonality in the incidence of type 1 diabetes has been described [1], but this is probably not of any relevance to the present findings, due to the overall low proportion of women who would be expected to have autoimmune diabetes in our material.

5. Conclusions

Based on a universally performed OGTT in the twenty-eighth week of pregnancy, seasonality in the proportion of women diagnosed with GDM was observed, with a peak in the summer. The mean 2-h glucose concentration in the OGTT followed the same seasonal trend. The findings may be related to the increased ambient temperature in the summer. Further studies are needed to determine whether our results are reproducible and if they are, to investigate the cause(s) of seasonality, as such variations may have implications for the diagnostic procedure and for interpretation of the results.

Disclosure

An earlier version of this work was presented as an abstract at 2016 European Association for the Study of Diabetes (EASD) annual conference in Munich.

Competing Interests

The authors declare that they have no competing interests.

Authors' Contributions

Kerstin Berntorp conceived the study. All the authors contributed to the study design and interpretation of data. Kerstin Berntorp wrote the initial draft of the manuscript, and Anastasia Katsarou and Rickard Claesson contributed equally to the subsequent draft. Claes Ignell helped analyse data. Claes Ignell and Nael Shaat critically reviewed and edited the manuscript. All the authors read and approved the final manuscript.

Acknowledgments

The authors thank Eva Anderberg, who coordinated the Mamma Study and collected the OGTT data for this study. They are indebted to Helene Jacobsson, biostatistician at the Skåne R&D Centre, University Hospital, Lund, Sweden, for statistical support. The study was supported by grants from the Research Funds of Skåne University Hospital and from the Skåne County Council Research and Development Foundation.

References

[1] C. C. Patterson, E. Gyürüs, J. Rosenbauer et al., "Seasonal variation in month of diagnosis in children with type 1 diabetes registered in 23 European centers during 1989–2008: little short-term influence of sunshine hours or average temperature," *Pediatric Diabetes*, vol. 16, no. 8, pp. 573–580, 2015.

[2] P. Doró, R. Benko, M. Matuz, and G. Soós, "Seasonality in the incidence of type 2 diabetes: a population-based study," *Diabetes Care*, vol. 29, no. 1, p. 173, 2006.

[3] W. W. Liang, "Seasonal changes in preprandial glucose, A1C, and blood pressure in diabetic patients," *Diabetes Care*, vol. 30, no. 10, pp. 2501–2502, 2007.

[4] A. Kershenbaum, A. Kershenbaum, J. Tarabeia, N. Stein, I. Lavi, and G. Rennert, "Unraveling seasonality in population averages: an examination of seasonal variation in glucose levels in diabetes patients using a large population-based data set," *Chronobiology International*, vol. 28, no. 4, pp. 352–360, 2011.

[5] C.-L. Tseng, M. Brimacombe, M. Xie et al., "Seasonal patterns in monthly hemoglobin A1c values," *American Journal of Epidemiology*, vol. 161, no. 6, pp. 565–574, 2005.

[6] M. Sohmiya, I. Kanazawa, and Y. Kato, "Seasonal changes in body composition and blood HbA1c levels without weight change in male patients with type 2 diabetes treated with insulin," *Diabetes Care*, vol. 27, no. 5, pp. 1238–1239, 2004.

[7] M. I. Schmidt, M. C. Matos, L. Branchtein et al., "Variation in glucose tolerance with ambient temperature," *The Lancet*, vol. 344, no. 8929, pp. 1054–1055, 1994.

[8] A. O. Akanji and R. N. Oputa, "The effect of ambient temperature on glucose tolerance," *Diabetic Medicine*, vol. 8, no. 10, pp. 946–948, 1991.

[9] A. O. Akanji, M. Bruce, K. Frayn, T. D. R. Hockaday, and G. M. Kaddaha, "Oral glucose tolerance and ambient temperature in non-diabetic subjects," *Diabetologia*, vol. 30, no. 6, pp. 431–433, 1987.

[10] R. Moses and R. Griffiths, "Is there a seasonal variation in the incidence of gestational diabetes?" *Diabetic Medicine*, vol. 12, no. 7, pp. 563–565, 1995.

[11] M. Janghorbani, E. Stenhouse, R. B. Jones, and A. Millward, "Gestational diabetes mellitus in Plymouth, U.K.: prevalence, seasonal variation and associated factors," *Journal of Reproductive Medicine*, vol. 51, no. 2, pp. 128–134, 2006.

[12] K. J. Hunt and K. L. Schuller, "The increasing prevalence of diabetes in pregnancy," *Obstetrics and Gynecology Clinics of North America*, vol. 34, no. 2, pp. 173–199, 2007.

[13] E. Anderberg, K. Källén, K. Berntorp, A. Frid, and A. Åberg, "A simplified oral glucose tolerance test in pregnancy: compliance and results," *Acta Obstetricia et Gynecologica Scandinavica*, vol. 86, no. 12, pp. 1432–1436, 2007.

[14] R. W. Burnett, P. D'Orazio, N. Fogh-Andersen et al., "IFCC recommendation on reporting results for blood glucose," *Clinica Chimica Acta*, vol. 307, no. 1-2, pp. 205–209, 2001.

[15] World Health Organization, *Definition, Diagnosis and Classification of Diabetes Mellitus and its Complications. Report of a WHO Consultation. Part 1: Diagnosis and Classification of Diabetes Mellitus*, World Health Organization, Geneva, Switzerland, 1999.

[16] K. Berntorp, E. Anderberg, R. Claesson, C. Ignell, and K. Källén, "The relative importance of maternal body mass index and glucose levels for prediction of large-for-gestational-age births," *BMC Pregnancy and Childbirth*, vol. 15, article 280, 2015.

[17] K. N. Frayn, P. L. Whyte, H. A. Benson, D. J. Earl, and H. A. Smith, "Changes in forearm blood flow at elevated ambient temperature and their role in the apparent impairment of glucose tolerance," *Clinical Science*, vol. 76, no. 3, pp. 323–328, 1989.

[18] E. A. H. McGuire, J. H. Helderman, J. D. Tobin, R. Andres, and M. Berman, "Effects of arterial versus venous sampling on analysis of glucose kinetics in man," *Journal of Applied Physiology*, vol. 41, no. 4, pp. 565–573, 1976.

[19] R. G. Moses, M. J. Patterson, J. M. Regan, R. Chaunchaiyakul, N. A. S. Taylor, and A. B. Jenkins, "A non-linear effect of ambient temperature on apparent glucose tolerance," *Diabetes Research and Clinical Practice*, vol. 36, no. 1, pp. 35–40, 1997.

[20] R. G. Moses, V. C. K. Wong, K. Lambert, G. J. Morris, and F. San Gil, "Seasonal changes in the prevalence of gestational diabetes mellitus," *Diabetes Care*, vol. 39, no. 7, pp. 1218–1221, 2016.

[21] P. E. Verburg, G. Tucker, W. Scheil, J. J. Erwich, G. A. Dekker, and C. T. Roberts, "Seasonality of gestational diabetes mellitus: a South Australian Population Study," *BMJ Open Diabetes Research & Care*, vol. 4, no. 1, Article ID e000286, 2016.

[22] K. Schousboe, J. E. Henriksen, K. O. Kyvik, T. I. A. Sørensen, and P. Hyltoft Petersen, "Reproducibility of S-insulin and B-glucose responses in two identical oral glucose tolerance tests," *Scandinavian Journal of Clinical and Laboratory Investigation*, vol. 62, no. 8, pp. 623–630, 2002.

[23] C. M. Balion, P. S. Raina, H. C. Gerstein et al., "Reproducibility of impaired glucose tolerance (IGT) and impaired fasting glucose (IFG) classification: a systematic review," *Clinical Chemistry and Laboratory Medicine*, vol. 45, no. 9, pp. 1180–1185, 2007.

[24] J. M. Mooy, P. A. Grootenhuis, H. De Vries et al., "Intra-individual variation of glucose, specific insulin and proinsulin concentrations measured by two oral glucose tolerance tests in a general Caucasian population: the Hoorn Study," *Diabetologia*, vol. 39, no. 3, pp. 298–305, 1996.

[25] World Health Organization and International Diabetes Federation, *Definition and Diagnosis of Diabetes Mellitus and Intermediate Hyperglycaemia: A Report of a WHO/IDF Consultation*, World Health Organization, Geneva, Switzerland, 2006.

[26] B. Carstensen, J. Lindström, J. Sundvall, K. Borch-Johnsen, and J. Tuomilehto, "Measurement of blood glucose: comparison between different types of specimens," *Annals of Clinical Biochemistry*, vol. 45, no. 2, pp. 140–148, 2008.

[27] C. Zhang, C. Qiu, F. B. Hu et al., "Maternal plasma 25-hydroxyvitamin D concentrations and the risk for gestational diabetes mellitus," *PLOS ONE*, vol. 3, no. 11, Article ID e3753, 2008.

[28] P. Doró, W. B. Grant, R. Benko, M. Matuz, T. Tóth, and G. Soós, "Vitamin D and the seasonality of type 2 diabetes," *Medical Hypotheses*, vol. 71, no. 2, pp. 317–318, 2008.

[29] A. Dornhorst and M. Roosi, "Risk and prevention of type 2 diabetes in women with gestational diabetes," *Diabetes Care*, vol. 21, supplement 2, pp. B43–B49, 1998.

[30] C. Nilsson, D. Ursing, C. Törn, A. Åberg, and M. Landin-Olsson, "Presence of GAD antibodies during gestational diabetes mellitus predicts type 1 diabetes," *Diabetes Care*, vol. 30, no. 8, pp. 1968–1971, 2007.

[31] A. Papadopoulou, K. F. Lynch, E. Anderberg et al., "HLA-DQB1 genotypes and islet cell autoantibodies against GAD65 and IA-2 in relation to development of diabetes post partum in women with gestational diabetes mellitus," *Diabetes Research and Clinical Practice*, vol. 95, no. 2, pp. 260–264, 2012.

21

Vitamin D, Gestational Diabetes, and Measures of Glucose Metabolism in a Population-Based Multiethnic Cohort

Åse Ruth Eggemoen,[1] **Christin Wiegels Waage**,[1] **Line Sletner**,[2] **Hanne L. Gulseth**,[3,4] **Kåre I. Birkeland**,[5,6] **and Anne Karen Jenum**[7]

[1]*Department of General Practice, Institute of Health and Society, University of Oslo, Oslo, Norway*
[2]*Department of Child and Adolescence Medicine, Akershus University Hospital, Lørenskog, Norway*
[3]*Department of Endocrinology, Morbid Obesity and Preventive Medicine, Oslo University Hospital, Oslo, Norway*
[4]*Department of Noncommunicable Diseases, Norwegian Institute of Public Health, Oslo, Norway*
[5]*Department of Transplantation Medicine, Oslo University Hospital, Oslo, Norway*
[6]*Institute of Clinical Medicine, Faculty of Medicine, University of Oslo, Oslo, Norway*
[7]*General Practice Research Unit (AFE), Department of General Practice, Institute of Health and Society, University of Oslo, Oslo, Norway*

Correspondence should be addressed to Åse Ruth Eggemoen; a.r.eggemoen@medisin.uio.no

Academic Editor: Eusebio Chiefari

Objective. We explored associations between maternal 25-hydroxyvitamin D (25(OH)D) status during pregnancy and gestational diabetes (GDM) and other measures of glucose metabolism. *Methods.* We analysed 25(OH)D at 15 and 28 gestational weeks (GW) in 745 multiethnic pregnant women attending antenatal care units in Oslo, Norway, between 2008 and 2010. GDM was diagnosed with a 75 g oral glucose tolerance test at 28 GW. Separate regression analyses were performed to investigate associations between 25(OH)D and GDM and measures of glucose metabolism. *Results.* A higher proportion of ethnic minority women had GDM ($p < 0.01$) and low 25(OH)D ($p < 0.01$) compared to Europeans. In logistic regression analyses, 25(OH)D < 50 nmol/L was associated with GDM after adjusting for age, parity, education, and season (OR 1.6; 95% CI 1.1–2.2). After additional adjustments for variables reflecting fat mass (skinfolds or BMI) and ethnicity, the association disappeared with ethnicity having a much stronger effect than the adiposity variables. We got similar results exploring effects on other measures of glucose metabolism and when change in 25(OH)D from inclusion to 28 GW was taken into account. *Conclusions.* Vitamin D deficiency was not associated with GDM or glucose metabolism in a multiethnic population-based study, after adjustments for confounding factors, in particular ethnicity.

1. Introduction

Although the role of vitamin D in calcium metabolism and bone health is undisputed, other long-term health consequences of low vitamin D are still debated [1, 2]. During the last decade, many observational studies have reported an association between low levels of vitamin D and impaired glucose metabolism and type 2 diabetes [1, 3], although results from trials so far have not confirmed a causal relationship [1, 4]. Observational studies have indicated that vitamin D deficiency may be a modifiable risk factor also for gestational diabetes mellitus (GDM) [5], and some studies have found associations with other measures of glucose metabolism in pregnancy [6]. Several reviews and meta-analyses have recently assessed the relation between vitamin D and GDM in observational studies [7–12]. A modest increase in odds of GDM has been found, with a range from 1.38 to 1.61 in women with low levels of vitamin D [5]. Subgroup analyses have found differences based on countries, analytical methods for vitamin D, definition of GDM, maternal age, sample size, adjustment for confounders, and study quality [8], confirming the complexity of interactions among individual, lifestyle, and geographical factors [5].

Vitamin D deficiency in pregnancy is widespread [13], and in Europe, women in ethnic minority groups from South Asia, the Middle East and Africa are at highest risk [14–16]. Possible biological mechanisms of the association between vitamin D and GDM are through effects on insulin-sensitive tissues, calcium pool dysregulation in the pancreas, genetic variations, or inflammation [5, 6]. In addition, β-cells may directly convert vitamin D into its active form as both the vitamin D receptor and the 1α-hydroxylase enzyme have been found expressed in a pancreatic islet [17]. During pregnancy, irrespective of the prepregnant level, insulin resistance increases about 50–60% [18, 19] but is exaggerated by excessive gestational weight gain. GDM reflects both increased insulin resistance and β-cell dysfunction, and both these components have been found to be associated with vitamin D levels [6]. Further, we have previously found a high prevalence of vitamin D deficiency [14], GDM [20] and measures of glucose metabolism, especially in ethnic minority groups, making us capable of exploring relations between vitamin D deficiency, ethnicity, and GDM. Therefore, in the present study, we aimed to assess associations between maternal 25-hydroxyvitamin D (25(OH)D) and GDM and measures of glucose metabolism, insulin resistance, and β-cell function, before and after adjusting for potentially confounding factors.

2. Materials and Methods

2.1. Design, Setting, and Study Population. Data are from a population-based, prospective cohort of 823 presumably healthy women attending maternal and child health clinics for antenatal care in Groruddalen, Oslo, Norway, between May 2008 and March 2010 (the STORK Groruddalen study) [21, 22]. The majority (75–85%) of pregnant women residing in this area, situated at a latitude of 60°N, attended the child health clinics for antenatal care. The study design has been described in detail elsewhere [21, 22]. In short, information material and questionnaires were translated into Arabic, English, Sorani, Somali, Tamil, Turkish, Urdu, and Vietnamese and quality checked by bilingual health professionals. Women were eligible if they (1) lived in the district, (2) planned to give birth at one of the two study hospitals, (3) were in <20 gestational weeks (GW), (4) were not suffering from diseases necessitating intensive hospital follow-up during pregnancy, (5) could communicate in Norwegian or any of the specified languages, and (6) were able to provide written consent. In total, 59% of the included women had an ethnic minority background. The participation rate was 74%, and the participating women were found representative of the main ethnic groups [20]. Maternal data were collected at 15 and 28 GW, through interviews by study personnel, assisted by professional interpreters when needed. Clinical measurements and blood samples were collected according to the study protocol.

2.2. Ethics. The Regional Committee for Medical and Health Research Ethics for Southeast Norway (ref. REK 2007/894) and the Norwegian Data Inspectorate approved the study protocol.

Participation was based on informed written consent.

2.3. Study Sample. Of the 823 women included in the STORK Groruddalen project at 15 GW, 772 met at 28 GW and 768 of these women had valid data on GDM status by the WHO 2013 criteria. Thirteen women were excluded because of missing data on 25(OH)D at inclusion (15 GW), and ten women from South or Central America were excluded due to low numbers from this geographic region, leaving a study sample of 745 (91%) women (flow chart, Supplementary Figure S1). For secondary outcomes, the sample size was 731 due to some missing values for C-peptide.

2.4. Variables

2.4.1. Outcome Variables. The primary outcome in this particular analysis was GDM by the WHO 2013 criteria (fasting plasma glucose (FPG) ≥ 5.1 or 2 h glucose ≥ 8.5 mmol/L) by vitamin D status [20, 23]. We used a modified version of the WHO 2013 criteria as 1-hour PG ≥ 10 mmol/L was not collected. A standard 75 g oral glucose tolerance test was performed at 28 GW [20], and venous blood glucose was measured on-site with a plasma-calibrated HemoCue glucose 201+ (Angelholm, Sweden).

Secondary outcome variables were FPG, 2-hour PG, insulin resistance (measured by homeostasis model assessment of insulin resistance (HOMA-IR)), β-cell function (HOMA-B), fasting serum insulin, and C-peptide, all measured at the follow-up visit at 28 GW [19]. C-peptide and insulin were measured at the Hormone Laboratory, Oslo University Hospital, by noncompetitive immunofluorometric assays (DELFIA, PerkinElmer Life Sciences, Wallac Oy, Turku, Finland). HOMA-IR and HOMA-B were estimated by the Oxford University HOMA Calculator 2.2 from the glucose and C-peptide concentrations [24]. Plasma glucose values used in the calculations of a homeostatic model were measured at the Akershus University Hospital from venous blood on gel tubes (VITROS 5,1 FS, Ortho Clinical Diagnostics, slide-adapted colorimetric method).

2.4.2. Main Exposure Variable. Serum 25(OH)D was analysed by competitive RIA (DiaSorin) at the Hormone Laboratory, Oslo University Hospital, at 16 and 28 GW. The method measures total 25(OH)D (both 25(OH)D_2 and D_3), with interassay coefficients of variation (CV) of 13–16%. The laboratory is accredited by the International Organization for Standardization and is part of the Vitamin D Quality Assessment Scheme, DEQAS. Concentrations of 25(OH)D < 12 nmol/L were replaced with "11 nmol/L" in the calculations ($n = 17$) so as to not overestimate the effect of low-vitamin D status. The laboratory's reference range was 37–131 nmol/L based on the ethnic Norwegian population from the Oslo Health Study [25]. Preplanned, and according to the protocol, women with 25(OH)D less than the laboratory's lower reference range (<37 nmol/L) at 15 and 28 GW were provided written information about their

25(OH)D concentration and recommended to consult their general practitioner for treatment [14].

2.4.3. Confounders. We performed a search of the literature for relevant confounders, set up a directed acyclic graph (DAG), and selected variables available in our cohort. Maternal age at inclusion was self-reported. Parity was categorised as nulliparous, uniparous, or multiparous (≥2), referring to status before the current pregnancy. Education level was categorised as completed primary education or less (<10 years), completed high school education (10–12 years), and completed ≥4 years college/university education. Season for 25(OH)D measurements at inclusion (15 GW) was categorised as summer (June to November) and winter (December to May) [14]. Specially trained study personnel performed maternal anthropometric measurements at 15 and 28 GW [21]. Each measurement was taken twice, and the mean used. We here report "sum of skinfolds," which is the sum of the triceps, the subscapular, and the suprailiac skinfold. A change in the sum of skinfolds was calculated as the difference between "sum of skinfolds" at 15 and 28 GW. Ethnic origin was defined by the pregnant participant's mother's country of birth [26]. Ethnic origin was further categorised as Europe (primarily from Norway and Sweden) and ethnic minority women, consisting of South Asia (primarily from Pakistan and Sri Lanka), Middle East including North Africa (primarily Turkey, Iraq, Afghanistan, and Morocco), Sub-Saharan Africa (primarily from Somalia, Eritrea, and Ethiopia), and East Asia (primarily from Vietnam and the Philippines). Prepregnancy BMI was calculated from self-reported weight before pregnancy and height measured at inclusion. Weight gain was calculated as the difference between self-reported prepregnant weight and measured weight at 28 GW. Dietary clusters were derived from four clusters reported earlier [27] and dichotomized as healthy (cluster 4) and unhealthy (clusters 1, 2, and 3).

2.5. Statistical Analyses. Descriptive statistics are presented as frequencies with proportions, mean values with standard deviations or 95% confidence intervals, and medians with interquartile range. All continuous response variables were assessed for normality. Nonparametric correlation coefficients between 25(OH)D at inclusion and secondary outcomes, assessed at 28 GW, were analysed. Differences between GDM and non-GDM women were tested by *t*-tests for continuous variables and chi-square test or Fischer's exact test for categorical variables. Logistic regression analyses were performed to investigate associations between 25(OH)D and GDM. Separate generalised linear models were performed to assess the relationship between the concentration of 25(OH)D and the secondary outcomes found significant in the correlation analysis (FPG, HOMA-IR, fasting insulin, and C-peptide). Maternal 25(OH)D was analysed as a continuous variable and categorised according to deficiency status (<50 nmol/L or ≥50 nmol/L). As treatment was recommended when 25(OH)D < 37 nmol/L, we further categorised the 25(OH)D status during pregnancy: consistently sufficient level (≥37 nmol/L at 15 and 28 GW), consistently deficient level (<37 nmol/L at 15 and 28 GW), increasing level (<37 nmol/L at 15 GW and ≥37 nmol/L at 28 GW), and decreasing level (≥37 nmol/L at 15 GW and <37 nmol/L at 28 GW). Guided by a DAG (Figure 1), we chose to account for the following *potential* confounders in the regression analyses: age, parity, education, season for measurement of 25(OH)D at 15 GW, sum of skinfolds at 15 GW, change in skinfolds from 15 GW to 28 GW, and ethnicity/geographic origin. Interactions between 25(OH)D and season and between 25(OH)D and ethnicity were examined graphically and by adding interaction terms into the models. We performed sensitivity analysis including prepregnant BMI and weight gain from 15 to 28 GW instead of "sum of skinfolds" at inclusion and change in "sum of skinfolds" to explore the impact of different measures of adiposity. We also included the variable of dietary clusters in the final model as a sensitivity analysis. As insulin, C-peptide, and HOMA-IR values were skewed, these variables were log-transformed, and we repeated the regression analyses with these variables. Results from regression analysis are presented as odds ratio (OR) and coefficients (β) with 95% CI. p values < 0.05 were considered statistically significant. SPSS software (version 22; IBM SPSS Statistics) and Stata/Se14.1 were used for statistical analysis.

3. Results

Sample characteristics for the total cohort are presented in Table 1 and stratified by ethnic groups in Supplementary Table 1. Age, sociodemographic and anthropometric variables, the prevalence of GDM, and 25(OH)D levels differed by ethnicity. The concentration of 25(OH)D ranged from <12 to 148 nmol/L at 15 GW, with large ethnic differences; only 35 women from Europe and 1 woman from the Middle East had values > 100 nmol/L (Figure 2). The proportion with vitamin D deficiency (25(OH)D < 50 nmol/L) was significantly higher among women with GDM than among non-GDM women (60% versus 49%, $p < 0.01$) (Table 1). Similarly, the proportion with severe deficiency (25(OH)D < 25 nmol/L) tended to be higher among GDM women (Supplementary Table 2). At 28 GW, the proportion with 25(OH)D < 50 nmol/L was reduced, but differences between GDM and non-GDM women remained significant (Supplementary Table 2). A higher proportion of women with consistent vitamin D deficiency and with levels increasing from low to sufficient were found among GDM women compared to non-GDM women (both $p < 0.01$) (Table 1). A higher proportion of ethnic minority women had GDM (Figure 3(a)) and low 25(OH)D (Figure 3(b)) compared to European women. In addition, a higher proportion of vitamin D-deficient women had GDM compared with women with a consistently sufficient level of vitamin D during pregnancy (Figure 4).

In univariate analyses, vitamin D deficiency (<50 nmol/L) at 15 GW and the categories consistently deficient and increasing of vitamin D status during pregnancy were significantly associated with GDM, but analysed as a continuous variable, 25(OH)D was not significantly associated with GDM ($p = 0.07$). Significant inverse correlations were found

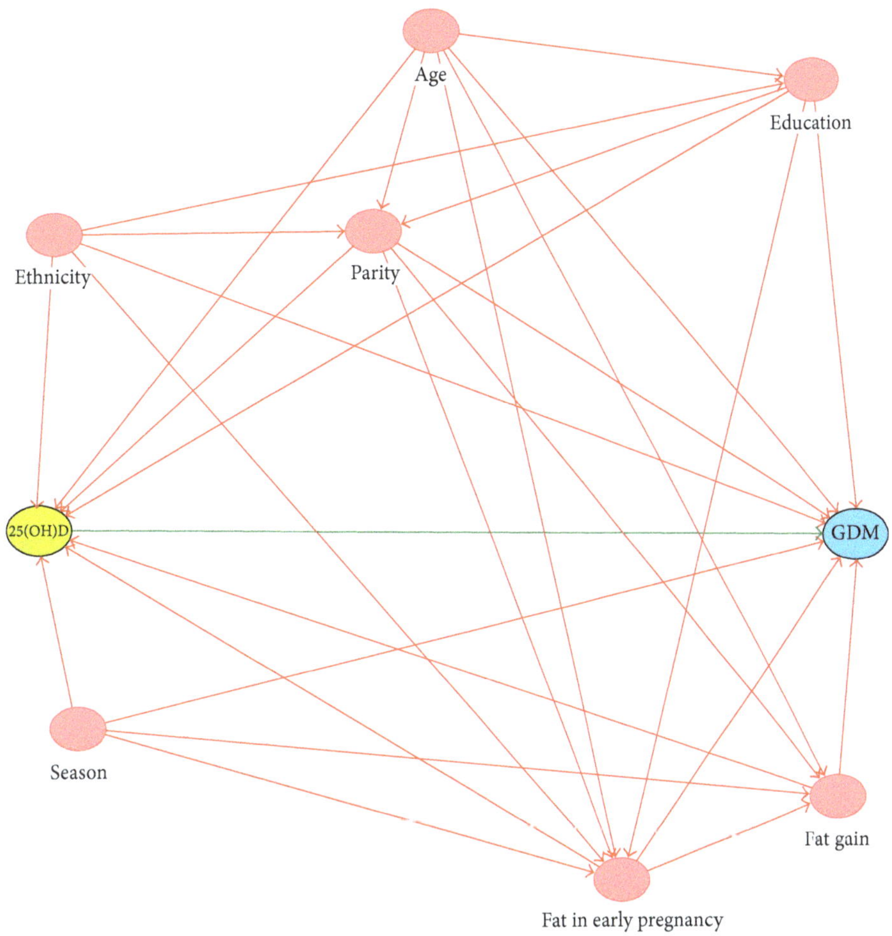

Figure 1: Directed acyclic graph of confounders between vitamin D (25(OH)D) and gestational diabetes mellitus (GDM).

between 25(OH)D in early pregnancy and FPG, HOMA-IR, fasting insulin, and fasting C-peptide but not with HOMA-B or 2-hour PG (Supplementary Table 3).

Possible confounders for the relation between 25(OH)D and GDM are presented in Table 1. After adjustments for age, parity, education, and season, vitamin D deficiency was still associated with GDM (model 1; OR 1.6; 95% CI 1.1–2.2) (Table 2). The OR was slightly reduced and the association was no longer significant after additional adjustments for the "sum of skinfolds" and change in the "sum of skinfolds" (model 2). Including ethnicity into the model, the OR was even more attenuated (model 3). Similarly, we found no association with GDM using vitamin D status during pregnancy after adjustments for confounders (Table 2). Based on the correlation analyses, we performed linear regression models for FPG, HOMA-IR, fasting insulin, and C-peptide (Table 3). All significant associations present in unadjusted analyses and model 1 disappeared after adjustments for confounders, with ethnicity having a much stronger effect than the adiposity variables.

3.1. Sensitivity Analyses. Using the same approach, but adjusting for prepregnant BMI and weight gain from 15 to 28 GW instead of the "sum of skinfolds" at 15 GW and change in the "sum of skinfolds" in model 2, the association was still significant (results not shown). Including dietary clusters into the models had no effect on the estimates. Using the log-transformed outcome variables in the regression models, we found exactly the same pattern of associations.

4. Discussion

In this population-based multiethnic cohort of pregnant women with a high proportion with vitamin D deficiency during the first and second trimesters of pregnancy, we found that the crude prevalence of vitamin D deficiency was higher in women with GDM compared to normoglycemic women. We also found significant inverse correlations between 25(OH)D in early pregnancy and FPG, HOMA-IR, fasting insulin, and fasting C-peptide. However, in fully adjusted regression models, taking into account a number of possible confounders, low levels of 25(OH)D did not predict the development of GDM or deterioration in glucose metabolism observed from 15 to 28 GW.

Strengths of the present study include its population-based longitudinal design, the high attendance rate with minor loss to follow-up, and the relatively large sample size in a multiethnic European context. We also performed universal screening for GDM in 28 GW and assessed GDM by two definitions. A broad data set was collected that made

TABLE 1: 25-Hydroxyvitamin D (25(OH)D) status and confounding variables in the total sample and stratified by gestational diabetes mellitus (GDM) status, WHO 2013 criteria. Values are mean (95% confidence interval) or (numbers (%)).

		GDM (WHO 2013)		
	$n = 745$	Yes $n = 235$	No $n = 510$	p
Status at inclusion (15 GW[i])				
Overall mean 25(OH)D (nmol/L)	50.2 (48.3, 52.1)	47.7 (44.0, 51.3)	51.4 (49.2, 53.7)	0.07
25(OH)D < 50 nmol/L (n (%))	389 (52)	141 (60)	248 (49)	**0.01**
25(OH)D status during pregnancy[a]				
Consistently sufficient (n (%))	417 (57)	109 (47)	308 (61)	**<0.01**
Decreasing (n (%))	63 (8.6)	22 (9.6)	41 (8.1)	0.50
Increasing (n (%))	145 (20)	55 (24)	90 (18)	0.06
Consistently deficient (n (%))	111 (15)	44 (19)	67 (13)	**0.03**
Prepregnancy maternal status				
Age (years)	29.8 (29.5, 30.2)	30.3 (29.6, 30.9)	29.6 (29.2, 30.1)	0.12
Ethnicity (n (%))				
Europe	346 (46.4)	82 (35)	264 (52)	**<0.01**
South Asia	191 (25.6)	81 (35)	110 (22)	**<0.01**
Middle East and North Africa	115 (15.4)	41 (17)	74 (15)	0.49
Sub-Saharan Africa	53 (7.1)	20 (8.5)	33 (6.5)	0.32
East Asia	40 (5.4)	11 (4.7)	29 (5.7)	0.57
Parity (n (%))				
Para 0	340 (46)	104 (44)	236 (46)	0.61
Para 1	256 (34)	73 (31)	183 (36)	0.18
Para ≥ 2	149 (20)	58 (25)	91 (18)	**0.03**
Education (years) (n (%))[a]				
<10	122 (16)	50 (21)	72 (14)	**0.02**
10–12	293 (40)	100 (43)	193 (38)	0.20
>12	324 (44)	84 (36)	240 (48)	**<0.01**
Prepregnancy BMI[ii] (kg/m^2)[a]	24.5 (24.2, 24.9)	25.9 (25.2, 26.6)	23.9 (23.5, 24.3)	**<0.01**
Status at inclusion				
Gestational week	15.1 (14.9, 15.4)	15.2 (14.7, 15.6)	15.1 (14.8, 15.4)	0.74
Sum of skinfolds (mm)[b]	72.0 (70.6, 73.5)	77.0 (74.3, 79.8)	69.8 (68.1, 71.5)	**<0.01**
Season for 25(OH)D measurement (n (%))				
Summer	347 (47)	130 (55)	217 (43)	**<0.01**
Winter	398 (53)	105 (45)	293 (57)	**<0.01**
Status at 28 GW				
Gestational week[c]	28.3 (28.2, 28.4)	28.2 (28.0, 28.3)	28.3 (28.2, 28.4)	0.20
ΔSum of skinfolds (15 to 28 GW) (mm)[d]	5.8 (4.8, 6.8)	6.2 (4.5, 7.9)	5.6 (4.3, 6.8)	0.58
Weight gain (prepregnant to 28 GW) (kg)	8.7 (8.3, 9.0)	8.8 (8.1, 9.4)	8.6 (8.2, 9.0)	0.71
Dietary clusters (n (%))[a]				
Healthy	239 (33)	54 (23)	185 (37)	**<0.01**
Unhealthy	493 (67)	179 (77)	314 (63)	**<0.01**

[i]GW: gestational week derived from the 1st day of the woman's last menstrual period; [ii]BMI: body mass index; [a]missing information of 5–13 women; [b]$n = 681$; [c]missing information of 1–4 women; [d]$n = 649$. Consistently sufficient: 25(OH)D ≥ 37 nmol/L at 15 and 28 GW. Decreasing: 25(OH)D ≥ 37 nmol/L at 15 GW and <37 nmol/L at 28 GW. Increasing: 25(OH)D < 37 nmol/L at 15 GW and ≥37 nmol/L at 28 GW. Consistently deficient: 25(OH)D < 37 nmol/L at 15 and 28 GW. p values for the differences between GDM and non-GDM. Bold numbers indicate p values < 0.05. Independent t-test or two-sample test of proportions.

us able to explore relations between 25(OH)D and several measures of glucose metabolism, and we adjusted for a range of possible confounders after drawing a DAG. Fore ethical reasons, women with 25(OH)D < 37 nmol/L were recommended vitamin D supplementation. As the main exposure variable 25(OH)D was measured at two time points in pregnancy, we were able to describe vitamin D levels during the first two trimesters (categories), where

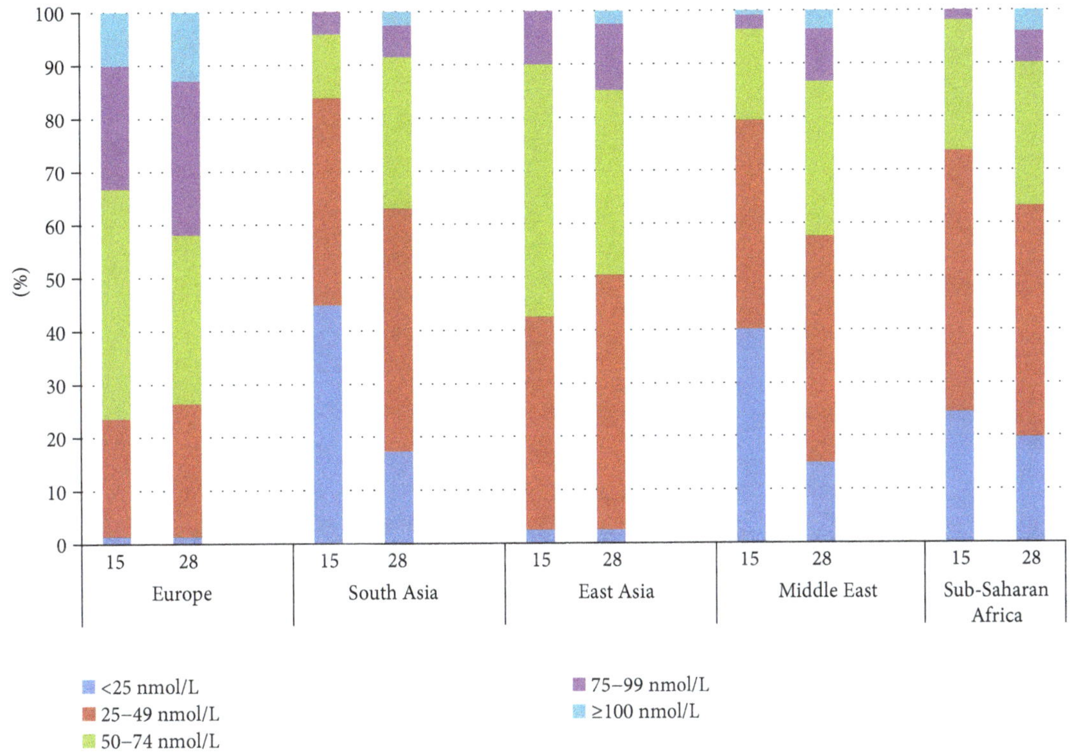

FIGURE 2: Proportion of participants (%) in categories of serum 25(OH)D concentrations at 15 and 28 weeks of gestation.

those who were recommended supplements can be followed. We measured 25(OH)D with standardized methods at the same high-quality laboratory, and half of the sample had vitamin D deficiency, many with severe deficiency.

The main limitation of our study is that the "gold standard" methods to quantify insulin resistance and β-cell function were not feasible in our primary care setting. The HOMA indexes are surrogate measures of insulin resistance and β-cell function estimated from FPG and fasting C-peptide concentrations. However, since HOMA-B is calculated from fasting values only, and the response over time after a glucose load, it has limited ability to detect chronic β-cell dysfunction, but HOMA is feasible in large studies and has been validated in pregnancy [28]. In addition, method-related differences in the measurement of 25(OH)D are widespread, although results from the Hormone Laboratory were found reliable compared with the gold standard of measuring 25(OH)D (standardized liquid chromatography-tandem mass spectrometry) [29]. Another limitation is that the categorisation of 25(OH)D may not be optimal as we do not separate women with a large increase in 25(OH)D from those with only a small increase from just below to above 37 nmol/L. Only very few women had levels above 100 nmol/L, and nearly all are from Europe, making comparison with 25(OH)D ≥ 100 nmol/L as reference impossible [30].

First, comparing studies may be hampered by different criteria of GDM, different definitions of vitamin D deficiency, and different methods of 25(OH)D measurements, and some studies have very low prevalence of vitamin D deficiency among the women included [7, 8]. We identified no other study exploring 25(OH)D at several time points during pregnancy in relation to GDM. In contrast to our population-based cohort study, several other observational studies have found an association between 25(OH)D and GDM [7, 8]. These studies are for the most part either cross-sectional or case-control/nested case-control studies, some are small, and some may represent selected groups. Another important issue in observational studies is adjustment for confounders. While most studies adjusted for age and BMI and some for season of blood drawn, some studies did not adjust for any confounders [10, 11]. In line with our study, some other studies did not find an association after adjusting for confounders [7, 8]. We used 50 nmol/L as the cutoff point for 25(OH)D, as this is the most used in literature. However, during pregnancy the conversion of 25(OH)D to $1,25(OH)_2D$ may be optimized at higher levels (>100 nmol/L) [30]. Some studies report that 25(OH)D < 100 nmol/L was associated with adverse pregnancy outcomes, such as preeclampsia and preterm birth [31–33]. In our study, we were not able to analyse this relation as very few women had high levels, making comparison with 25(OH)D > 100 nmol/L as a reference impossible. However, linear regression analyses did not indicate any nonlinear relationships between 25(OH)D and measures of glucose metabolism, so our results do not suggest any specific cutoff points. If the variation of serum levels of 25(OH)D is small, it might be difficult to find an association with GDM. A strength of our study is a large range in serum levels and, in particular, many women with low values, in contrast to some other studies. To account for the range in 25(OH)D concentrations, we also analysed 25(OH)D as a continuous variable in regression models. Importantly,

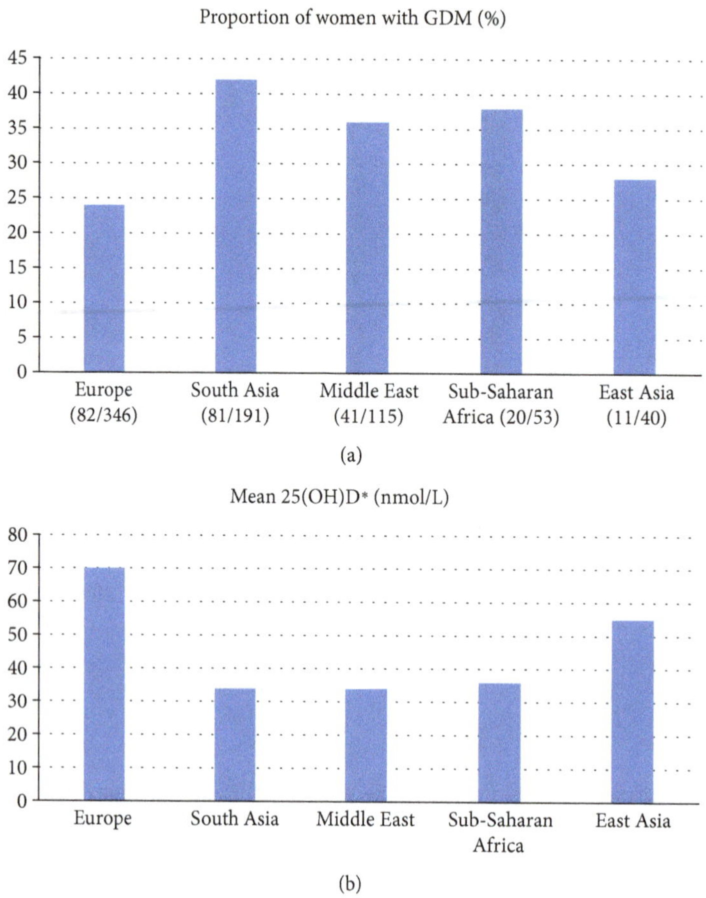

FIGURE 3: (a) Ethnic variation in gestational diabetes (GDM). (b) Ethnic variation in serum 25(OH)D concentrations. 25(OH)D: 25-hydroxyvitamin D; *15 gestational week.

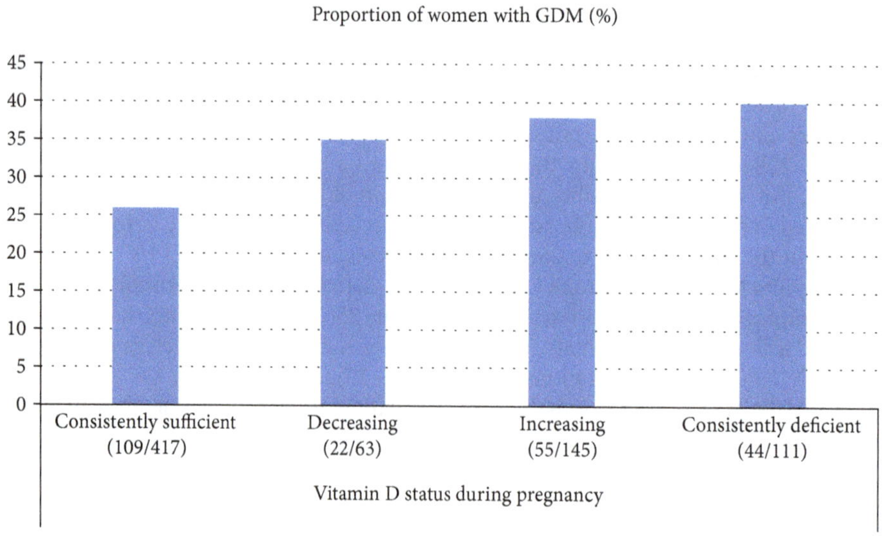

FIGURE 4: Consistently sufficient: 25(OH)D $\geq$ 37 nmol/L at 15 and 28 gestational weeks (GW). Decreasing: 25(OH)D $\geq$ 37 nmol/L at GW 15 and <37 nmol/L at 28 GW. Increasing: 25(OH)D < 37 nmol/L at GW 15 and $\geq$37 nmol/L at 28 GW. Consistently deficient: 25(OH)D < 37 nmol/L at 15 and 28 GW.

25(OH)D was not significantly associated with GDM or other measures of glucose metabolism in these analyses. However, as mentioned, there were relatively few women with high levels (>100 nmol/L), which may have limited our possibility to assess these associations across the full range of 25(OH)D levels.

Table 2: Univariate and multiple regressions between 25-hydroxyvitamin D (25(OH)D) and gestational diabetes mellitus (GDM)[a] (odds ratios and 95% confidence intervals). Associations according to vitamin D deficiency at inclusion (25(OH)D < 50 nmol/L) and vitamin D status during pregnancy (consistently sufficient or deficient, increasing or decreasing).

		Univariate analysis			Multiple analysis (model 1)			Multiple analysis (model 2)			Multiple analysis (model 3)		
	n	OR	(95% CI)	p	OR	(95% CI)	p	OR	(95% CI)	p	OR	(95% CI)	p
					$n = 739$, $R^2 = 0.064$			$n = 645$, $R^2 = 0.113$			$n = 645$, $R^2 = 0.130$		
25(OH)D sufficiency (≥50 nmol/L) at inclusion (15 GW) (ref)	745												
25(OH)D < 50 nmol/L		1.6	(1.2, 2.2)	**<0.01**	1.6	(1.1, 2.2)	**<0.01**	1.4	(0.95, 2.0)	0.09	1.1	(0.69, 1.6)	0.79
					$n = 730$, $R^2 = 0.065$			$n = 640$, $R^2 = 0.108$			$n = 640$, $R^2 = 0.127$		
25(OH)D consistently sufficient (ref)	736												
Decreasing		1.5	(0.86, 2.7)	0.15	1.4	(0.77, 2.5)	0.29	1.3	(0.68, 2.4)	0.49	1.1	(0.60, 2.1)	0.69
Increasing		1.7	(1.2, 2.6)	**<0.01**	1.8	(1.2, 2.7)	**<0.01**	1.4	(0.87, 2.2)	0.18	1.0	(0.60, 1.7)	0.97
Consistently deficient		1.9	(1.2, 2.9)	**<0.01**	1.7	(1.0, 2.7)	**0.04**	1.3	(0.74, 2.2)	0.39	0.88	(0.49, 1.6)	0.68

[a]Logistic regression analysis with GDM as dependent variable. ref: referent value; GW: gestational week; R^2: coefficient of determination. Model 1: adjusted for age, parity, education, and season. Model 2: the same as model 1, with additional adjustment for the sum of skinfolds at visit 1 and change in skinfolds from visit 1 to visit 2. Model 3: the same as model 2, with additional adjustment for ethnicity/geographic origin. Consistently sufficient: 25(OH)D ≥ 37 nmol/L at 15 and 28 GW. Decreasing: 25(OH)D ≥ 37 nmol/L at 15 GW and <37 nmol/L at 28 GW. Increasing: 25(OH)D < 37 nmol/L at 15 GW and ≥37 nmol/L at 28 GW. Consistently deficient: 25(OH)D < 37 nmol/L at 15 and 28 GW.

TABLE 3: Separate generalised linear models between 25-hydroxyvitamin D (25(OH)D) and each of the following dependent variables: fasting plasma glucose (FPG), HOMA-IR, fasting insulin, and C-peptide (regression coefficients and 95% confidence intervals). Associations according to vitamin D deficiency at inclusion (25(OH)D < 50 nmol/L) with vitamin D sufficiency (25(OH)D ≥ 50 nmol/L) as reference.

		Univariate analysis			Multiple analysis (model 1)			Multiple analysis (model 2)			Multiple analysis (model 3)[a]		
	n	B	(95% CI)	p	B	(95% CI)	p	B	(95% CI)	p	B	(95% CI)	p
FPG[a]	745	0.13	(0.04, 0.21)	**<0.01**	0.13	(0.04, 0.22)	**<0.01**	0.10	(0.01, 0.20)	**0.04**	0.017	(−0.10, 0.13)	0.77
HOMA-IR[b]	731	0.16	(0.04, 0.28)	**<0.01**	0.19	(0.07, 0.32)	**<0.01**	0.14	(0.01, 0.27)	**0.03**	0.045	(−0.10, 0.20)	0.54
Insulin[c] (fasting)	731	16	(6.4, 25)	**<0.01**	15.2	(5.6, 25)	**<0.01**	10	(0.39, 20)	**0.04**	−0.13	(−11, 11)	0.98
C-peptide[d] (fasting)	731	70	(14, 125)	**0.01**	84	(26, 141)	**<0.01**	63	(5.2, 122)	**0.03**	21	(−45, 87)	0.54

Model 1: adjusted for age, parity, education, and season. Model 2: the same as model 1, with additional adjustment for the sum of skinfolds at visit 1 and change in skinfolds from visit 1 to visit 2. Model 3: the same as model 2, with additional adjustment for ethnicity/geographic origin. [a]FPG: $n = 645$, AIC (Akaike' information criterion) = 1182; [b]HOMA-IR: $n = 635$, AIC = 1482; [c]Insulin: $n = 635$, AIC = 6971; [d]C-peptide: $n = 635$, AIC = 9259.

An association between vitamin D and body fat has been found in several studies [34, 35]. As body fat and weight gain are risk factors for GDM [18, 36], it is important to adjust for body fat as a confounder of the association between vitamin D and GDM. Asians are known to have a body composition with more visceral and central fat and more fat per BMI unit compared with Western subjects which contribute to an increased insulin resistance, particularly seen in South Asians [37]. Therefore, BMI is not a good measure of body fat across populations. Many of the studies have adjusted for BMI or prepregnant BMI, although BMI is affected by physiological changes during pregnancy, with increased body fluid, and weight of the foetus and placenta. In our study in a pregnant population, we measured the sum of skinfolds in addition to BMI, in early pregnancy and at the time of GDM diagnosis. In our primary analyses, we adjusted for sum of skinfolds and change in sum of skinfolds accounting for increasing fat deposits from inclusion to 28 GW by including change in sum of skinfolds [8]. We identified only two studies adjusting for weight gain or other measures of increasing fat deposits during pregnancy [38, 39]. In the sensitivity analysis, adjusting for prepregnant BMI and weight gain, vitamin D deficiency and GDM were still significantly associated. However, when adjusting for a more direct measure of fat deposits, the association was attenuated and no longer significant, probably reflecting that sum of skinfolds is a better measure of fat deposits in multiethnic pregnant populations. Furthermore, of the studies that found an association, only a few studies adjusted for socioeconomic status and demographics such as ethnicity. Many of these are studies from the USA primarily representing groups with African American and Hispanic ethnicities in addition to European-origin populations [7]. Studies from other countries representing other populations provide divergent results as one study from Iran [40] and one study from China [41] found an association, while a study from India did not [42].

Studies exploring relations between 25(OH)D and other measures of glucose metabolism are fewer, results are inconsistent, and studies are often hampered with methodological flaws, as few used a longitudinal design and adjustment for confounding factors. Many studies report only correlations, primarily with FPG, insulin, and different measures of HOMA, most showing inverse correlations with 25(OH)D. In studies adjusting for confounders, results are inconsistent [38, 40, 43–46].

The most striking finding in our study was that the association with 25(OH)D disappeared after adjusting for ethnicity both for the primary and secondary outcomes. We can only speculate about the reason for this. Ethnicity obviously reflects numerous factors; some may be related to vitamin D and some to GDM, but not necessarily to both. For example, skin pigmentation and use of concealing clothes and minimal sun exposure of the skin are associated with some ethnic groups and vitamin D status, but not necessarily with GDM, although these factors may be related to low levels of physical activity. Lifestyle factors, such as a low fibre-high simple carbohydrate diet and a low physical activity level, are strongly related to ethnicity and GDM, but not necessarily vitamin D. We have also found a strong relation with early life factors and GDM explaining some of the excess susceptibility for GDM in ethnic minority groups [47], but the relation with these factors and 25(OH)D is less clear. Further, genes involved in vitamin D metabolism or GDM, but probably not the same genes, could be differentially expressed depending on ethnic origin. Hence, ethnicity is an important confounder, but the effects on the exposure and the outcome are probably mediated through different mechanisms and could represent cultural, social, genetic, or other unmeasured factors.

Generally, most of the observational studies seem to be hampered by poor methodological design and probably residual confounding. Two reviews of trials concluded that vitamin D supplementation did not influence the incidence of GDM, but few and very small trials were found [48, 49]. Well-designed randomized controlled trials in multiethnic populations with low vitamin D status and high risk of GDM are considered necessary to determine the effect of vitamin D supplementation on prevention of GDM.

5. Conclusion

Vitamin D deficiency was not associated with GDM or glucose metabolism in a multiethnic population-based study, after adjustments for confounding factors. Our findings indicate that confounding by fat deposits and ethnicity explained most of the observed associations in unadjusted analysis.

Abbreviations

25(OH)D: 25-Hydroxyvitamin D
BMI: Body mass index
FPG: Fasting plasma glucose
DAG: Directed acyclic graph
GDM: Gestational diabetes mellitus
GW: Gestational week
HOMA: Homeostasis model assessment
HOMA-IR: Homeostasis model assessment of insulin resistance
HOMA-B: Homeostasis model assessment of β-cell function
PG: Plasma glucose.

Conflicts of Interest

The authors declare that there is no conflict of interest that could be perceived as prejudicing the impartiality of the research reported.

Acknowledgments

The authors would like to thank the midwives and research staff at the Grorud, Bjerke, and Stovner child health clinics and the women who participated in the STORK Groruddalen study. The authors would also like to thank Ragnhild S. Falk at the Oslo Center for Biostatistics and Epidemiology, Oslo University Hospital, for statistical advice. The authors would also like to thank the Hormone Laboratory at the Oslo University Hospital for the analyses of serum. The Norwegian Research Fund for General Practice has funded the PhD fellowship for Åse Ruth Eggemoen. The data collection was supported by the Norwegian Research Council, the Southern and Eastern Norway Regional Health Authority, the Norwegian Directorate of Health, and collaborative partners in the Stovner, Grorud, and Bjerke administrative districts of the city of Oslo.

Supplementary Materials

Supplementary 1. Supplementary Table 1: characteristics of the cohort by geographic origin. Values are mean (standard deviation), numbers (%), or median (interquartile range (IQR)).

Supplementary 2. Supplementary Table 2: 25-hydroxyvitamin D (25(OH)D) status in the total sample and stratified by gestational diabetes mellitus (GDM) status, WHO 2013 criteria. Values are mean (95% confidence interval) or numbers (%).

Supplementary 3. Supplementary Table 3: Spearman's rank correlation coefficients between 25-hydroxyvitamin D (25(OH)D) at inclusion (15 GW) and measures of glucose metabolism at 28 GW.

References

[1] C. J. Rosen, J. S. Adams, D. D. Bikle et al., "The non-skeletal effects of vitamin D: an Endocrine Society scientific statement," *Endocrine Reviews*, vol. 33, no. 3, pp. 456–492, 2012.

[2] P. Pludowski, M. F. Holick, S. Pilz et al., "Vitamin D effects on musculoskeletal health, immunity, autoimmunity, cardiovascular disease, cancer, fertility, pregnancy, dementia and mortality—a review of recent evidence," *Autoimmunity Reviews*, vol. 12, no. 10, pp. 976–989, 2013.

[3] H. L. Gulseth, I. M. Gjelstad, K. I. Birkeland, and C. A. Drevon, "Vitamin D and the metabolic syndrome," *Current Vascular Pharmacology*, vol. 11, no. 6, pp. 968–984, 2013.

[4] J. Mitri, M. D. Muraru, and A. G. Pittas, "Vitamin D and type 2 diabetes: a systematic review," *European Journal of Clinical Nutrition*, vol. 65, no. 9, pp. 1005–1015, 2011.

[5] S. Triunfo, A. Lanzone, and P. G. Lindqvist, "Low maternal circulating levels of vitamin D as potential determinant in the development of gestational diabetes mellitus," *Journal of Endocrinological Investigation*, vol. 40, no. 10, pp. 1049–1059, 2017.

[6] M. Alzaim and R. J. Wood, "Vitamin D and gestational diabetes mellitus," *Nutrition Reviews*, vol. 71, no. 3, pp. 158–167, 2013.

[7] M. X. Zhang, G. T. Pan, J. F. Guo, B. Y. Li, L. Q. Qin, and Z. L. Zhang, "Vitamin D deficiency increases the risk of gestational diabetes mellitus: a meta-analysis of observational studies," *Nutrients*, vol. 7, no. 12, pp. 8366–8375, 2015.

[8] M. Lu, Y. Xu, L. Lv, and M. Zhang, "Association between vitamin D status and the risk of gestational diabetes mellitus: a meta-analysis," *Archives of Gynecology and Obstetrics*, vol. 293, no. 5, pp. 959–966, 2016.

[9] Y. H. Poel, P. Hummel, P. Lips, F. Stam, T. van der Ploeg, and S. Simsek, "Vitamin D and gestational diabetes: a systematic review and meta-analysis," *European Journal of Internal Medicine*, vol. 23, no. 5, pp. 465–469, 2012.

[10] S. Q. Wei, H. P. Qi, Z. C. Luo, and W. D. Fraser, "Maternal vitamin D status and adverse pregnancy outcomes: a systematic review and meta-analysis," *The Journal of Maternal-Fetal & Neonatal Medicine*, vol. 26, no. 9, pp. 889–899, 2013.

[11] S. Q. Wei, "Vitamin D and pregnancy outcomes," *Current Opinion in Obstetrics and Gynecology*, vol. 26, no. 6, pp. 438–447, 2014.

[12] F. Aghajafari, T. Nagulesapillai, P. E. Ronksley, S. C. Tough, M. O'Beirne, and D. M. Rabi, "Association between maternal serum 25-hydroxyvitamin D level and pregnancy and neonatal outcomes: systematic review and meta-analysis of observational studies," *BMJ*, vol. 346, article f1169, 2013.

[13] C. L. Wagner, S. N. Taylor, A. Dawodu, D. D. Johnson, and B. W. Hollis, "Vitamin D and its role during pregnancy in attaining optimal health of mother and fetus," *Nutrients*, vol. 4, no. 12, pp. 208–230, 2012.

[14] A. R. Eggemoen, R. S. Falk, K. V. Knutsen et al., "Vitamin D deficiency and supplementation in pregnancy in a multiethnic population-based cohort," *BMC Pregnancy and Childbirth*, vol. 16, no. 1, p. 7, 2016.

[15] I. M. van der Meer, N. S. Karamali, A. J. Boeke et al., "High prevalence of vitamin D deficiency in pregnant non-Western women in The Hague, Netherlands," *The American Journal of Clinical Nutrition*, vol. 84, no. 2, pp. 350–353, 2006.

[16] C. Toher, K. Lindsay, M. McKenna et al., "Relationship between vitamin D knowledge and 25-hydroxyvitamin D levels amongst pregnant women," *Journal of Human Nutrition and Dietetics*, vol. 27, no. 3, pp. 261–269, 2014.

[17] L. Rejnmark, L. S. Bislev, K. D. Cashman et al., "Non-skeletal health effects of vitamin D supplementation: a systematic review on findings from meta-analyses summarizing trial data," *PLoS One*, vol. 12, no. 7, article e0180512, 2017.

[18] P. M. Catalano, "Obesity, insulin resistance, and pregnancy outcome," *Reproduction*, vol. 140, no. 3, pp. 365–371, 2010.

[19] K. Morkrid, A. K. Jenum, L. Sletner et al., "Failure to increase insulin secretory capacity during pregnancy-induced insulin resistance is associated with ethnicity and gestational diabetes," *European Journal of Endocrinology*, vol. 167, no. 4, pp. 579–588, 2012.

[20] A. K. Jenum, K. Morkrid, L. Sletner et al., "Impact of ethnicity on gestational diabetes identified with the WHO and the modified International Association of Diabetes and Pregnancy Study Groups criteria: a population-based cohort study," *European Journal of Endocrinology*, vol. 166, no. 2, pp. 317–324, 2012.

[21] A. K. Jenum, L. Sletner, N. Voldner et al., "The STORK Groruddalen research programme: a population-based cohort study of gestational diabetes, physical activity, and obesity in pregnancy in a multiethnic population. Rationale, methods, study population, and participation rates," *Scandinavian Journal of Public Health*, vol. 38, Supplement 5, pp. 60–70, 2010.

[22] A. R. Eggemoen, A. K. Jenum, I. Mdala, K. V. Knutsen, P. Lagerlov, and L. Sletner, "Vitamin D levels during pregnancy and associations with birth weight and body composition of the newborn: a longitudinal multiethnic population-based study," *British Journal of Nutrition*, vol. 117, no. 07, pp. 985–993, 2017.

[23] WHO, *Diagnostic Criteria and Classifiction of Hyperglycemia First Detected in Pregnancy*, World Health Organization, 2013, http://apps.who.int/iris/bitstream/10665/85975/1/WHO_NMH_MND_13.2_eng.pdf.

[24] T. M. Wallace, J. C. Levy, and D. R. Matthews, "Use and abuse of HOMA modeling," *Diabetes Care*, vol. 27, no. 6, pp. 1487–1495, 2004.

[25] H. E. Meyer, J. A. Falch, A. J. Sogaard, and E. Haug, "Vitamin D deficiency and secondary hyperparathyroidism and the association with bone mineral density in persons with Pakistani and Norwegian background living in Oslo, Norway: The Oslo Health Study," *Bone*, vol. 35, no. 2, pp. 412–417, 2004.

[26] R. Bhopal, "Glossary of terms relating to ethnicity and race: for reflection and debate," *Journal of Epidemiology & Community Health*, vol. 58, no. 6, pp. 441–445, 2004.

[27] C. Sommer, L. Sletner, A. K. Jenum et al., "Ethnic differences in maternal dietary patterns are largely explained by socio-economic score and integration score: a population-based study," *Food & Nutrition Research*, vol. 57, no. 1, article 21164, 2013.

[28] T. Radaelli, K. A. Farrell, L. Huston-Presley et al., "Estimates of insulin sensitivity using glucose and C-peptide from the hyperglycemia and adverse pregnancy outcome glucose tolerance test," *Diabetes Care*, vol. 33, no. 3, pp. 490–494, 2010.

[29] K. D. Cashman, K. G. Dowling, Z. Skrabakova et al., "Standardizing serum 25-hydroxyvitamin D data from four Nordic population samples using the Vitamin D Standardization Program protocols: shedding new light on vitamin D status in Nordic individuals," *Scandinavian Journal of Clinical and Laboratory Investigation*, vol. 75, no. 7, pp. 549–561, 2015.

[30] B. W. Hollis, D. Johnson, T. C. Hulsey, M. Ebeling, and C. L. Wagner, "Vitamin D supplementation during pregnancy: double-blind, randomized clinical trial of safety and effectiveness," *Journal of Bone and Mineral Research*, vol. 26, no. 10, pp. 2341–2357, 2011.

[31] C. L. Wagner, C. Baggerly, S. McDonnell et al., "Post-hoc analysis of vitamin D status and reduced risk of preterm birth in two vitamin D pregnancy cohorts compared with South Carolina March of Dimes 2009–2011 rates," *The Journal of Steroid Biochemistry and Molecular Biology*, vol. 155, Part B, pp. 245–251, 2016.

[32] S. L. McDonnell, K. A. Baggerly, C. A. Baggerly et al., "Maternal 25(OH)D concentrations ≥40 ng/mL associated with 60% lower preterm birth risk among general obstetrical patients at an urban medical center," *PLoS One*, vol. 12, no. 7, article e0180483, 2017.

[33] H. Mirzakhani, A. A. Litonjua, T. F. McElrath et al., "Early pregnancy vitamin D status and risk of preeclampsia," *The Journal of Clinical Investigation*, vol. 126, no. 12, pp. 4702–4715, 2016.

[34] J. Wortsman, L. Y. Matsuoka, T. C. Chen, Z. Lu, and M. F. Holick, "Decreased bioavailability of vitamin D in obesity," *The American Journal of Clinical Nutrition*, vol. 72, no. 3, pp. 690–693, 2000.

[35] S. Cheng, J. M. Massaro, C. S. Fox et al., "Adiposity, cardiometabolic risk, and vitamin D status: the Framingham Heart Study," *Diabetes*, vol. 59, no. 1, pp. 242–248, 2010.

[36] B. E. Metzger, T. A. Buchanan, D. R. Coustan et al., "Summary and recommendations of the Fifth International Workshop-Conference on Gestational Diabetes Mellitus," *Diabetes Care*, vol. 30, Supplement 2, pp. S251–S260, 2007.

[37] A. K. Jenum, C. Sommer, L. Sletner, K. Morkrid, A. Baerug, and A. Mosdol, "Adiposity and hyperglycaemia in pregnancy and related health outcomes in European ethnic minorities of Asian and African origin: a review," *Food & Nutrition Research*, vol. 57, no. 1, article 18889, 2013.

[38] C. K. Kramer, B. Swaminathan, A. J. Hanley et al., "Vitamin D and parathyroid hormone status in pregnancy: effect on insulin sensitivity, β-cell function, and gestational diabetes mellitus," *The Journal of Clinical Endocrinology & Metabolism*, vol. 99, no. 12, pp. 4506–4513, 2014.

[39] H. H. Burris, S. L. Rifas-Shiman, K. Kleinman et al., "Vitamin D deficiency in pregnancy and gestational diabetes mellitus," *American Journal of Obstetrics & Gynecology*, vol. 207, no. 3, pp. 182.e1–182.e8, 2012.

[40] Z. Maghbooli, A. Hossein-Nezhad, F. Karimi, A. R. Shafaei, and B. Larijani, "Correlation between vitamin D_3 deficiency and insulin resistance in pregnancy," *Diabetes/Metabolism Research and Reviews*, vol. 24, no. 1, pp. 27–32, 2008.

[41] O. Wang, M. Nie, Y. Y. Hu et al., "Association between vitamin D insufficiency and the risk for gestational diabetes mellitus in pregnant Chinese women," *Biomedical and Environmental Sciences*, vol. 25, no. 4, pp. 399–406, 2012.

[42] H. J. Farrant, G. V. Krishnaveni, J. C. Hill et al., "Vitamin D insufficiency is common in Indian mothers but is not associated with gestational diabetes or variation in newborn size," *European Journal of Clinical Nutrition*, vol. 63, no. 5, pp. 646–652, 2009.

[43] E. C. O'Brien, E. J. O'Sullivan, M. T. Kilbane, A. A. Geraghty, M. J. McKenna, and F. M. McAuliffe, "Season and vitamin D status are independently associated with glucose homeostasis in pregnancy," *Nutrition & Metabolism*, vol. 14, no. 1, p. 50, 2017.

[44] D. S. McLeod, J. V. Warner, M. Henman, D. Cowley, K. Gibbons, and H. D. McIntyre, "Associations of serum vitamin D concentrations with obstetric glucose metabolism in a subset of the Hyperglycemia and Adverse Pregnancy Outcome (HAPO) study cohort," *Diabetic Medicine*, vol. 29, no. 8, pp. e199–e204, 2012.

[45] M. Lacroix, M. C. Battista, M. Doyon et al., "Lower vitamin D levels at first trimester are associated with higher risk of developing gestational diabetes mellitus," *Acta Diabetologica*, vol. 51, no. 4, pp. 609–616, 2014.

[46] R. J. Clifton-Bligh, P. McElduff, and A. McElduff, "Maternal vitamin D deficiency, ethnicity and gestational diabetes," *Diabetic Medicine*, vol. 25, no. 6, pp. 678–684, 2008.

[47] K. Morkrid, A. K. Jenum, S. Berntsen et al., "Objectively recorded physical activity and the association with gestational diabetes," *Scandinavian Journal of Medicine & Science in Sports*, vol. 24, no. 5, pp. e389–e397, 2014.

[48] F. R. Perez-Lopez, V. Pasupuleti, E. Mezones-Holguin et al., "Effect of vitamin D supplementation during pregnancy on maternal and neonatal outcomes: a systematic review and meta-analysis of randomized controlled trials," *Fertility and Sterility*, vol. 103, no. 5, pp. 1278–1288.e4, 2015.

[49] L. M. De-Regil, C. Palacios, L. K. Lombardo, and J. P. Pena-Rosas, "Vitamin D supplementation for women during pregnancy," *Cochrane Database of Systematic Reviews*, no. 1, article CD008873, 2016.

22

Quality of Life in Women with Gestational Diabetes Mellitus

Daniela Marchetti,[1] Danilo Carrozzino,[1,2] Federica Fraticelli,[3] Mario Fulcheri,[1] and Ester Vitacolonna[3]

[1]*Department of Psychological Health and Territorial Sciences, "G. d'Annunzio" University of Chieti-Pescara, Chieti, Italy*
[2]*Psychiatric Research Unit, Psychiatric Centre North Zealand, Copenhagen University Hospital, Hillerød, Denmark*
[3]*Department of Medicine and Aging, "G. d'Annunzio" University of Chieti-Pescara, Chieti, Italy*

Correspondence should be addressed to Ester Vitacolonna; e.vitacolonna@unich.it

Academic Editor: Rosa Corcoy

Background and Objective. Diagnosis of Gestational Diabetes Mellitus (GDM) could significantly increase the likelihood of health problems concerning both potential risks for the mother, fetus, and child's development and negative effects on maternal mental health above all in terms of a diminished Quality of Life (QoL). The current systematic review study is aimed at further contributing to an advancement of knowledge about the clinical link between GDM and QoL. *Methods.* According to PRISMA guidelines, PubMed, Web of Science, Scopus, and Cochrane databases were searched for studies aimed at evaluating and/or improving levels of QoL in women diagnosed with GDM. *Results.* Fifteen research studies were identified and qualitatively analyzed by summarizing results according to the following two topics: GDM and QoL and interventions on QoL in patients with GDM. Studies showed that, in women with GDM, QoL is significantly worse in both the short term and long term. However, improvements on QoL can be achieved through different intervention programs by enhancing positive diabetes-related self-management behaviors. *Conclusion.* Future studies are strongly recommended to further examine the impact of integrative programs, including telemedicine and educational interventions, on QoL of GDM patients by promoting their illness acceptance and healthy lifestyle behaviors.

1. Introduction

Gestational Diabetes Mellitus (GDM) is defined as "diabetes diagnosed in the second or third trimester of pregnancy that was not clearly overt diabetes prior to gestation" [1]. GDM is one of the most frequent metabolic diseases during pregnancy and approximately affects 7% (range: 2–18%) of all pregnancies [2–5]. This clinical condition potentially affects not only negative medical outcomes but also the mental health status with additional adverse consequences on psychological well-being and Quality of Life (QoL) [6, 7].

Pregnancy is a particular time for all women. This condition becomes even more delicate when there is a diagnosis of GDM which makes necessary controls and therapies that will inevitably affect the woman's life. GDM can lead to potential risks for the mother, fetus, and child's development, as well as clinically relevant negative effects on maternal mental health, above all in terms of a diminished QoL [8, 9].

Health-related QoL was extensively accepted as a highly relevant outcome in different clinical trials [10]. QoL potentially operates as a unifying concept that comprises many domains such as general, physical, and psychological health, positive social relationships, environmental mastery, purpose in life, self-acceptance, autonomy, and personal growth factors [3, 11]. However, it may act by a core mechanism of subjective appraisal of own health status [12] resulting in specific diagnostic and therapeutic implications [13]. That is, QoL dimension can explain the different individual response to a standard medical treatment leading to an incomplete recovery in terms of health perception [14].

This concept was further highlighted by the World Health Organization criteria [15], which stressed the clinical relevance to promote the health status by not only treating physical symptoms but also instilling a positive mental state [16]. In this regard, the current systematic review study is aimed at further contributing to an advancement of knowledge about the clinical link between GDM and QoL.

2. Materials and Methods

2.1. Information Sources and Searches. According to Preferred Reporting Items for Systematic Reviews and Meta-Analyses (PRISMA) guidelines [17], a comprehensive electronic search strategy was used to identify peer-reviewed articles assessing QoL experienced by pregnant women diagnosed with GDM up to 19 October 2016. The following keywords were used: "gestational diabetes OR gestational hyperglycemia OR hyperglycemic pregnancy" combined using AND Boolean operator with "quality of life OR well-being". After the initial search was performed, studies were screened for eligibility; their relevance was initially assessed using titles and abstracts and finally the full review of papers. Searching and eligibility of target responses were carried out independently by two investigators (DM and DC); any type of disagreements was resolved by consensus among these primary raters and a senior investigator (EV).

Electronic research-literature databases searched included PubMed, Web of Science, Scopus, and Cochrane databases. In order to detect any missed articles during the literature search, reference lists of candidate articles were reviewed for further studies not yet identified. For each excluded study, we determined which elements of the electronic search were not addressed.

2.2. Eligibility Criteria. Papers were eligible for inclusion if they were research reports in English language describing data on QoL domains in relation to GDM diagnosis during pregnancy. We focused on studies examining QoL in women with *GDM* directly or evaluating the link between QoL and well-being alternatively by specifically using measures testing QoL. Based on this inclusion criterion, we selected studies referring to QoL or well-being related to QoL by consequently excluding research reports assessing well-being through measures on negative mental health (i.e., depression, anxiety, bipolar mood, and distress) or by focusing on a medical definition of well-being (health status, wellness, physical health, etc.). Also studies aimed at evaluating the effectiveness of programs targeted for GDM patients providing effects on QoL were included.

We excluded peer-reviewed single-case studies, reviews, meta-analyses, letters to the editor and commentaries, conference abstracts, books, and papers that were clearly irrelevant. In order to generate conclusions specific to GDM, we excluded research reports aimed at addressing levels of QoL in diabetic patients, without reporting specific data for GDM subgroup (e.g., considering diabetic pregnant women those with preexisting diabetes and those receiving the first diagnosis of GDM during pregnancy). No limit was set with regard to publication date.

2.3. Analysis and Data Synthesis. The heterogeneous nature of the identified studies (in terms of design and measures) did not permit a formal meta-analysis. Hence, narrative synthesis approach was judged to be the most appropriate method for the review.

Studies were categorized based on the object of the study, differentiated as those that aimed at assessing association and those that evaluated interventions. Significant information for each study was summarized and compared.

3. Results

The search of PubMed, Web of Science, Scopus, and Cochrane databases, including additional manual search, initially provided a total of 906 articles, as shown in the PRISMA flowchart (see Figure 1). Fifteen research studies were identified as clearly relevant and qualitatively analyzed in the systematic review. Pertinent results were summarized according to the following two specific chapters: (a) GDM and QoL (Table 1) and (b) interventions on QoL in patients with GDM (Table 2). Criteria for the diagnosis of GDM used in reviewed studies are illustrated in Table 3. In all but two studies [9, 26], standardized measures of QoL were used (see Tables 1 and 2 for details).

3.1. GDM and QoL. When combining an evaluation of levels of illness acceptance with an assessment of the QoL, Bień et al. [3] have found that illness acceptance was significantly correlated with all QoL related scores ($p < 0.05$) with R values ranging from 0.20 to 0.54. Similarly, GDM participants who did not report an individual illness interference with everyday life obtained significantly higher scores compared to those stating an illness limitation on specific QoL factors. That is, statistical differences between groups were observed on general QoL ($p = 0.006$), perceived general health ($p = 0.006$), and physical ($p = 0.003$), psychological ($p = 0.01$), and environmental ($p = 0.0001$) domains. Moreover, further examining QoL dimensions, the psychological domain was slightly worse than other QoL domains [3].

A similar study from Kopec et al. [19] evidenced that 171 respondents (i.e., 87.3% of the total sample specifically used for statistical analyses) reported a negative impact of GDM on their social life. Results also showed that higher levels of distress were significantly reported by women who tested glucose levels more frequently and those under treatment with insulin. In addition, patients perceiving insufficient information about their GDM symptoms reported higher levels of distress than those perceiving adequate information [19].

Another recent study from Danyliv et al. [18] compared levels of health-related QoL (HRQoL) of GDM patients with those of women with normal glucose tolerance (NGT) during pregnancy. They found significantly lower scores on HRQoL dimension for the group of GDM patients. However, when adjusting for the effects of other clinical covariates by performing a pooled multivariate analysis, the authors [18] showed that GDM per se did not influence HRQOL levels.

Similarly, a study of Dalfrà et al. [8] compared levels of QoL between GDM patients, pregnant women with type 1 diabetes, and healthy pregnant participants. GDM respondents scored significantly lower than healthy controls on the SF-36 general health perception subscale ($p < 0.05$) as

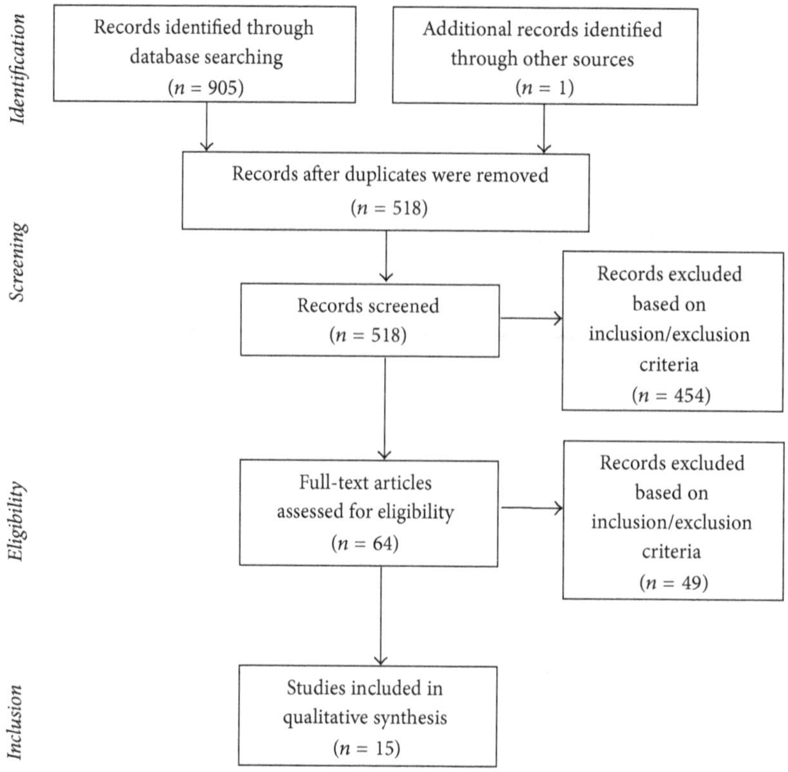

FIGURE 1: Flowchart of the systematic search.

evaluated during pregnancy at the third trimester. Moreover, whereas the SF-36 domains of QoL significantly improved after delivery among all three groups, rates of the SF-36 general health perception subscale remained significantly lower in GDM patients than in healthy controls [8].

Results in contrast with aforementioned findings were obtained from a previous research study aimed at evaluating impact of GDM on HRQOL after delivery. The authors [21] revealed no statistically significant differences between GDM patients and the healthy control group on the HRQOL dimensions. Similar results were previously reported also by Mautner et al. [22]. Their study underlined no clinically relevant differences between women with GDM and the healthy control group as concerns HRQoL levels.

Different results were later obtained from Trutnovsky et al. [20] who demonstrated significantly diminished levels of QoL among GDM patients. Specifically, GDM participants showed, from mid to late pregnancy, a significant reduction of physical, psychological, social, and global scores on the World Health Organization Quality of Life subscales (WHOQOL-BREF).

Results in line with above reported data were addressed by Rumbold and Crowther [24] when evidencing that women positively screened for GDM showed lower health perceptions than those with negative screening ($p < 0.05$). However, these statistical differences between positive and negative screened women for GDM were not significant late in pregnancy [24].

Similar results were provided in a study from Kim et al. [23]. This research highlighted that women with a diagnosis of GDM were significantly more prone to report poor physical function and a worse self-rated health status compared to healthy pregnant women. The same result was further supported after delivery with a greater proportion of GDM pregnant women reporting a lower self-rated health status than healthy controls. In addition, self-rated health status further worsened in the third trimester among women with GDM compared to healthy pregnant women without GDM. Surprisingly, GDM clinical condition was not significantly associated with declines in any other SF-36 health status subscales in the third trimester [23].

Finally, Lapolla et al. [9] indirectly revealed a worsening level of QoL among GDM women when demonstrating that this diagnosis resulted in the development of anxiety symptoms.

3.2. Interventions on QoL in Patients with GDM. When comparing QoL levels in GDM women attending different treatment programs (i.e., metformin alone, insulin alone, or a combination of both treatments), Latif et al. [25] showed that the negative influence on overall QoL was less with metformin compared to insulin. Nevertheless, the treatment combining metformin with insulin resulted in a greater negative impact on the QoL. Concerning the evaluation of treatment outcomes, Elnour et al. [28] observed statistically significant ($p < 0.05$) improvements in the HRQoL among patients attending a pharmacological care program.

A study, testing the effect of a telemedicine intervention, by Dalfrà and colleagues [27] found a significant improvement of the SF-36 general health perception, energy/vitality,

Table 1: Characteristics of included studies assessing the impact of GDM on Quality of Life.

Study	Country/setting/year	Study design	Aim	*N*	Measure of Quality of Life
Bień et al. [3]	Poland Three hospitals 2016	Observational study without control group	To assess the factors affecting QoL (and illness acceptance) in pregnant women diagnosed with GDM.	114 pregnant women with GDM	WHOQOL-BREF
Danyliv et al. [18]	Ireland Five antenatal centers involved in The Atlantic Diabetes in Pregnancy (DIP) initiative 2015	Observational study with control group	To compare QoL between GDM and NGT women 2 to 5 years after pregnancy. To explore participants characteristics which may influence their QoL.	234 women diagnosed with GDM during pregnancy 108 women with a history of healthy pregnancy	Visual Analog Scale of the EQ-5D-3L
Kopec et al. [19]	Poland University-affiliated GDM clinic 2015	Observational study without control group (longitudinal)	To assess, among other objectives, factors affecting the QoL of pregnant women with GDM.	205 pregnant women diagnosed with GDM	SF-8
Trutnovsky et al. [20]	Austria University GDM clinic 2012	Observational study without control group (prospective)	To evaluate, among other outcomes, QoL of women treated for GDM.	45 pregnant women affected by GDM, divided based on type of treatment: 27 diet-treated women 18 diet plus insulin women	WHOQOL-BREF
Lapolla et al. [9]	Italy Ten diabetes centers specialized in the care of pregnant women 2012	Observational study without control group	To evaluate QoL, wishes, and needs of Italian and immigrant women diagnosed with GDM.	286 pregnant women affected by GDM, divided into two groups: 198 Italian women 88 immigrant women	QoL is only indirectly evaluated with questions covering feelings and concerns related to the diagnosis of GDM and its treatment
Dalfrà et al. [8]	Italy Twelve diabetes clinics 2012	Observational study with control group	To examine the impact of diabetes on QoL among pregnant women with diabetes (GDM and T1DM) compared with pregnant women with a normal glucose tolerance.	245 women divided into three groups: 176 pregnant women with GDM 30 pregnant women with T1DM 39 healthy controls (pregnant women with negative GCT or OGTT findings)	SF-36
Halkoaho et al. [21]	Finland University hospital 2010	Observational study with control group	To evaluate the effects of GDM on women's QoL after delivery.	77 women diagnosed with GDM during pregnancy 54 healthy controls (women with normal glucose tolerance tests during pregnancy)	15D HRQoL

Table 1: Continued.

Study	Country/setting/year	Study design	Aim	*N*	Measure of Quality of Life
Mautner et al. [22]	Austria Public hospital 2009	Observational study with control group (longitudinal)	To explore QoL (and the incidence of depressive symptoms) in women during pregnancy and after delivery, comparing women with GDM, hypertensive disorders, and risk for preterm delivery with a control group characterized by uncomplicated pregnancy.	90 pregnant women, divided into four groups: 18 women affected by hypertensive disorders 11 women affected by GDM 32 women at risk of preterm delivery 29 healthy controls (pregnancy without complications)	WHOQOL-BREF
Kim et al. [23]	California, USA Six hospitals 2005	Observational study with control group (prospective)	To investigate the influence of GDM (and PIH) on maternal health status, testing the hypothesis that, among others, women with GDM would have a great likelihood to report declines in health status than women without GDM, with at least a partial mediation by cesarean birth or preterm delivery.	1445 pregnant women divided into three groups: 64 women with GDM 148 women with PIH 1233 healthy women	Physical functioning scale, vitality scale, and self-rated health item of the SF-36
Rumbold and Crowther [24]	South Australia Hospital with a high-risk pregnancy service and neonatal intensive care unit 2002	Observational study with control group (prospective)	To survey pregnant women on their experience of being screened for GDM, testing the hypothesis that women with a GDM diagnosis would experience a reduction in QoL (perception of the pregnancy, their health, and that of their baby) compared with women with a negative screening result.	145 pregnant women divided into two groups 21 with positive OGTT (GDM group) 124 with negative OGTT	SF-36

GDM: Gestational Diabetes Mellitus; NGT: normal glucose tolerance; OGTT: oral glucose tolerance test; QoL: Quality of Life; PIH: pregnancy-induced hypertension; T1DM: type 1 diabetes mellitus; EQ-5D-3L: 3-level version of the EuroQol 5-Dimension; 15D HRQoL: 15-Dimensional Health-Related Quality of Life; SF-36: 36-Item Short-Form Health Survey; SF-8: 8-Item Short-Form Health Survey; WHOQOL-BREF: World Health Organization Quality of Life-BREF.

TABLE 2: Characteristics of included studies assessing the impact of treatments on Quality of Life among GDM pregnant women.

Study	Country/setting/year	Study design	Aim	*N*	Measure of Quality of Life
Latif et al. [25]	England Two hospitals 2013	Quasi-experimental study Three conditions: (1) Treatment with metformin (2) Treatment with insulin (3) Treatment with metformin + insulin	To examine QoL (and treatment satisfaction) of women affected by GDM receiving metformin alone, insulin alone, or a combination of both treatments.	128 women diagnosed with GDM during pregnancy assigned to one of three conditions: 68 treated with metformin 32 treated with insulin 28 treated with metformin + insulin	ADDQoL
Petkova et al. [26]	Bulgaria Antenatal clinic 2011	Quasi-experimental study Two conditions: (1) Education group (intervention) (2) Control group	To investigate the effectiveness of an educational program for pregnant women with GDM on their QoL (and other outcomes).	30 pregnant women affected by GDM assigned to one of two conditions: 15 assigned to the intervention condition (education program) 15 assigned to the control condition	Five items measuring QoL
Dalfrà et al. [27]	Italy Twelve diabetes clinics 2009	Quasi-experimental study Two conditions: (1) Telemedicine condition (intervention) (2) Usual care condition (control)	To assess the effect of a telemedicine intervention on QoL (and other outcomes) among pregnant women with diabetes (GDM and T1DM).	235 pregnant women divided into two groups: 203 women with GDM 32 women with T1DM Participants of each group were sequentially assigned to one of two conditions: 88 women affected by GDM and 17 women affected by T1DM assigned to the telemedicine condition 115 women affected by GDM and 15 women affected by T1DM assigned to the control condition	SF-36

Table 2: Continued.

Study	Country/setting/year	Study design	Aim	*N*	Measure of Quality of Life
Elnour et al. [28]	United Arab Emirates Hospital 2008	Experimental study (RCT) Two conditions: (1) Pharmaceutical care program (intervention) (2) Usual care (control)	To evaluate the effect of a pharmaceutical care intervention programme for women with GDM on QoL (and other outcomes) both during pregnancy and after delivery.	180 pregnant women diagnosed with GDM randomly assigned to one of two conditions: 108 assigned to the intervention condition 72 assigned to the control condition	SF-36
Crowther et al. [29]	New South Wales; Queensland; South Australia; England; Wales Eighteen antenatal clinics 2005	Experimental study (RCT) Two conditions: (1) Intervention group (2) Routine-care group (control)	To examine the effect of an intervention (including dietary advice, blood glucose monitoring, and insulin therapy) for women with GDM on QoL (and other primary and secondary outcomes).	1000 pregnant women with GDM, randomly assigned to one of two conditions: 490 assigned to the intervention condition 510 assigned to the control condition	SF-36

GDM: Gestational Diabetes Mellitus; QoL: Quality of Life; T1DM: type 1 diabetes mellitus; ADDQoL: Audit of Diabetes-Dependent Quality of Life; SF-36: 36-Item Short-Form Health Survey.

Table 3: Diagnostic criteria for GDM of included studies.

Study	Time and methods of diagnosis	Diagnostic criteria
Bień et al. [3]	Diabetes first diagnosed during pregnancy, in accordance with the current guidelines of the Polish Diabetology Society: for pregnant women with risk factors, the 75 g OGTT is required. If glycemia is normal, the test should be readministered at 24–28 weeks of pregnancy or when first symptoms indicative of diabetes are observed. For women without risk factors, the 75 g OGTT is administered at 24–28 weeks of pregnancy	75-g OGTT: FPG levels of 92–125 mg/dl and/or 1 h PG level ≥180 mg/dl and/or 2 h PG level of 153–199 mg/dl
Danyliv et al. [18]	Pregnant women were offered screening at 24–28 weeks' gestation using a 75 g OGTT	75 g OGTT in accordance with the IADPSG criteria
Kopec et al. [19]	GDM was diagnosed by a two-step approach. The oral GCT administered between 24 and 28 weeks of pregnancy. Women with 1 h PG level >180 mg/dl (10.0 mmol/l) in the OGCT were classified as having GDM. Women with PG levels between 140 mg/dl (7.8 mmol/l) and 180 mg/dl (10.0 mmol/l) were referred for a diagnostic 75 g OGTT	Two-step approach: 50 g GCT followed, if positive, by 75 g OGTT interpreting the results according to the WHO diagnostic criteria
Latif et al. [25]	GDM was diagnosed at 28 weeks of pregnancy	A 2 h 75 g OGTT according to the WHO diagnostic criteria
Trutnovsky et al. [20]	Diagnosed GDM based on the results of an elevated 75 g OGTT	Diagnostic criteria not fully specified
Lapolla et al. [9]	GDM was diagnosed according to Carpenter and Coustan's criteria	Carpenter and Coustan's criteria
Dalfrà et al. [8]	Screening for GDM was done with a GCT between the 24th and 28th weeks of gestation, and the diagnosis was confirmed with a 100 g OGTT, interpreting the results according to the Recommendations of the 4th International Workshop Conference on GDM	Carpenter and Coustan's criteria
Petkova et al. [26]	Women, suspected to have GDM, were subjected to 2 h 75 g GCT. Those with sugar level around 140 mg/dl (7.8 mmol/L) or above were requested for OGTT recommended by WHO	Two-step approach: GCT + OGTT interpreting the results according to the WHO diagnostic criteria

Table 3: Continued.

Study	Time and methods of diagnosis	Diagnostic criteria
Halkoaho et al. [21]	The diagnosis of GDM is based on a 2 h glucose tolerance test generally administered during the 24th–28th weeks of pregnancy to women with GDM risk factors	Diagnostic criteria not fully specified
Mautner et al. [22]	The group "gestational diabetes" included women diagnosed with a pathological oral glucose tolerance test requiring insulin therapy at the end of the second and the beginning of the third trimester. The diagnosis of GDM is based on a pathological OGTT	Diagnostic criteria not fully specified
Dalfrà et al. [27]	Screening for GDM was done with a GCT between the 24th and 28th weeks of gestation, and the diagnosis was confirmed with a 100 OGTT	Carpenter and Coustan's criteria
Elnour et al. [28]	Women within the first 20 weeks of gestation confirmed diagnosis of GDM	Diagnostic criteria not specified
Kim et al. [23]	GDM was diagnosed according to Carpenter and Coustan's criteria between 24–28 weeks of gestation	Carpenter and Coustan's criteria
Crowther et al. [29]	Pregnancy between 16 and 30 weeks' gestation with one or more risk factors for gestational diabetes on selective screening or a positive 50 g GCT and a 75 g OGTT at 24 to 34 weeks' gestation in accordance with the WHO diagnostic criteria	Two-step or one-step approach: 50 g GCT: 1 h PG level ≥140 mg/dl (7.8 mmol/l) + 75 g OGTT: 2 h PG level of 140–198 (7.8–11.0 mmol/l) or selective screening: 75 g OGTT interpreting the results according to the WHO diagnostic criteria
Rumbold and Crowther [24]	Universal antenatal screening for GDM by either a random blood sample or a 50 g GCT at 24 to 28 weeks' gestation. Women who screen positive are offered a diagnostic 75 g OGTT	Two-step approach: random blood sample or 50 g GCT followed, if positive, by 75 g OGTT interpreting the results according to the WHO diagnostic criteria

GCT: glucose challenge test; GDM: Gestational Diabetes Mellitus; IADPSG: International Association of Diabetes and Pregnancy Study Groups; OGTT: oral glucose tolerance test; WHO: World Health Organization.

and mental health subscales among participants attending the intervention group. Similar results were later obtained from Petkova et al. [26]. They found a significant improvement in QoL of women with GDM involved in an intervention program aimed at educating about diet, exercise, self-monitoring, and insulin treatment.

Finally, Crowther et al. [29] randomly assigned women with GDM to a specific intervention group aimed to provide dietary advice, blood glucose monitoring, and insulin therapy. At three months after delivery, participants reported a significant improvement in their QoL by obtaining higher scores on the SF-36.

4. Discussion

QoL is a clinically relevant concept determining the individual evaluation of own health status. This subjective appraisal seems to act, above all physical and treatment components of diabetes during pregnancy, as a psychological factor affecting medical outcomes in GDM. Based on current research studies, we have found that QoL could be significantly compromised, both short term and long term, when women cope with pregnancy complicated by GDM. However, GDM per se does not seem to act as unique clinical variable negatively affecting different levels of QoL among women with GDM. That is, the relationship between GDM medical symptoms and QoL domains could be mediated by a complex interaction of several factors whose unifying psychological element can be identified through the concept of the illness experience [30]. The potential underlying psychological factor, operating as core variable to clinically explain the different QoL status among patients with GDM, may consist of the varying individual way to respond to own bodily symptoms. Such psychological component conceived as general health perception was originally investigated by Mechanic and Volkart [31]. In this regard, they provided a definition of "the ways in which symptoms may be differentially perceived, evaluated, and acted upon by different kinds of persons" [30]. A relatively recent review study of Lawrence [32] has further underlined how perceptions and expectations of women with GDM may significantly affect their psychological and behavioral response during and after pregnancy.

To the very best of our knowledge, this is the first review study systematically analyzing the impact of GDM and its symptoms on QoL levels. Indeed, only a previous recently published systematic review study, evaluating the health status and QoL in postpartum women, was fulfilled by Van Der Woude et al. [33]. However, the authors neglected the assessment of such psychological mechanisms in women with GDM.

Based on additional relevant results from a review study examining the influence of QoL in the treatment outcomes of diabetes [34], specific implications can be identified. The medical evaluation of GDM should comprise a clinically valid psychological assessment of QoL in order to attempt monitoring its potential effects on GDM prognosis from first diagnosis, during the treatment, and after delivery. Specifically, the gold standard should comprise self-rating scales as screening measures for identifying psychological comorbidities potentially leading to adverse and negative clinical consequences during diabetes [35].

As regards the intervention studies examining the impact of specific treatments on QoL dimensions among women with GDM, promising results were found. The five studies retrieved [25–29] clearly indicate the efficacy of different therapeutic programs to improve QoL by enhancing positive diabetes self-management behaviors such as balanced diet, exercise, self-monitoring, and insulin control. Despite this, much more studies are largely needed when taking into account heterogeneity in subjects and study design as well as the evidence that the control group and experimental group were not consistent across studies we have qualitatively examined.

Further research should be conducted to test the effect of integrative programs on QoL focusing on pharmacological care mixed up with advanced practices based on information and communication technologies (e.g., telemedicine and/or games for health) [36, 37]. In this regard, the major aim is to educate patients on healthier lifestyle habits (healthy diet and physical activity domains) [38, 39] and to facilitate the process of illness acceptance [40] after a diagnosis of GDM.

Finally, our review shows some noteworthy points: (1) the positive effect of a telemedicine intervention on both diabetes-related medical outcomes and general health perception, energy/vitality, and mental health; (2) a significant improvement in QoL of women with GDM attending an educational program. In the future, these considerations should be taken into account for the management of diabetes during pregnancy.

Competing Interests

The authors declare that they have no competing interests to disclose.

References

[1] American Diabetes Association, "2. Classification and diagnosis of diabetes," *Diabetes Care*, vol. 40, supplement 1, pp. S11–S24, 2017.

[2] H. Alptekin, A. Çizmecioäÿlu, H. Işik, T. Cengiz, M. Yildiz, and M. S. Iyisoy, "Predicting gestational diabetes mellitus during the first trimester using anthropometric measurements and HOMA-IR," *Journal of Endocrinological Investigation*, vol. 39, no. 5, pp. 577–583, 2016.

[3] A. Bień, E. Rzońca, A. Kańczugowska, and G. Iwanowicz-Palus, "Factors affecting the quality of life and the illness acceptance of pregnant women with diabetes," *International Journal of Environmental Research and Public Health*, vol. 13, no. 1, article 68, 2015.

[4] B. S. Buckley, J. Harreiter, P. Damm et al., "Gestational diabetes mellitus in Europe: prevalence, current screening practice and barriers to screening. A review," *Diabetic Medicine*, vol. 29, no. 7, pp. 844–854, 2012.

[5] K. Strawa-Zakoscielna, M. Lenart-Lipinska, A. Szafraniec, G. Rudzki, and B. Matyjaszek-Matuszek, "A new diagnostic perspective—hyperglycemia in pregnancy—as of the year, 2014," *Current Issues in Pharmacy and Medical Sciences*, vol. 27, no. 4, pp. 246–249, 2014.

[6] R. Guglani, S. Shenoy, and J. S. Sandhu, "Effect of progressive pedometer based walking intervention on quality of life and general well being among patients with type 2 diabetes," *Journal of Diabetes & Metabolic Disorders*, vol. 13, article 110, 2014.

[7] J. Lewko, J. Kochanowicz, W. Zarzycki, Z. Mariak, M. Górska, and E. Krajewska-Kulak, "Poor hand function in diabetics. Its causes and effects on the quality of life," *Saudi Medical Journal*, vol. 33, no. 4, pp. 429–435, 2012.

[8] M. G. Dalfrà, A. Nicolucci, T. Bisson, B. Bonsembiante, and A. Lapolla, "Quality of life in pregnancy and post-partum: a study in diabetic patients," *Quality of Life Research*, vol. 21, no. 2, pp. 291–298, 2012.

[9] A. Lapolla, G. Di Cianni, A. Di Benedetto et al., "Quality of life, wishes, and needs in women with gestational diabetes: Italian DAWN pregnancy study," *International Journal of Endocrinology*, vol. 2012, Article ID 784726, 6 pages, 2012.

[10] C. W. Topp, S. D. Østergaard, S. Søndergaard, and P. Bech, "The WHO-5 well-being index: a systematic review of the literature," *Psychotherapy and Psychosomatics*, vol. 84, no. 3, pp. 167–176, 2015.

[11] C. D. Ryff, "Psychological well-being revisited: advances in the science and practice of eudaimonia," *Psychotherapy and Psychosomatics*, vol. 83, no. 1, pp. 10–28, 2014.

[12] G. A. Fava and P. Bech, "The Concept of Euthymia," *Psychotherapy and Psychosomatics*, vol. 85, no. 1, pp. 1–5, 2016.

[13] A. Rodriguez-Urrutia, F. J. Eiroa-Orosa, A. Accarino, C. Malagelada, and F. Azpiroz, "Incongruence between clinicians' assessment and self-reported functioning is related to psychopathology among patients diagnosed with gastrointestinal disorders," *Psychotherapy and Psychosomatics*, vol. 85, no. 4, pp. 244–245, 2016.

[14] N. Sonino and G. A. Fava, "Improving the concept of recovery in endocrine disease by consideration of psychosocial issues," *The Journal of Clinical Endocrinology & Metabolism*, vol. 97, no. 8, pp. 2614–2616, 2012.

[15] World Health Organization, *Construction in Basic Documents*, World Health Organization, Geneva, Switzerland, 1948.

[16] P. Bech, D. Carrozzino, S. F. Austin, S. B. Møller, and O. Vassend, "Measuring euthymia within the Neuroticism Scale from the NEO Personality Inventory: a Mokken analysis of the Norwegian general population study for scalability," *Journal of Affective Disorders*, vol. 193, pp. 99–102, 2016.

[17] D. Moher, A. Liberati, J. Tetzlaff, and D. G. Altman, "Preferred reporting items for systematic reviews and meta-analyses: the PRISMA statement," *Journal of Clinical Epidemiology*, vol. 62, no. 10, pp. 1006–1012, 2009.

[18] A. Danyliv, P. Gillespie, C. O'Neill et al., "Health related quality of life two to five years after gestational diabetes mellitus: cross-sectional comparative study in the ATLANTIC DIP cohort," *BMC Pregnancy and Childbirth*, vol. 15, article 274, 2015.

[19] J. A. Kopec, J. Ogonowski, M. M. Rahman, and T. Miazgowski, "Patient-reported outcomes in women with gestational diabetes: a longitudinal study," *International Journal of Behavioral Medicine*, vol. 22, no. 2, pp. 206–213, 2015.

[20] G. Trutnovsky, T. Panzitt, E. Magnet, C. Stern, U. Lang, and M. Dorfer, "Gestational diabetes: women's concerns, mood state, quality of life and treatment satisfaction," *Journal of Maternal-Fetal and Neonatal Medicine*, vol. 25, no. 11, pp. 2464–2466, 2012.

[21] A. Halkoaho, M. Kavilo, A.-M. Pietilä, H. Huopio, H. Sintonen, and S. Heinonen, "Does gestational diabetes affect women's health-related quality of life after delivery?" *European Journal of Obstetrics & Gynecology and Reproductive Biology*, vol. 148, no. 1, pp. 40–43, 2010.

[22] E. Mautner, E. Greimel, G. Trutnovsky, F. Daghofer, J. W. Egger, and U. Lang, "Quality of life outcomes in pregnancy and postpartum complicated by hypertensive disorders, gestational diabetes, and preterm birth," *Journal of Psychosomatic Obstetrics & Gynecology*, vol. 30, no. 4, pp. 231–237, 2009.

[23] C. Kim, P. Brawarsky, R. A. Jackson, E. Fuentes-Afflick, and J. S. Haas, "Changes in health status experienced by women with gestational diabetes and pregnancy-induced hypertensive disorders," *Journal of Women's Health*, vol. 14, no. 8, pp. 729–736, 2005.

[24] A. R. Rumbold and C. A. Crowther, "Women's experiences of being screened for gestational diabetes mellitus," *Australian and New Zealand Journal of Obstetrics and Gynaecology*, vol. 42, no. 2, pp. 131–137, 2002.

[25] L. Latif, S. Hyer, and H. Shehata, "Metformin effects on treatment satisfaction and quality of life in gestational diabetes," *British Journal of Diabetes and Vascular Disease*, vol. 13, no. 4, pp. 178–182, 2013.

[26] V. Petkova, M. Dimitrov, and S. Geourgiev, "Pilot project for education of gestational diabetes mellitus (GDM) patients—can it be beneficial?" *African Journal of Pharmacy and Pharmacology*, vol. 5, no. 10, pp. 1282–1286, 2011.

[27] M. G. Dalfrà, A. Nicolucci, A. Lapolla et al., "The effect of telemedicine on outcome and quality of life in pregnant women with diabetes," *Journal of Telemedicine and Telecare*, vol. 15, no. 5, pp. 238–242, 2009.

[28] A. A. Elnour, I. T. El Mugammar, T. Jaber, T. Revel, and J. C. McElnay, "Pharmaceutical care of patients with gestational diabetes mellitus," *Journal of Evaluation in Clinical Practice*, vol. 14, no. 1, pp. 131–140, 2008.

[29] C. A. Crowther, J. E. Hiller, J. R. Moss, A. J. McPhee, W. S. Jeffries, and J. S. Robinson, "Effect of treatment of gestational diabetes mellitus on pregnancy outcomes," *New England Journal of Medicine*, vol. 352, no. 24, pp. 2477–2486, 2005.

[30] L. Sirri, G. A. Fava, and N. Sonino, "The unifying concept of illness behavior," *Psychotherapy and Psychosomatics*, vol. 82, no. 2, pp. 74–81, 2013.

[31] D. Mechanic and E. H. Volkart, "Illness behavior and medical diagnoses," *Journal of Health and Human Behavior*, vol. 1, no. 2, pp. 86–94, 1960.

[32] J. M. Lawrence, "Women with diabetes in pregnancy: different perceptions and expectations," *Best Practice and Research: Clinical Obstetrics and Gynaecology*, vol. 25, no. 1, pp. 15–24, 2011.

[33] D. A. A. Van Der Woude, J. M. A. Pijnenborg, and J. De Vries, "Health status and quality of life in postpartum women: a systematic review of associated factors," *European Journal of Obstetrics Gynecology and Reproductive Biology*, vol. 185, pp. 45–52, 2015.

[34] L. D. F. Gusmai, T. D. S. Novato, and L. D. S. Nogueira, "The influence of quality of life in treatment adherence of diabetic patients: a systematic review," *Revista da Escola de Enfermagem da USP*, vol. 49, no. 5, pp. 839–846, 2015.

[35] C. Conti, D. Carrozzino, C. Patierno, E. Vitacolonna, and M. Fulcheri, "The clinical link between type D personality and diabetes," *Frontiers in Psychiatry*, vol. 7, article no. 113, 2016.

[36] T. M. Rasekaba, J. Furler, I. Blackberry, M. Tacey, K. Gray, and K. Lim, "Telemedicine interventions for gestational diabetes mellitus: a systematic review and meta-analysis," *Diabetes Research and Clinical Practice*, vol. 110, no. 1, pp. 1–9, 2015.

[37] Y. L. Theng, J. W. Y. Lee, P. V. Patinadan, and S. S. B. Foo, "The use of videogames, gamification, and virtual environments in the self-management of diabetes: a systematic review of evidence," *Games for Health Journal*, vol. 4, no. 5, pp. 352–361, 2015.

[38] D. Marchetti, F. Fraticelli, F. Polcini et al., "Preventing adolescents' diabesity: design, development, and first evaluation of "Gustavo in Gnam's Planet"," *Games for Health Journal*, vol. 4, no. 5, pp. 344–351, 2015.

[39] M. Tabak, M. Dekker-van Weering, H. van Dijk, and M. Vollenbroek-Hutten, "Promoting daily physical activity by means of mobile gaming: a review of the state of the art," *Games for Health Journal*, vol. 4, no. 6, pp. 460–469, 2015.

[40] N. C. Chilelli, M. G. Dalfrà, and A. Lapolla, "The emerging role of telemedicine in managing glycemic control and psychobehavioral aspects of pregnancy complicated by diabetes," *International Journal of Telemedicine and Applications*, vol. 2014, Article ID 621384, 7 pages, 2014.

23

Risk Factors for the Requirement of Antenatal Insulin Treatment in Gestational Diabetes Mellitus

Mayu Watanabe,[1,2] Akihiro Katayama,[1] Hidetoshi Kagawa,[2] Daisuke Ogawa,[1,2] and Jun Wada[1]

[1]*Department of Nephrology, Rheumatology, Endocrinology and Metabolism, Okayama University Graduate School of Medicine, Dentistry and Pharmaceutical Sciences, Okayama 700-8558, Japan*
[2]*Department of Internal Medicine, Japanese Red Cross Society Himeji Hospital, Himeji, Hyogo 670-8540, Japan*

Correspondence should be addressed to Mayu Watanabe; mitahamamamaka@yahoo.co.jp

Academic Editor: Kazuya Yamagata

Poor maternal glycemic control increases maternal and fetal risk for adverse outcomes, and strict management of gestational diabetes mellitus (GDM) is recommended to prevent neonatal and maternal complications. However, risk factors for the requirement of antenatal insulin treatment (AIT) are not well-investigated in the pregnant women with GDM. We enrolled 37 pregnant women with GDM and investigated the risk for AIT by comparing the patients with AIT (AIT group; $n = 10$) and without insulin therapy (Diet group; $n = 27$). The 1-h and 2-h plasma glucose levels and the number of abnormal values in 75 g OGTT were significantly higher in AIT group compared with Diet group. By logistic regression analysis, plasma glucose level at 1-h was significant predictor for AIT and the odds ratios were 1.115 (1.004–1.239) using forward selection method and 1.192 (1.006–1.413) using backward elimination method. There were no significant differences in obstetrical outcomes and neonatal complications. 1-h plasma glucose levels in 75 g OGTT are useful parameters in predicting the requirement for AIT in GDM. Both maternal and neonatal complications are comparable in GDM patients with and without insulin therapy.

1. Introduction

International Association of Diabetes and Pregnancy Study Groups (IADPSG) published criteria for the universal screening and diagnosis for gestational diabetes mellitus (GDM) based on Hyperglycemia and Adverse Pregnancy Outcome (HAPO) study [1]. After the release, the criteria for GDM were also updated in Japan [2] and they were characterized by two major revisions. First, GDM is diagnosed if one or more of the following criteria are met in the 75 g oral glucose tolerance test (OGTT) and threshold values were defined as a fasting plasma glucose level of 5.1 mmol/L (92 mg/dl), a 1-h plasma glucose level of 10.0 mmol/L (180 mg/dl), and a 2-h plasma glucose level of 8.5 mmol/L (153 mg/dl). Second, the new criteria exclude overt diabetes in pregnancy from GDM. By these new diagnostic criteria, the total incidence was 17.8% and FPG plus 1-h plasma glucose levels identified a large majority of these individuals [1].

Poor maternal glycemic control can significantly increase maternal and fetal risk for adverse outcomes [3] and strict management of GDM is recommended to prevent neonatal and maternal complications. Several studies have shown the treatment interventions, including dietary treatment, self-monitoring blood glucose levels, and insulin therapy if required, reduced prenatal complications [4, 5]. Crowther et al. found that 20 percent of women with GDM need antenatal insulin treatment (AIT) to achieve good glycemic control [6], while other studies also showed that 10.8~52.8 percent of GDM patients required AIT [7–11]. In addition, Baptiste-Roberts et al. reviewed that the AIT was the risk factor for the development of type 2 diabetes [12]. However, the risk factors for the requirement of AIT are not well-investigated and this prompted us to investigate the clinical characteristics of the patients with GDM to identify risk factors for AIT.

2. Materials and Methods

2.1. Subjects. The current clinical investigation is a noninterventional and retrospective study enrolling 37 pregnant women with GDM. They were diagnosed at 35.2 ± 4.7 years of age at their estimated 20.9 ± 3.8 gestational weeks and admitted between 2010 and 2016 at Himeji Red Cross Hospital, Hyogo, Japan. GDM was diagnosed according to IADPSG criteria [1]. Data collected included gestational age at diagnosis, gestational weeks at diagnosis, twins, family history of diabetes mellitus, pregestational body mass index (BMI), infertility treatments such as timed intercourse, *in vitro* fertilization, and egg donation, hospitalization for threatened premature delivery and intravenous ritodrine hydrochloride, prior gestational diabetes, primipara, plasma glucose levels of 75 g OGTT (fasting, 1-h, and 2-h), number of abnormal values of 75 g OGTT, glycosylated hemoglobin A1c (HbA1c), weeks of gestation at start of insulin therapy, the maximum of insulin dose, obstetrical outcome such as weeks of gestation at delivery, preterm delivery, cesarean section, pregnancy-induced hypertension (PIH), and neonatal characteristics such as birth weight, neonatal plasma glucose levels, hypoglycemia defined as plasma glucose levels of less than 45 mg/dL, transient tachypnea of the newborn (TTN), and respiratory distress syndrome (RDS). We excluded the patients with overt diabetes in pregnancy, with known type 1 or type 2 diabetes before pregnancy, or having not undergone 75 g OGTT. Furthermore, pregnant women were classified as normal weight (BMI < 25 kg/m^2), overweight (25 ≤ BMI < 30 kg/m^2), and obese (30 ≤ BMI kg/m^2) according to pregestational BMI. The study protocol was approved by the institutional review boards of Himeji Red Cross Hospital.

2.2. Treatments. The patients received dietary education from registered dietitians with 30 kcal/kg weight of ideal body weight based on BMI 22 kg/m^2 supplemented with 200 to 250 kcal, and they were instructed to take three meals and one to three snacks. They also received instructions for the procedures to perform self-monitoring of blood glucose (SMBG) and measured daily both preprandial and 2-hour postprandial glucose levels. If targeted glucose levels with preprandial glucose less than 5.6 mmol/L (100 mg/dl) and 2-hour postprandial glucose less than 6.7 mmol/L (120 mg/dl) were not achieved three times or more after breakfast, lunch, and dinner during seven days, AIT was initiated before breakfast, lunch, and dinner, respectively. We classified the patients into two groups, the patients who received AIT (AIT group; n = 10) and the patients without insulin therapy (Diet group; n = 27).

2.3. Statistical Analysis. All data were presented as the mean ± standard deviation. For univariate analysis, we used Student's t-test and χ-square test for categorical data. For multivariate logistic regression analysis after controlling simultaneously for potential confounders, we selected independent variables which were significantly higher in AIT group compared with Diet group for univariate analysis, such as postprandial PG at 1-hr and 2-hr in 75 g OGTT and number of abnormal values in 75 g OGTT. We also used the forward selection and backward elimination methods. Logistic regression analyses with each independent variable to explore risk factors contributing to AIT were also performed. We performed receiver-operating characteristic (ROC) curve to identify clinical factors to predict the requirement for AIT. We determined a cut-off value by the point on the ROC curve closest to the upper left corner. P values of less than 0.05 were considered statistically significant. The data were analyzed with IBM SPSS Statistics Ver. 22.0 and IBM SPSS Regression (IBM).

3. Results

3.1. Characteristics of GDM. Maternal age, number of twins, family history of DM, pregestational BMI, infertility treatment, prior gestational diabetes, primipara, fasting plasma glucose levels at 75 g OGTT, and HbA1c levels demonstrated no significant differences between AIT and Diet groups. The gestational age at diagnosis was lower in AIT group (18.9 ± 2.0 weeks) compared with Diet group (21.6 ± 4.1 weeks), but it did not reveal significant differences (P = 0.053). The 1-h and 2-h plasma glucose levels and number of abnormal values in 75 g OGTT were significantly higher in AIT group compared with Diet group (Table 1). The maximal glucose level during ritodrine treatment in AIT group was higher compared to Diet group, the intravenous injection of ritodrine to treat preterm delivery was more frequently administered in AIT group (40.0%) compared with Diet group (14.8%), but it was not statistically significant (Table 1).

3.2. Risk Factors for AIT. By logistic regression analysis, plasma glucose level at 1-h was significant predictor for AIT and the odds ratios were 1.115 (1.004–1.239) using forward selection method and 1.192 (1.006–1.413) using backward elimination method (Table 2). In logistic analyses using each independent variable, plasma glucose levels at 1-h and 2-h and the number of abnormal values in 75 g OGTT were only significant predictors for AIT and the odds ratios were 1.128 (1.022–1.246), 1.054 (1.006–1.104), and 10.950 (1.959–61.218), respectively (Table 3). ROC curves were used to determine the cut-off values of 1-h and 2-h plasma glucose levels and the number of abnormal values to predict the AIT (Figure 1). The cut-off values of 1-h and 2-hr plasma glucose levels and the number of abnormal values in 75 g OGTT were 10.25 mmol/L (AUC 0.872, sensitivity 100%, and specificity of 77.8%), 8.75 mmol/L (AUC 0.756, sensitivity 70%, specificity 70.4%), and 1.5 (AUC 0.783, sensitivity 80%, and specificity 74.1%), respectively (Table 4).

3.3. Obstetrical Outcomes and Neonatal Characteristics. The rate of cesarean section and PIH was higher in AIT group compared with Diet group, but it was not statistically significant (Table 5). There were no differences in the rate of preterm delivery; however, gestational age at delivery was significantly lower in AIT group (36.4 ± 2.0 weeks) compared with Diet group (38.2 ± 2.4 weeks) (Table 5). There was no stillbirth, Apgar score at 5 minutes less than 8, shoulder dystopia, and birth weight more than 4000 grams. TTN occurred more often in AIT group compared with Diet group without significant differences (Table 6). There was no difference in the rate of RDS between two groups. Birth weight, neonatal

TABLE 1: Characteristics of GDM.

	AIT group (n = 10)	Diet group (n = 27)	P value
Gestational age at diagnosis (years)	33.8 ± 7.0	35.7 ± 3.6	0.284†
Gestational weeks at diagnosis (weeks)	18.9 ± 2.0	21.6 ± 4.1	0.053†
Twins, n (%)	2 (20.0)	1 (3.7)	0.107‡
Family history of diabetes mellitus, n (%)	7 (70.0)	16 (59.3)	0.550‡
Pregestational BMI (kg/m^2)	24.5 ± 4.8	23.0 ± 4.4	0.383†
95% CI	21.0–27.9	21.3–24.7	
<20.0 (%)	20.0	14.8	
20–24.9 (%)	40.0	59.3	
25–29.9 (%)	30.0	18.5	
≥30.0 (%)	10.0	7.4	
Infertility treatment, n (%)	4 (40.0)	12 (44.4)	0.809‡
Treatment of preterm labor with ritodrine, n (%)	4 (40.0)	4 (14.8)	0.098‡
Maximal glucose levels during ritodrine treatment (mmol/L)	9.0 ± 1.2	7.3 ± 0.7	0.062†
Prior gestational diabetes, n (%)	1 (10.0)	5 (18.5)	0.532‡
Primipara, n (%)	5 (50.0)	12 (44.4)	0.763‡
Plasma glucose level (mmol/L)			
Fasting¶	4.82 ± 0.49	4.69 ± 0.46	0.465†
At 1 hr$	10.86 ± 0.62	9.19 ± 1.57	0.003†
At 2 hr$	9.43 ± 1.56	7.96 ± 1.37	0.008†
Number of abnormal values, n	1.9 ± 0.6	1.26 ± 0.4	0.001†
HbA1c (%)	5.3 ± 0.3	5.2 ± 0.4	0.234†
Gestational weeks at start of AIT (weeks)	26.1 ± 5.9		
The maximum of insulin dose (units/day)	10 ± 5.5		

AIT, antenatal insulin treatment; BMI, body mass index; CI, confidence interval; and HbA1c, hemoglobin A1c.
Data are shown as mean ± SD or n.
†By Student's t-test.
‡By Chi-square test.
¶At the time of the 75 g oral glucose tolerance test.
$After the administration of 75 g of glucose.

TABLE 2: Logistic regression analysis after controlling simultaneously for potential confounders of predictors for antenatal insulin treatment (AIT).

Independent variables	β-Coefficient	Odds ratio (95% CI)	P values
Postprandial PG at 1-hr in 75 g OGTT	0.165	1.179 (0.988–1.407)	0.067
Postprandial PG at 2-hr in 75 g OGTT	0.053	1.054 (0.987–1.126)	0.113
Number of abnormal values in 75 g OGTT	0.420	1.521 (0.207–11.201)	0.680
Forward selection method (conditional)			
Postprandial PG at 1-hr in 75 g OGTT	0.109	1.115 (1.004–1.239)	0.043
Number of abnormal values in 75 g OGTT	1.451	4.267 (0.669–27.228)	0.125
Backward elimination method (conditional)			
Postprandial PG at 1-hr in 75 g OGTT	0.176	1.192 (1.006–1.413)	0.042
Postprandial PG at 2-hr in 75 g OGTT	0.059	1.061 (0.998–1.127)	0.057

AIT, antenatal insulin treatment; PG, plasma glucose; 75 g OGTT, 75 g oral glucose tolerance test, BMI, body mass index, and HbA1c, hemoglobin A1c.

TABLE 3: Logistic regression analysis with each independent variable of predictors for antenatal insulin treatment (AIT).

	β-Coefficient	Odds ratio (95% CI)	P values
Postprandial PG at 1-hr in 75 g OGTT	0.121	1.128 (1.022–1.246)	0.017
Postprandial PG at 2-hr in 75 g OGTT	0.053	1.054 (1.006–1.104)	0.026
Number of abnormal values in 75 g OGTT	2.393	10.950 (1.959–61.218)	0.006

AIT, antenatal insulin treatment; PG, plasma glucose; and 75 g OGTT, 75 g oral glucose tolerance test.

TABLE 4: The cut-off values of 1-h and 2-h plasma glucose levels and the number of abnormal values to predict antenatal insulin treatment (AIT).

	Cut-off point	Sensitivity	Specificity	AUC
Postprandial PG at 1-hr in 75 g OGTT	10.25 mmol/L	100%	77.8%	0.872
Postprandial PG at 2-hr in 75 g OGTT	8.75 mmol/L	70%	70.4%	0.756
Number of abnormal values in 75 g OGTT	1.5	80%	74.1%	0.783

AUC, area under the curve; PG, plasma glucose; and 75 g OGTT, 75 g oral glucose tolerance test.

TABLE 5: Obstetrical outcomes.

	AIT group (n = 10)	Diet group (n = 27)	P values
Gestational age at delivery (week)	36.4 ± 2.0	38.2 ± 2.4	0.046[†]
Maternal weight gain (kg)	6.24 ± 5.46	7.27 ± 3.93	0.531[†]
Preterm delivery, n (%)	3 (30.0)	5 (18.5)	0.451[‡]
Cesarean section, n (%)	7 (70.0)	10 (37.0)	0.074[‡]
PIH, n (%)	3 (30.0)	2 (7.4)	0.074[‡]

Data are shown as mean ± standard deviation (SD) or number (n). AIT, antenatal insulin; PIH, pregnancy-induced hypertension; [†]Student's t-test; and [‡]χ-square test.

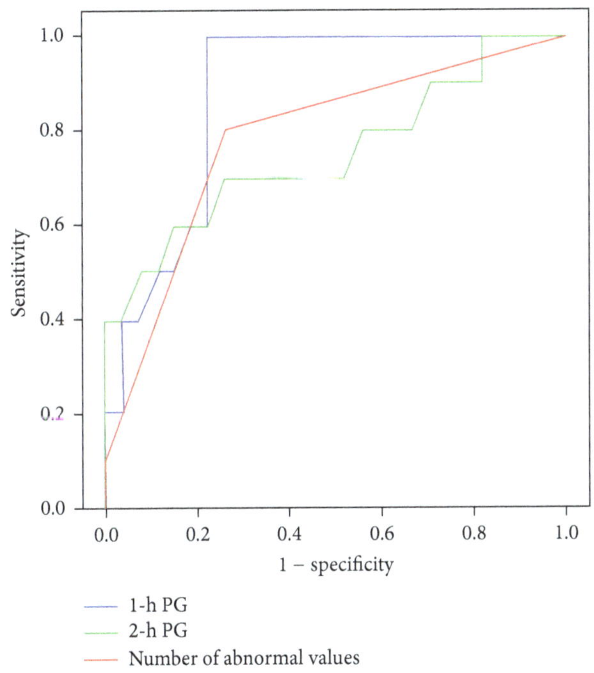

FIGURE 1

plasma glucose levels, and the rate of hypoglycemia were similar in both groups (Table 6).

4. Discussion

The main finding in the current investigation is that 1-h and 2-h plasma glucose levels and the number of abnormal values in 75 g OGTT predict the requirement for AIT in GDM patients. The number of abnormal OGTT values was 1.5; therefore two or three of abnormal values in 75 g OGTT are a predictor for need of AIT with sensitivity of 90% and specificity 35.5%. Ikenoue et al. evaluated the insulin sensitivity, insulin secretion, and β cell function with insulin secretion-sensitivity index-2 (ISSI-2) in women between one and two or three abnormal OGTT values. The insulin sensitivity of women with two or three abnormal values deteriorated significantly compared with one abnormal value, although the insulin secretions were similar between two groups. Consequently, ISSI-2 levels of women with two or three abnormal values were significantly lower compared to one abnormal value. They also found that women with two or three abnormal OGTT values required more frequently AIT compared to one abnormal value [13]. Saisho et al. found that Japanese women with GDM failed to increase insulin secretion to compensate decreased insulin sensitivity compared to women with normal glucose tolerance [14]. Therefore, the number of abnormal OGTT values might reflect insulin sensitivity and β cell function of women with GDM.

Previous studies reported diverse possible factors predicting the need for AIT including HbA1c, plasma glucose levels in OGTT, pregestational BMI, maternal age, gestational age at diagnosis, and family history of diabetes [7–11], but they were not associated with the requirement for AIT in the current study. The differences in risk factors among the previous and current studies may be derived from the clinical characteristics of the participants. For example, several studies showed that fasting glucose level could be predictor for AIT among women with GDM [7, 9–11, 15]. The mean of pregestational BMI among women who required AIT was reported as 31.6 kg/m^2 [11] and 29.9 kg/m^2 [7]. The proportion of overweight and obese women in AIT group was 72.9 percent [7]. In the current study, the mean of pregestational BMI among women who required AIT was 24.5 kg/m^2. The proportion of overweight and obese women in AIT group was 40 percent; the current study included overweight and obese woman, but prevalence was less compared to the previous studies. Black et al. found the association between BMI and fasting glucose levels, and obese women with GDM had significantly higher mean fasting glucose levels compared to

Table 6: Neonatal characteristics.

	AIT group (n = 10)	Diet group (n = 27)	P values
Birth weight (g)	2703.2 ± 526.0	2827.6 ± 534.3	0.532†
Neonatal plasma glucose level (mmol/L)	2.3 ± 1.3	3.0 ± 1.0	0.099†
Hypoglycemia, n (%)	4 (40)	5 (18.5)	0.176‡
TTN, n (%)	3 (30.0)	2 (7.4)	0.074‡
RDS, n (%)	2 (20.0)	1 (3.7)	0.107‡

Data are shown as mean ± standard deviation (SD) or number (n). AIT, antenatal insulin; TTN, transient tachypnea of the newborn; RDS, respiratory distress syndrome; †Student's t-test; and $^{\ddagger}\chi$-square test.

Table 7

	AIT group (n = 10)		
	Pregestational BMI < 25.0 (kg/m^2) (n = 6)	Pregestational BMI ≥ 25.0 (kg/m^2) (n = 4)	P value
Fasting plasma glucose level (mmol/L)¶	4.6 ± 0.4	5.2 ± 0.5	0.071†
	Diet group (n = 27)		
	Pregestational BMI < 25.0 (kg/m^2) (n = 20)	Pregestational BMI ≥ 25.0 (kg/m^2) (n = 7)	P value
Fasting plasma glucose level (mmol/L)¶	4.6 ± 0.4	5.0 ± 0.4	0.031†

AIT, antenatal insulin treatment; BMI, body mass index.
Data are shown as mean ± SD.
†By Student's t-test.
¶At the time of the 75 g oral glucose-tolerance test.

overweight and normal weight women with GDM [16]. In the current study, indeed fasting glucose levels were significantly different between overweight or obese and normal weight women in Diet group, but fasting glucose levels were not significantly different between overweight, obese women and normal weight women in AIT group (Table 7). In the current study, the proportion of overweight and obese women of participants was less and fasting glucose level was not important risk factor for AIT.

β-Adrenergic agonist (ritodrine) infusion has been used as tocolytic; however it has some maternal side effects such as hyperglycemia. Even in nondiabetic pregnancy in women with normal glucose tolerance, it raised blood glucose levels additional 2.2 mmol/L (40 mg/dl) [17] and the continuous ritodrine infusion increased plasma glucose levels during first 24 hours after beginning of ritodrine [18]. In contrast, the Canadian preterm labor investigators group reported that the incidences of hyperglycemia were similar between ritodrine and placebo infusion group [19]. In the current study there were four women to treat preterm labor with ritodrine in each group (Table 1), and there was one woman with twin in Diet group, as well as two women with twin in AIT group. Twin was risk factor of preterm labor [20]. In the current study, all three women with twin had treatment of preterm labor with ritodrine (Table 1). That was one of the reasons that AIT group had higher frequency of ritodrine, although there were no significant differences in the number of the women given ritodrine to arrest preterm delivery between AIT and Diet group.

There are some limitations in the current study. First, the number of participants was small to assess the predictors of requirement for AIT and it underestimated other important factors. Second, current study was single-center retrospective investigation. The prospective cohort study in larger participants is needed to further determine risk factors to predict AIT.

In conclusion, 1-h and 2-h plasma glucose levels and number of abnormal values in 75 g OGTT are useful parameters in predicting the requirement for AIT in GDM. Both maternal and neonatal complications are comparable in GDM patients with and without insulin therapy.

Competing Interests

The authors declare that they have no conflict of interests.

Authors' Contributions

Mayu Watanabe, Akihiro Katayama, Daisuke Ogawa, and Jun Wada contributed to the conception and design of current clinical study. Hidetoshi Kagawa, Daisuke Ogawa, and Jun Wada contributed to the acquisition, analysis, and interpretation of data. Mayu Watanabe and Jun Wada drafted the manuscript and Akihiro Katayama, Hidetoshi Kagawa, and Daisuke Ogawa critically revised the manuscript. All authors approved and agreed to be accountable for all aspects of the work.

Acknowledgments

Jun Wada receives speaker honoraria from Astellas, Boehringer Ingelheim, Novartis, and Tanabe Mitsubishi and receives grant support from Astellas, Bayer, Chugai, Daiichi Sankyo, Kissei, Kyowa Hakko Kirin, MSD, Otsuka, Teijin, Torii, Pfizer, Takeda, and Taisho Toyama.

References

[1] International Association of Diabetes and Pregnancy Study Groups Consensus Panel, "International association of diabetes and pregnancy study groups recommendations on the diagnosis and classification of hyperglycemia in pregnancy," *Diabetes Care*, vol. 33, no. 3, pp. 676–682, 2010.

[2] The Committee of the Japan Diabetes Society on the Diagnostic Criteria of Diabetes Mellitus, Y. Seino, K. Nanjo et al., "Report of the committee on the classification and diagnostic criteria of diabetes mellitus," *Journal of Diabetes Investigation*, vol. 1, no. 5, pp. 212–228, 2010.

[3] E. A. Garrison and S. Jagasia, "Inpatient management of women with gestational and pregestational diabetes in pregnancy," *Current Diabetes Reports*, vol. 14, no. 2, p. 457, 2014.

[4] M. B. Landon, C. Y. Spong, E. Thom et al., "A multicenter, randomized trial of treatment for mild gestational diabetes," *The New England Journal of Medicine*, vol. 361, no. 14, pp. 1339–1348, 2009.

[5] O. Langer, D. A. Rodriguez, E. M. Xenakis, M. B. McFarland, M. D. Berkus, and F. Arrendondo, "Intensified versus conventional management of gestational diabetes," *American Journal of Obstetrics & Gynecology*, vol. 170, no. 4, pp. 1036–1047, 1994.

[6] C. A. Crowther, J. E. Hiller, J. R. Moss, A. J. McPhee, W. S. Jeffries, and J. S. Robinson, "Effect of treatment of gestational diabetes mellitus on pregnancy outcomes," *The New England Journal of Medicine*, vol. 352, no. 24, pp. 2477–2486, 2005.

[7] V. W. Wong and B. Jalaludin, "Gestational diabetes mellitus: who requires insulin therapy?" *Australian and New Zealand Journal of Obstetrics and Gynaecology*, vol. 51, no. 5, pp. 432–436, 2011.

[8] A. D. Sapienza, R. P. V. Francisco, T. C. Trindade, and M. Zugaib, "Factors predicting the need for insulin therapy in patients with gestational diabetes mellitus," *Diabetes Research and Clinical Practice*, vol. 88, no. 1, pp. 81–86, 2010.

[9] T. Pertot, L. Molyneaux, K. Tan, G. P. Ross, D. K. Yue, and J. Wong, "Can common clinical parameters be used to identify patients who will need insulin treatment in gestational diabetes mellitus?" *Diabetes Care*, vol. 34, no. 10, pp. 2214–2216, 2011.

[10] S. Meshel, E. Schejter, T. Harel et al., "Can we predict the need for pharmacological treatment according to demographic and clinical characteristics in gestational diabetes?" *The Journal of Maternal-Fetal & Neonatal Medicine*, vol. 29, no. 13, pp. 2062–2066, 2016.

[11] O. Bakiner, "Risk factors that can predict antenatal insulin need in gestational diabetes," *Journal of Clinical Medicine Research*, vol. 5, no. 5, pp. 381–388, 2013.

[12] K. Baptiste-Roberts, B. B. Barone, T. L. Gary et al., "Risk Factors for type 2 diabetes among women with gestational diabetes: a systematic review," *American Journal of Medicine*, vol. 122, no. 3, pp. 207.e4–214.e4, 2009.

[13] S. Ikenoue, K. Miyakoshi, Y. Saisho et al., "Clinical impact of women with gestational diabetes mellitus by the new consensus criteria: two year experience in a single institution in Japan," *Endocrine Journal*, vol. 61, no. 4, pp. 353–358, 2014.

[14] Y. Saisho, K. Miyakoshi, M. Tanaka et al., "Beta cell dysfunction and its clinical significance in gestational diabetes," *Endocrine Journal*, vol. 57, no. 11, pp. 973–980, 2010.

[15] B. Akinci, A. Celtik, S. Yener, and S. Yesil, "Is fasting glucose level during oral glucose tolerance test an indicator of the insulin need in gestational diabetes?" *Diabetes Research and Clinical Practice*, vol. 82, no. 2, pp. 219–225, 2008.

[16] M. H. Black, D. A. Sacks, A. H. Xiang, and J. M. Lawrence, "The relative contribution of prepregnancy overweight and obesity, gestational weight gain, and IADPSG-defined gestational diabetes mellitus to fetal overgrowth," *Diabetes Care*, vol. 36, no. 1, pp. 56–62, 2013.

[17] M. Ogawa, Y. Matsuda, A. Kobayashi et al., "Ritodrine should be carefully administered during antenatal glucocorticoid therapy even in nondiabetic pregnancies," *ISRN Obstetrics and Gynecology*, vol. 2013, Article ID 120735, 4 pages, 2013.

[18] M. Hirai, I. Yasuhi, T. Ishimaru, T. Yamabe, and K. Kubota, "Effect of prolonged intravenous ritodrine tocolysis on diurnal glucose profiles in pregnant women with normal carbohydrate tolerance," *Nihon Sanka Fujinka Gakkai Zasshi*, vol. 48, no. 7, pp. 488–494, 1996.

[19] The Canadian Preterm Labor Investigators Group, "Treatment of preterm labor with the beta-adrenergic agonist ritodrine," *The New England Journal of Medicine*, vol. 327, no. 5, pp. 308–312, 1992.

[20] H. Minakami and I. Sato, "Reestimating date of delivery in multifetal pregnancies," *The Journal of the American Medical Association*, vol. 275, no. 18, pp. 1432–1434, 1996.

24

High Fasting Plasma Glucose during Early Pregnancy: A Review about Early Gestational Diabetes Mellitus

E. Cosson,[1,2] L. Carbillon,[3] and P. Valensi[1]

[1]*Department of Endocrinology-Diabetology-Nutrition, AP-HP, Jean Verdier Hospital, Paris 13 University, Sorbonne Paris Cité, CRNH-IdF, CINFO, Bondy, France*
[2]*Sorbonne Paris Cité, UMR U1153 Inserm/U1125 Inra/Cnam/Université Paris 13, Bobigny, France*
[3]*Department of Gynecology-Obstetrics, AP-HP, Jean Verdier Hospital, Paris 13 University, Sorbonne Paris Cité, Bondy, France*

Correspondence should be addressed to E. Cosson; emmanuel.cosson@aphp.fr

Academic Editor: Patrizio Tatti

Fasting plasma glucose (FPG) is nowadays routinely measured during early pregnancy to detect preexisting diabetes (FPG ≥ 7 mmol/L). This screening has concomitantly led to identify early intermediate hyperglycemia, defined as FPG in the 5.1 to 6.9 mmol/L range, also early gestational diabetes mellitus (eGDM). Early FPG has been associated with poor pregnancy outcomes, but the recommendation by the IADPSG to refer women with eGDM for immediate management is more pragmatic than evidence based. Although eGDM is characterized by insulin resistance and associated with classical risk factors for type 2 diabetes and incident diabetes after delivery, it is not necessarily associated with preexisting prediabetes. FPG ≥ 5.1 mmol/L in early pregnancy is actually poorly predictive of gestational diabetes mellitus diagnosed after 24 weeks of gestation. An alternative threshold should be determined but may vary according to ethnicity, gestational age, and body mass index. Finally, observational data suggest that early management of intermediate hyperglycemia may improve prognosis, through reduced gestational weight gain and potential early introduction of hypoglycemic agents. Considering all these issues, we suggest an algorithm for the management of eGDM based on early FPG levels that would be measured in case of risk factors. Nevertheless, interventional randomized trials are still missing.

1. Introduction

Gestational diabetes mellitus (GDM) was historically defined as "any degree of glucose intolerance with onset or first recognition during pregnancy," whatever the treatment course and postpartum evolution [1]. Chronic insulin resistance in the second half of pregnancy is a central component of the pathophysiology of GDM [2, 3]. Diagnostic criteria were therefore established for 24–28 weeks of gestation (WG) including both glucose values during an oral glucose tolerance test (OGTT) and incident events [1]. The International Association of Diabetes Pregnancy Study Group (IADPSG) proposed the following diagnostic criteria: fasting plasma glucose (FPG) value ≥ 5.1 mmol/L and/or 1-hour glucose value ≥ 10.0 mmol/L and/or 2-hour glucose value ≥ 8.5 mmol/L. Although the National Institute for Health and Care Excellence (NICE) did not (http://www.nice.org.uk/guidance/ng3/evidence), these diagnostic criteria have been adopted worldwide, for example, by the American Diabetes Association (ADA) [4], the American Association of Clinical Endocrinologists [5], the Société Francophone du Diabète and the Collège National des Gynécologues et Obstétriciens Français [6], the International Federation of Gynecology and Obstetrics (FIGO) [7], and the Italian National Institute of Health (ISS) (http://www.salute.gov.it). The IADPSG criteria for the diagnosis of GDM are therefore now commonly called the 2013 WHO criteria for GDM (http://apps.who.int/iris/bitstream/10665/85975/1/WHO_NMH_MND_13.2_eng.pdf).

As the proportion of patients with unknown type 2 diabetes has been increasing, a new category of glucose disorder was introduced with the IADPSG recommendations. Women are considered to have overt diabetes [1] or diabetes in pregnancy (DIP (WHO criteria)) if their plasma glucose values are above the thresholds defining diabetes outside of pregnancy: FPG value ≥ 7 mmol/L and/or 2-hour glucose value ≥ 11.1 mmol/L and/or HbA1c ≥ 6.5%. Preconceptional diagnosis of diabetes or prediabetes would actually be useful to optimize glucose levels prior to conception but is rarely performed. On another hand, waiting for 24 WG to diagnose DIP would delay care in an unacceptable way and potentially lead to severe obstetric complications, as obstetric outcomes are quite similar for undiagnosed type 2 and type 1 diabetes [8]. Furthermore, the prevalence of fetal malformations was recently reported to be higher in women with DIP compared to women with GDM [9]. The incidence of other outcomes was similar in both groups [9].

Concomitantly, the IADPSG recommended using a FPG range 5.1–6.9 mmol/L before 24 WG to define early GDM (eGDM). Measurement was recommended at the first prenatal visit, or later if undone, especially in high-risk women [1]. The threshold of 5.1 mmol/L is arbitrary and was chosen as the same value as after 24 WG. Actually, FPG was described to be quite stable during pregnancy [10]. In this study, FPG levels were similar in the same women when measured at 17 WG then at 32 WG [10], despite an increase in insulin secretion and a propensity for earlier hypoglycemia during fasting as described a long time ago [11]. The IADPSG recommends that women with eGDM should be referred for immediate care, even if the level of proof for this recommendation is very low regarding to prognosis [12, 13]. Alternatively, some guidelines do not recommend to treat immediately women with high FPG levels in early pregnancy, such as the ADA [4]. Other advice for patients who have an early FPG between 5.6 and 6.9 mmol/L is to perform an OGTT at 16–18 WG and to monitor and treat abnormal results at this time (http://www.salute.gov.it).

2. Methods

References for this review were identified through searches of PubMed for articles published until March 2017, by use of the terms "early gestational diabetes mellitus" and "fasting plasma glucose and pregnancy." English and French articles resulting from these searches and relevant references cited in those articles were reviewed. We discuss here the prevalence, risk factors, and metabolic characteristics of eGDM, as well as its prognosis.

3. Results

3.1. Bibliography. Our search in Medline suggested 1800 references between January 2010 and March 2017. Of these articles, we selected and analysed around 100 articles. We additionally analysed around 20 articles that were cited in these papers. We also found 5 relevant ongoing studies in clinicaltrials.gov. We finally selected 49 references.

3.2. The Burden of eGDM

3.2.1. Diagnosis with Early FPG Measurement. A FPG level ≥ 5.0 mmol/L was reported in 11.9% of pregnant women during the first trimester of pregnancy (mean 9 WG) in Israel [14], where universal screening for FPG has been recommended at the first prenatal care visit. This prevalence was close to the prevalence of FPG above 5.1 mmol/L that was reported at the first prenatal visit in a multicenter study in China [15] and in one center in Italy [16] (11.4% and 7.2%, resp.), noting that almost all women were tested in these studies.

In France, where selective screening and using IADPSG criteria is recommended, data from the French National Interscheme Health Insurance Information System (SNIIRAM) showed that only 2.3% of 788,494 pregnant women in 2013 without known diabetes were treated for a dysglycemia diagnosed before 22 WG [17]. These women corresponded to 26.9% of all women with dysglycemia during their pregnancy. The French criteria for selective screening are maternal age ≥ 35 years, body mass index (BMI) ≥ 25 kg/m^2, history of diabetes in a first-degree relative, personal history of GDM, or having giving birth to a child with fetal macrosomia [6]. In the United States, implementing early screening nearly doubled the incidence of GDM as compared with a previous standard two-step approach [18].

3.2.2. Diagnosis with Early OGTT. A high prevalence of eGDM has also been reported when OGTT is performed in early pregnancy in selected populations with risk factors. The prevalence was 23.4% in pregnant women with a BMI at or above 29.0 kg/m^2 in early pregnancy as part of the enrollment into the DALI (Vitamin D And Lifestyle Intervention for GDM prevention) pilot and lifestyle Pan-European multicenter trials [19]. Additionally, the prevalence of eGDM in high-risk populations was recently reported to be 48.8% in Italy [20] and 27.3% in Australia [21].

To conclude this part, intermediate FPG levels in early pregnancy, also known as eGDM, have become a very common issue.

3.3. Risk Factors for Hyperglycemia in Early Pregnancy. Figure 1 shows that FPG ≥ 5.1 mmol/L during early pregnancy is more prevalent with aging [16, 19, 22], higher BMI [16, 19, 22], a family history of diabetes [19, 22], a personal history of GDM [19, 22] or newborn with macrosomia [19], and multiparity [23].

Studies using other definition for eGDM found similar risk factors [21, 23–26]. However, all those results should be interpreted with caution as screening is usually performed in already high-risk subjects.

3.4. Metabolic Characteristics of Women with eGDM. Bozkurt et al. have evaluated pathophysiological characteristics of pregnant women diagnosed with GDM according to IADPSG criteria [22]. Unlike patients with late (regular) GDM or normal glucose tolerant women, subjects with eGDM exhibited decreased insulin sensitivity, with lower oral glucose insulin sensitivity index and quantitative insulin sensitivity check index. The subgroups also differed in BMI, with significantly higher levels in patients with eGDM compared to subjects with late GDM and those with normal glucose tolerance (31.7 ± 6.4, 27.7 ± 4.4, and 27.3 ± 5.6 kg/m^2, resp., $p < 0.001$). However, differences in estimated insulin sensitivity remained significant after adjustment for BMI,

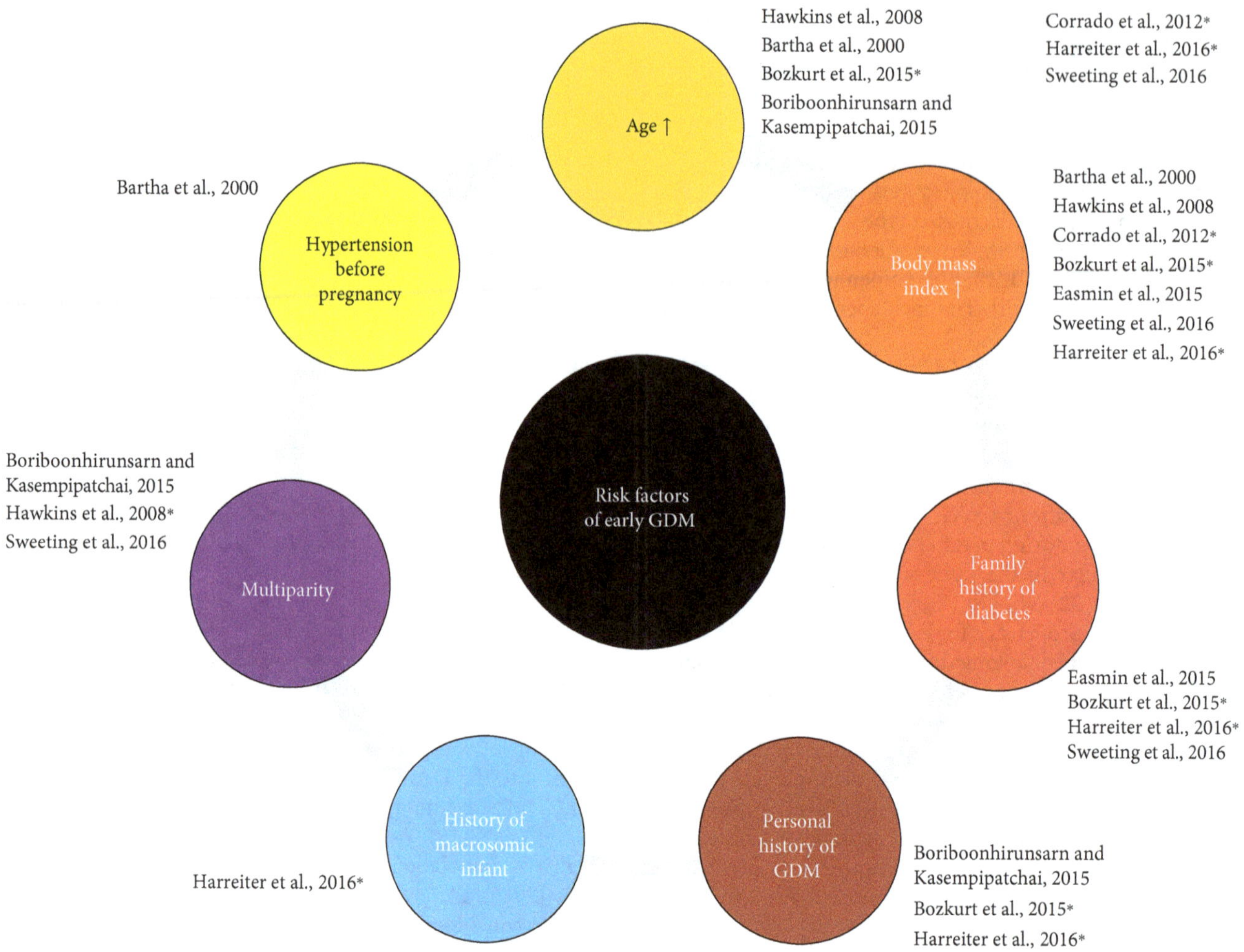

Figure 1: Risk factors for early gestational diabetes mellitus. GDM: gestational diabetes mellitus. * identifies references where early GDM is defined according to the IADPSG definition, that is, fasting plasma glucose value ≥ 5.1 mmol/L.

age, and history of GDM. In this study, subjects with either early or late GDM showed impairments in β-cell function (insulinogenic index) as compared with women without GDM [22].

In another study including women with BMI at or above 29 kg/m^2 who were screened in early pregnancy using a 75 g OGTT, various indexes of insulin sensitivity (oral glucose insulin sensitivity index, quantitative insulin sensitivity check index, and homeostasis model assessment of insulin resistance (HOMA-IR)) and secretion (Stumvoll first and second phases) decreased progressively in women with normal glucose tolerance, eGDM, and DIP [19]. Differences persisted after adjustment for age, pregestational BMI, gestational week, and fetal gender [19].

3.5. What Does eGDM Outside Pregnancy Mean? Mills et al. [27] have shown that there is a physiological reduction in FPG concentration in normal pregnancy. In their cohort of 361 healthy pregnant women, they showed that FPG levels decrease with advancing pregnancy with a plateau occurring around 10–20 WG [27]. Thereafter, insulin resistance increases and "late" GDM may occur [28]. As shown and explained in Figure 2 and as it was previously suggested [29], high FPG during early pregnancy could indicate unknown prediabetes (if eGDM) or diabetes (if DIP) before pregnancy as insulin resistance remains present in both cases. Although glycemic status before pregnancy is usually unknown, we may use several indicators, such as markers for glycemic exposure before pregnancy, early postdelivery glycemic status (which is usually considered to reflect glycemic status before pregnancy), and incidence of type 2 diabetes postpartum.

3.5.1. Marker for Long-Term Glycemic Exposure at the Time of eGDM Diagnosis. Skin autofluorescence, a measurement of cutaneous advanced glycation end products, can be used as a screening method in detecting unknown diabetes. Maury et al. have suggested that skin autofluorescence was a marker of metabolic memory in pregnant women. During pregnancy, forearm skin autofluorescence at 24–30 WG was reported to gradually decrease from patients with previous diabetes, to women with GDM and previous hyperglycemia, to those with GDM without previous hyperglycemia, and finally to normal subjects without diabetes or GDM [30]. In

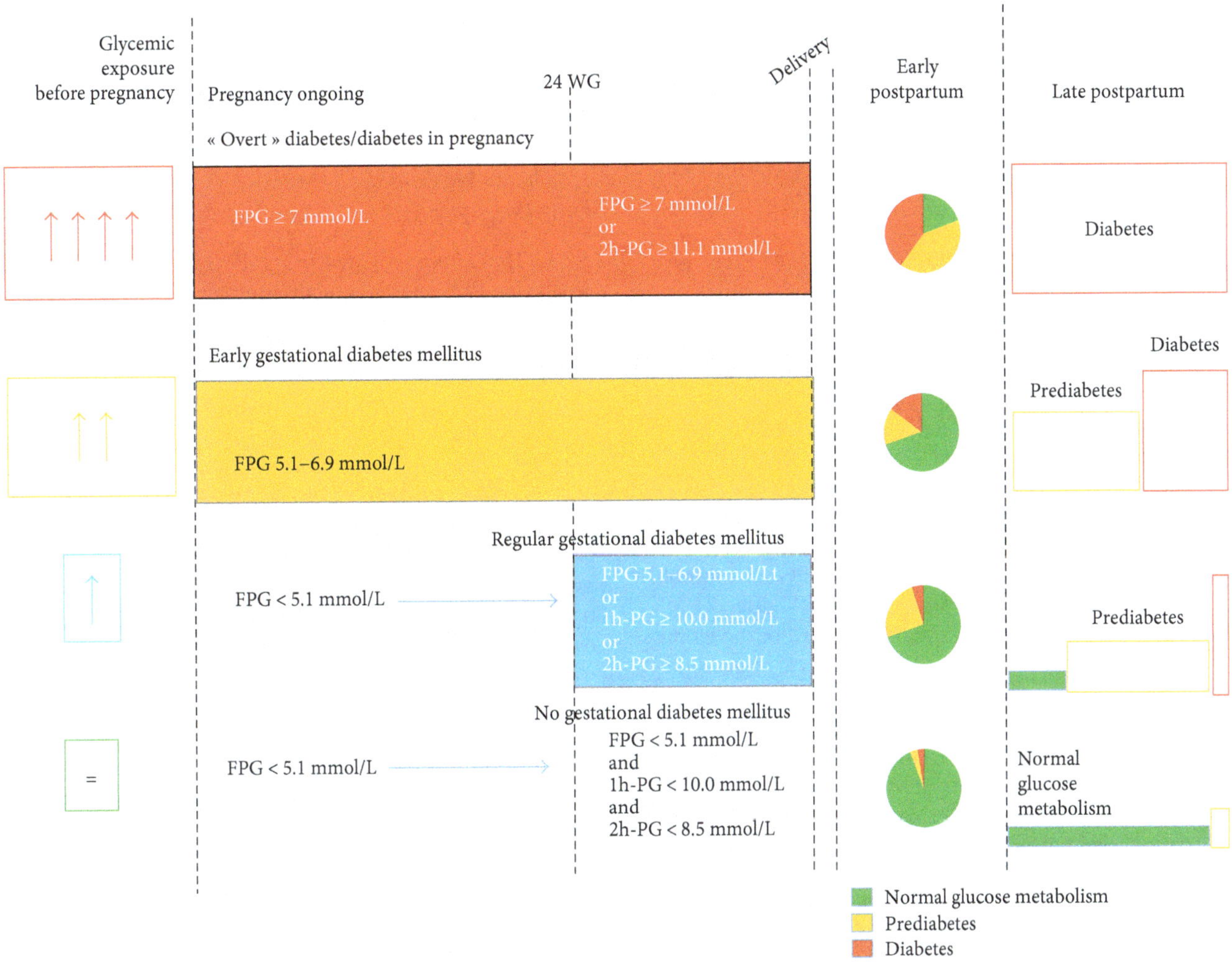

FIGURE 2: Does eGDM mean preexisting prediabetes? The hypothesis is when hyperglycemia has been present (but unknown) before pregnancy, then fasting plasma glucose (FPG) is already increased during early pregnancy while insulin resistance increases after 24 weeks of gestation (WG). Accordingly, oral glucose tolerance will reveal dysglycemia in early postpartum. 1h-PG and 2h-PG: plasma glucose 1 and 2 hours after 75 g oral glucose tolerance test; FPG: fasting plasma glucose; WG: weeks of gestation.

that study, previous hyperglycemia was defined as previous GDM or having given birth to a macrosomic infant or GDM diagnosed before 24 WG (eGDM) [30].

3.5.2. Data Based on OGTT in the Immediate Postpartum. Sweeting et al. have recently reported the results of postpartum OGTT according to the time of GDM diagnosis [21]. In this study, women were tested between 2001 and 2011, with early screening performed in women considered at high risk for GDM. The repartition of normal plasma glucose values, impaired glucose tolerance, and diabetes during OGTT performed three months postpartum significantly differed according to eGDM < 12 WG (normal glucose tolerance 79%, impaired glucose tolerance 11%, and diabetes 11%), GDM 12–23 WG (71, 24, and 5%, resp.), and GDM > 24 WG (85, 14, and 1%, resp.). However, the proportion of dysglycemia was only 22% in women with eGDM < 12 WG, suggesting that eGDM is not a good marker of preexisting dysglycemia. However, the implementation of a lifestyle change program during pregnancy and postpartum might partially account for this result.

3.5.3. Postpartum Development of Type 2 Diabetes. The presence of eGDM could also identify women with an increased risk to later develop type 2 diabetes. In a systematic review including 8 studies and 4026 women with GDM defined with numerous criteria, women with eGDM had a twofold increased risk of incident type 2 diabetes 6 weeks to 20 years after delivery compared to subjects with "late" GDM (relative risk (RR) 2.13 (95% CI 1.52–3.56)) [31]. IADPSG-diagnosed eGDM has also been reported to be a significant predictor of progression to abnormal glucose tolerance up to 5 years postpartum. In this study, the earlier the GDM was diagnosed, the higher was the rate of dysglycemia up to 5 years postpartum [32].

To conclude at this step, although eGDM is associated with a profile comparable to metabolic syndrome, with higher insulin resistance than in "regular GDM," it has not been consistently associated with prediabetes or diabetes during early postpartum. However, it is associated with more incident type 2 diabetes than regular GDM (Figure 2). Overall, this suggests that eGDM should be considered as a new intermediate entity between normal glucose metabolism and prediabetes/diabetes outside pregnancy.

3.6. The Meaning of an Early High FPG through Pregnancy

3.6.1. Persistence through Pregnancy. eGDM was initially supposed to be persistent through pregnancy. Therefore, it was hypothesized that early care for eGDM would improve prognosis and that was the reason why FPG in the range 5.1–6.9 mmol/L was recommended to diagnose GDM at any time during pregnancy [1]. However, data from Italy [16] and China [15] have challenged this recommendation. Actually, at least 50% of the women with eGDM have no GDM after 24 WG, despite the absence of specific care. In the Italian publication, 55% of women with FPG ≥ 5.1 mmol/L during early pregnancy had a normal OGTT after 24 WG [16]; in the Chinese study, less than one-third of the women still had a FPG ≥ 5.1 mmol/L between the first prenatal visit and 24–28 WG [15].

3.6.2. Does Early FPG Predict GDM after 24 WG? Smirnakis et al. showed in a prospective study that women in whom GDM was diagnosed at 24–28 WG (using the O'Sullivan and Mahan criteria of the American Diabetes Association) demonstrated higher levels of FPG (4.8 ± 0.6 versus 4.4 ± 0.4 mmol/L, $p < 0.05$) and HOMA-IR at 17 WG compared to women who had normoglycemic pregnancies [33]. Riskin-Mashia et al. have also shown that first-trimester FPG levels were positively associated with the risk of GDM after 24 WG, especially when values were ≥5.0 mmol/L [14]. In another study including overweight women at very high risk for GDM, the prevalence of IADPSG-defined GDM after 24 WG was 53% in those with early FPG ≥ 4.9 mmol/L whereas the prevalences were 15, 12, and 20% in those with early FPG ≤ 4.4, 4.41–4.6, and 4.61–4.89 mmol/L, respectively [34]. Therefore, FPG in early pregnancy can be considered as a tool to select the women at risk for GDM after 24 WG. For example, the sensitivity, specificity, positive, and negative predictive values of FPG > 4.4 mmol/L in early pregnancy to predict IADPSG-defined GDM in an Italian population were 80%, 66%, 77%, and 96%, respectively [35]. Therefore, using the recursive portioning and amalgamation method, it was suggested to consider a low FPG to avoid OGTT after 24 WG because of its high negative predictive value [35]. Actually, the negative predictive value was not so high in two other studies. First, in a Chinese population, the sensitivity, specificity, positive, and negative predictive values of FPG > 4.4 mmol/L to predict IADPSG-defined GDM were 78%, 38%, 21%, and 89%, respectively [15]. Second, in overweight women at very high risk of GDM, the negative predictive value of early FPG ≤ 4.4 mmol/L was only 85% [34].

Additionally, FPG concentration at first antenatal visit in 2284 women in China was higher in those who later developed GDM than in those who did not. However, early FPG was associated with late GDM when measured between 12 and 16 WG, 16–20 WG and 20–24 WG, but not before 12 WG. This suggested that the relationship between FPG and late GDM appeared during the second trimester [36].

3.7. Should We Consider Alternatives to FPG Measurement in Early Pregnancy

3.7.1. The Limits of Measuring FPG in Early Pregnancy. Analyzing FPG level is actually complex. First, FPG decreases with increasing gestational age [15]. For example, in a Chinese population [15], median FPG was 4.95 mmol/L at 4–6 WG, 4.70 at 10–12 WG, and 4.53 at 14–16 WG and was the lowest at 4.38 mmol/L at 20–24 WG.

Second, based on the receiving operating curves and area under the curve measurements, in another Chinese population, the optimal FPG cut-off values to predict GDM after 24 WG were different according to BMI categorization groups [37]. The FPG cut-off value was 4.77 mmol/L in prepregnancy underweight women, 4.92 mmol/L in prepregnancy normal weight women, 5.00 mmol/L in prepregnancy overweight women, and 5.05 mmol/L in prepregnancy obese women [37].

Overall, the threshold for FPG could be different according to WG and to BMI level. There is a need to investigate the best threshold for early FPG and the association with late GDM or poor pregnancy outcomes. The concordances of early OGTT, at 12–15 WG [38] or at 18–20 WG [39], are going to be compared to OGTT results at 24–28 WG in two studies, but no data are currently available yet.

3.7.2. OGTT. OGTT could be more sensitive than FPG alone to diagnose GDM during early pregnancy. For example, in pregnant women with obesity at 15.2 ± 3.0 WG and using IADPSG criteria, 1- and 2-hour glucose values led to diagnose 21.5% additional GDM as compared to FPG value during the OGTT [19]. However, data on 1- and 2-hour OGTT glucose values are rare in early pregnancy. Using IADPSG criteria is not evidence based in early pregnancy. Especially, thresholds that are used after 24 WG are too high for early pregnancy [10]. OGTT is time-consuming, inconvenient, and uncomfortable, inducing nausea and vomiting in some patients. Therefore, some women might refuse to repeat OGTT after 24 GW.

3.7.3. HbA1c Measurement. HbA1c measurement also warrants further evaluation [13]. HbA1c ≥ 5.9% has been reported to identify all cases of DIP and to be associated with poor pregnancy outcomes, including congenital anomalies, preeclampsia, shoulder dystocia, and perinatal deaths [40]. The association with poor outcomes appears to be independent of later GDM diagnosis [41]. However, HbA1c may vary with pregnancy hemodilution [42] and with the presence of hemoglobinopathy and/or anemia.

To conclude this part, FPG > 5.1 mmol/L persists in less than one-half of untreated women and we should define an alternative FPG threshold to define eGDM. However, it may differ according to BMI and WG.

3.8. Prognosis Related to Hyperglycemia in Early Pregnancy (Table 1)

3.8.1. Poor Pregnancy Prognosis Related to FPG in Early Pregnancy. A poor prognosis of high FPG levels during the first trimester was reported, with an increased risk of adverse pregnancy outcomes, including macrosomia [14, 36] and cesarean section [14].

Among the 788,494 women who delivered in France in 2013, women with early onset of GDM were more likely to have need for cesarean section (odds ratio 1.10 (95% confidence interval 1.05–1.15)) and large for gestational age infants (1.18 (1.12–1.24)) than women diagnosed between 22 and 30 WG [17].

3.8.2. Poor Prognosis Associated with eGDM Not Defined with FPG. Bartha et al. [24] have compared complications associated with GDM diagnosed in early (mainly during the first trimester) or late pregnancy. eGDM screening was performed only in case of risk factors, especially increased BMI, which was a bias as the presence of risk factors has been associated with a worse prognosis [43]. They reported that the group diagnosed earlier in pregnancy had higher rates of preeclampsia, neonatal hypoglycemia, and perinatal deaths and lower rate of oligohydramnios [24]. Preeclampsia, shoulder dystocia, macrosomia, and hyperbilirubinemia were reported to be more frequent in women with diet-treated GDM diagnosed before than after 24 WG, even after adjustment for maternal age, ethnicity, parity, weight, and blood glucose control [23]. Obstetric outcomes were also compared in early onset and late onset GDM in Bangladesh and showed a poorer prognosis associated with eGDM, including more preeclampsia, neonatal admission in intensive care unit, and neonatal hypoglycemia [26].

When using the Australasian Diabetes in Pregnancy Society diagnostic criteria in a large Australian multiethnic cohort of women considered at high risk for GDM, eGDM was also associated with poorer pregnancy outcomes [21]. In this study, the eGDM cohort was a preselected high-risk group and patients with eGDM diagnosed before 12 WG had an intermediate risk profile, standing between the risk of subjects with preexisting type 2 diabetes and the risk of patients diagnosed with eGDM between 12 and 23 WG. The outcomes in women who were diagnosed with GDM before 12 WG were quite comparable to those observed in subjects with preexisting diabetes despite early testing and current best practice treatment [21].

Further research is currently necessary to evaluate the effects of early metabolic changes on short- and long-term outcomes for the mother and the child and of the potential consequences on generational transmission of metabolic diseases.

3.9. Does the Treatment of Hyperglycemia in Early Pregnancy Improve Prognosis? (Table 1)

3.9.1. Argumentation from Retrospective Studies Comparing Women Cared for Early or Regular GDM. Early detection and treatment of women at high risk of eGDM might improve pregnancy outcomes: several studies have shown a similar prognosis in early and late GDM with treatment. For example, an Indian team assessed the merits of care given to women in whom GDM was diagnosed in different WG in order to find out the ideal period of screening in women with history of high-risk pregnancies. The babies born to GDM women diagnosed before 12 WG had a lower birth weight than the ones born to GDM women diagnosed after 30 WG. The authors concluded therefore that screening in the first trimester of pregnancy and institution of therapy was advisable in women with high-risk pregnancies [44]. In Thailand, the incidence of pregnancy complications was similar in women diagnosed with GDM early and late in pregnancy [25]. In this study, gestational weight gain and glycemic control, but not the time of diagnosis, were independently associated with macrosomia in women with GDM [25]. The authors suggested that the higher frequency of insulin treatment, as consistently reported [17, 18, 21, 24–26, 45], and the lower gestational weight gain [21, 24, 25] in women with eGDM compared to women with late GDM might explain a similar prognosis in both groups in these studies. However, although insulin initiation was also earlier in eGDM than in late GDM, with a higher maximum daily insulin dose in the study by Sweeting et al., the prognosis was worse in women with eGDM [46].

3.9.2. Argumentation from Retrospective Studies Comparing Strategies including Early Screening for Dysglycemia or Not. Alunni et al. compared two cohorts of pregnant women with GDM: those diagnosed via two-step screening (standard approach) versus those diagnosed via early screening diagnosis with additional screening after 24 WG if early screening was negative. The second approach doubled the incidence of GDM, but there was no significant difference in neonatal outcomes [18].

Hong et al. analyzed a retrospective cohort of women with singleton pregnancies diagnosed with GDM who had indications for early screening, defined as the presence of obesity, or GDM or macrosomia in a prior pregnancy. Women were classified as having been screened early (<20 WG) or routinely (>24 WG). The decision of whether or not a patient had early screening for GDM was at the discretion of the managing provider. Early screening was not associated with significant reduction in the risk of cesarean, preeclampsia, macrosomia, or birth injury. The authors concluded that the utility of early GDM screening still required an evaluation [45].

3.9.3. Future Randomized Trials. Randomized controlled trials evaluating the benefit-cost balance for screening and treating less severe hyperglycemia than DIP in early pregnancy are mandatory [13]. We have found several ongoing trials. One will compare the prognosis of pregnancies of 202 women with first trimester hyperglycemia (defined with FPG or HbA1c) when treatment begins before 15 WG versus after 28 WG (clinicaltrials.gov NCT01926457). The Early Gestational Diabetes Screening in the Gravid Obese Woman (EGGO, clinicaltrials.gov NCT01864564) and the Randomization of Early Diabetes Screening Among Obese Pregnant

Table 1: Data considering prognosis of early fasting plasma glucose, of early gestational diabetes mellitus, and of strategies including early screening for gestational diabetes mellitus or not.

Reference	*n*	Population	Screening methods for glycemic disorders	Predictive factors of eGDM	Care and differences during pregnancy (eGDM versus remaining)	Prognosis of eGDM (*adjusted)
Fasting plasma glycemia & prognosis						
Riskin-Mashiah et al., 2009 [14]	6129 women	Retrospective Israel	FPG measurement at 9.5 (7.6–11.6) GW classified in 7 HAPO categories	NA	NA	Late GDM development ↑* LGA/macrosomia ↑* Cesarean delivery ↑*
Liu et al., 2014 [36]	2284 women	Retrospective China	FPG at first antenatal visit (17.4 ± 4.6 GW)	NA	NA	Late GDM development ↑* Neonatal birth weight ↑*
eGDM & prognosis						
Bartha et al., 2000 [24]	50 eGDM versus 133 regular GDM (24–28 WG)	Retrospective Case control Spain	Women with risk factors O'Sullivan then 100 g OGTT	Age ↑ BMI ↑ Hypertension ↑	GWG ↓ Insulin therapy ↑	Total preeclampsia ↑ Oligohydramnios ↓ Neonatal hypoglycemia ↑ Perinatal death ↑ Prematurity, fetal anomalies, cesarean section, SGA, macrosomia, NICU =
Hawkins et al., 2008 [23]	339 eGDM (<24 WG) versus 2257 regular GDM	Retrospective Case control United States	Diet-treated GDM Early screening in women with risk factors O'Sullivan then 100 g OGTT	Age ↑ BMI ↑ Multiparity ↑	DIET ONLY (insulin-treated women were excluded) Better decrease in fasting plasma value during follow up for eGDM group	Preeclampsia ↑* Shoulder dystocia ↑ Macrosomia ↑ Hyperbilirubinemia ↑* Shoulder dystocia, cesarean section, NICU, neonatal death =
Seshiah et al., 2008 [44]	120 NGT versus 87 GDM < 12 WG versus 18 GDM 13–23 WG versus 15 GDM 24–30 WG versus 18 GDM > 30 WG	Retrospective Case control India	Women with family history of diabetes and bad obstetric history 75 g OGGT: 2 h PG > 140 mg/dL	FPG, 2 h PG, and HbA1c are the highest in women with GDM < 12 GW	Unknown	Birth weight GDM < 12 GW lower than birth weight GDM > 30 GW
Easmin et al., 2015 [26]	60 eGDM (<24 WG) versus 60 regular GDM (24–32 WG)	Prospective observational Case control Bangladesh	Unknown	BMI ↑ Family history of diabetes ↑	Insulin therapy ↑	Preeclampsia ↑ NICU ↑ Neonatal hypoglycemia ↑ Hyperbilirubinemia, asphyxia, perinatal death =
Boriboonhirunsarn and Kasempipatchai, 2015 [25]	142 women with eGDM (<20 GW) versus 120 women with regular GDM	Thailand 2014	Women with risk factors O'Sullivan then 100 g OGTT in early and late pregnancies	Age ↑ Previous history of GDM ↑ Multiparity ↑	GWG↓ Insulin therapy↑ Better glycemic control	Term, preeclampsia, cesarean delivery, macrosomia, hyperbilirubinemia =

Table 1: Continued.

Reference	*n*	Population	Screening methods for glycemic disorders	Predictive factors of eGDM	Care and differences during pregnancy (eGDM versus remaining)	Prognosis of eGDM (*adjusted)
Sweeting et al., 2016 [21]	3493 GDM ≥ 24 GW versus 1247 GDM 12–23 GW versus 68 GDM < 12 GW versus 65 preexisting diabetes	Retrospective Case control	Early screening only in women with risk factors ADIPS criteria	Age ↑ BMI ↑ Family history of diabetes ↑ Multiparity ↑	GWG↓ Insulin therapy↑ Earlier insulin therapy↑ Maximum daily insulin dose↑	Gradient in 4 groups Preterm delivery ↑ Cesarean section ↑ Hypertensive disorders ↑ Macrosomia ↑ Hyperbilirubinemia ↑ Respiratory distress syndrome ↑
Regnault et al., 2016 [17]	18,299 women with eGDM (<22 GW) versus 37,551 women with GDM (22–30 GW)	From the 788,494 women who delivered in France in 2013	Early and regular screening in case of risk factors IADPSG criteria	No data	Insulin therapy ↑	Cesarean delivery ↑ LGA ↑
Screening strategy including early screening & prognosis						
Alunni et al., 2015 [18]	First period: 147 women with GDM after 24 GW versus second period: 175 GDM women with early and, if negative screening, late screening	From 2652 women who delivered between 2010 and 2012 United States	First period: O'Sullivan and 100 g OGTT after 24 GW Second period: early screening FPG and HbA1c; 75 g OGTT (IADPSG)	BMI ↓ during the second period	Comparison between first and second periods Insulin = Comparison during the second period (eGDM versus regular GDM) Insulin therapy ↑	Term = Cesarean delivery = Macrosomia = SGA =
Hong et al., 2016 [45]	112 women screened early (including 85 with early GDM and 27 with regular GDM) versus 457 women with regular GDM who were not tested earlier	569 women with risk factors for GDM United States	Early screening only in case of risk factors In early and regular screening: O'Sullivan then 100 g OGTT	Early screening strategy Private insurance ↑ History of GDM ↑ Chronic hypertension ↑ BMI ↑	Insulin therapy ↑	Early screening strategy Cesarean section =* Preeclampsia =* SGA and LGA =* Birth injury =* Preterm delivery ↑*

2h-PG: 2-hour plasma glucose; ADIPS: Australasian Diabetes in Pregnancy Society; BMI: body mass index; eGDM: early gestational diabetes mellitus; GDM: gestational diabetes mellitus; GWG: gestational weight gain; HAPO: hyperglycemia and adverse pregnancy outcome; LGA: large for gestational age; NA: nonapplicable; NICU: neonatal intensive care unit; OGTT: oral glucose tolerance test; SGA: small for gestational age; WG: weeks of gestation; =: similar; ↓: decreased or lower; ↑: increased or higher. *References where multivariate analyses were performed.

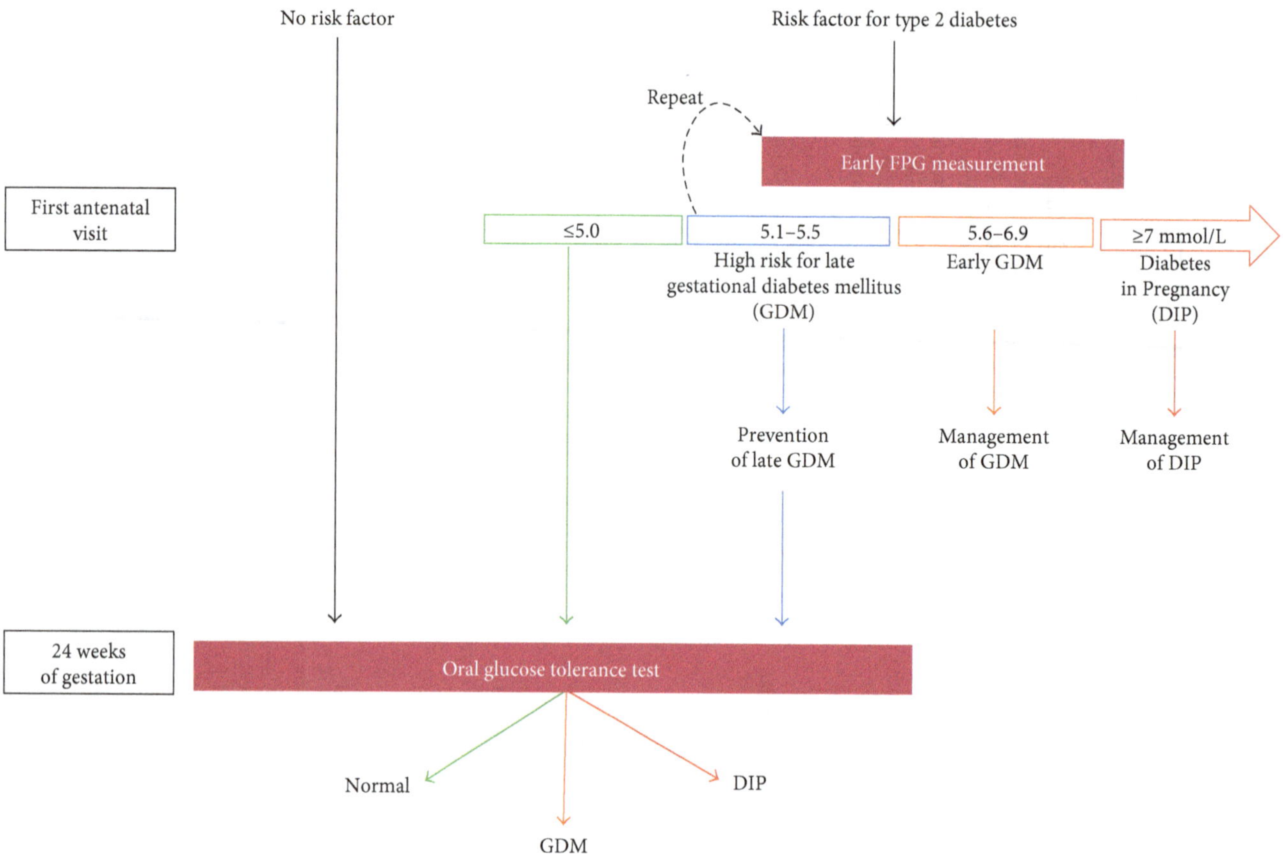

Figure 3: Proposals for a management algorithm according to the presence of risk factors and screening for dysglycemia during pregnancy. DIP: diabetes in pregnancy; FPG: fasting plasma glucose; GDM: gestational diabetes mellitus.

Women (REDSOAP, clinicaltrials.gov NCT03116009) studies will include 1150 and 600 obese women, respectively. They will compare the prognosis associated with screening strategies including or not a screening for dysglycemia during early pregnancy. Finally, the Early Diagnosis of Gestational Diabetes Mellitus Study (EDoGDM) will randomize 600 low-risk pregnant women with an OGTT performed at 18 to 20 WG versus 24 and 28 WG and will compare prognosis in both groups ([39], clinicaltrials.gov NCT02740283).

To conclude this part, high FPG during early pregnancy is associated with a poor prognosis, which might be improved with immediate care through diet and insulin therapy if necessary. However, the results of randomized trials are still lacking.

3.10. What Could Be Proposed in Clinical Practice at the Current Time? We propose the following algorithm of management according to early FPG (Figure 3). This proposal has not been validated by an expert consensus and should obviously not be considered as validated recommendations. The increasing number of subjects with undiagnosed type 2 diabetes mellitus before pregnancy justifies the screening of women with risk factors for preexisting diabetes by the first antenatal visit. We currently suggest to keep diagnosing DIP when FPG is 7.0 mmol/L or above. Actually, the incidence of macrosomia, preeclampsia, and neonatal hypoglycemia has been reported to be similar in treated women with DIP or GDM [9]. As eGDM is also associated with classical risk factors for type 2 diabetes, we suggest, for feasibility reasons, to screen early in pregnancy only the subjects considered to be at high risk. We suggest to test subjects with characteristics predisposing to type 2 diabetes according to the local frequency of abnormal glucose metabolism and according to local guidelines.

The current recommended FPG threshold (5.1 mmol/L) to define eGDM is an issue, as FPG depends on gestational age, ethnicity, and BMI categories [13, 15, 37]. We suggest to refer for care any subject with a FPG between 5.6 and 6.9 mmol/L as the risk of giving birth to a child with macrosomia increases with higher FPG [14, 36, 47]. We acknowledge that a FPG threshold at 5.6 mmol/L is also arbitrary as the association between early FPG and pregnancy outcomes appears to be a continuum [48]. However, Zhu et al. [15] showed that the positive predictive value of an abnormal OGTT at 24–28 weeks was 60% from an early FPG 5.7 mmol/L, and last but not the least, Riskin-Mashiah et al. [14] reported in 6129 women with early FPG that the risk of macrosomia and primary cesarean section almost tripled and doubled, respectively, from this same threshold. Accordingly and as shown in the FIGO report [7], FPG values between 5.6 and 6.9 mmol/L are considered as GDM in China, Latin America, and the UK.

Because women might have inadequately fasted before the first measurement and because the reproducibility of FPG is imperfect, we propose to recheck the level of FPG when it is between 5.1 and 5.5 mmol/L and to consider the lowest value among both FPG measurements. HbA1c measurement might be an alternative to the second FPG but warrants further evaluation [13]. If the level of FPG is confirmed to be between 5.1 and 5.5 mmol/L, we suggest lifestyle changes (nutrition and exercise). Actually, the prevention of GDM seems more effective when started before 15 WG [49]. These women should be screened again, with OGTT, after 24 WG.

We think that all the remaining women, even those with a low early FPG level, should be screened after 24 WG. Actually, an early FPG < 4.4 mmol/L had a very high negative predictive value for late GDM in one study [35] but this was not confirmed in two other studies [15, 34]. Therefore, we do propose to keep a late screening in these women. Noteworthily, the screening after 24 WG includes women without risk factor but we have previously reported that women with GDM, even without risk factor and with adequate management, have a poor prognosis [43].

4. Conclusions

Measuring FPG in early pregnancy appears to be crucial to diagnose DIP and treat this condition as early as possible. Intermediate FPG levels in early pregnancy, also known as eGDM, have become a frequent issue. eGDM appears to represent a new intermediate entity in the following continuum: normal glucose metabolism, late GDM, eGDM, DIP, and pregravidic diabetes. Indeed, women diagnosed with eGDM have more risk factors for prevalent type 2 diabetes compared to subjects diagnosed with GDM later in pregnancy. They also have more incident type 2 diabetes and are more insulin resistant. This might participate to a poorer prognosis. However, there are major remaining issues about this new entity. Indeed, (i) a FPG > 5.1 mmol/L has been reported to persist in less than one-half of untreated women and the definition of eGDM needs to be better determined and (ii) there is nowadays no clear evidence of the usefulness of its treatment.

Abbreviations

ADA: American Diabetes Association
BMI: Body mass index
DIP: Diabetes in pregnancy
eGDM: Early gestational diabetes mellitus
FIGO: International Federation of Gynecology and Obstetrics
FPG: Fasting plasma glucose
GDM: Gestational diabetes mellitus
HOMA-IR: Homeostasis model assessment of insulin resistance
IADPSG: International Association of Diabetes Pregnancy Study Group
NICE: National Institute for Health and Care Excellence
OGTT: Oral glucose tolerance test
WG: Weeks of gestation.

Conflicts of Interest

The authors declare that they have no conflicts of interest.

Acknowledgments

The authors thank Dr. Sylvie Picard for the English revision and useful advices about the manuscript.

References

[1] B. E. Metzger, S. G. Gabbe, B. Persson et al., "International Association of Diabetes and Pregnancy Study Groups recommendations on the diagnosis and classification of hyperglycemia in pregnancy," *Diabetes Care*, vol. 33, no. 3, pp. 676–682, 2010.

[2] P. M. Catalano, E. D. Tyzbir, R. R. Wolfe et al., "Carbohydrate metabolism during pregnancy in control subjects and women with gestational diabetes," *The American Journal of Physiology*, vol. 264, no. 1, Part 1, pp. E60–E67, 1993.

[3] L. A. Barbour, C. E. McCurdy, T. L. Hernandez, J. P. Kirwan, P. M. Catalano, and J. E. Friedman, "Cellular mechanisms for insulin resistance in normal pregnancy and gestational diabetes," *Diabetes Care*, vol. 30, Supplement 2, pp. S112–S119, 2007.

[4] American Diabetes Association, "Diagnosis and classification of diabetes mellitus," *Diabetes Care*, vol. 40, Supplement 1, pp. S11–S24, 2017.

[5] Y. Handelsman, J. I. Mechanick, L. Blonde et al., "American Association of Clinical Endocrinologists Medical Guidelines for Clinical Practice for developing a diabetes mellitus comprehensive care plan," *Endocrine Practice*, vol. 17, Supplement 2, pp. 1–53, 2011.

[6] Gestational diabetes, "Summary of expert consensus," *Diabetes & Metabolism*, vol. 36, no. 6, Part 2, pp. 695–699, 2010.

[7] M. Hod, A. Kapur, D. A. Sacks et al., "The International Federation of Gynecology and Obstetrics (FIGO) initiative on gestational diabetes mellitus: a pragmatic guide for diagnosis, management, and care," *International Journal of Gynaecology and Obstetrics*, vol. 131, Supplement 3, pp. S173–S211, 2015.

[8] A. McGrogan, J. Snowball, and C. S. de Vries, "Pregnancy losses in women with type 1 or type 2 diabetes in the UK: an investigation using primary care records," *Diabetic Medicine*, vol. 31, no. 3, pp. 357–365, 2014.

[9] F. Corrado, B. Pintaudi, R. D'Anna, A. Santamaria, L. Giunta, and A. Di Benedetto, "Perinatal outcome in a Caucasian population with gestational diabetes and preexisting diabetes first diagnosed in pregnancy," *Diabetes & Metabolism*, vol. 42, no. 2, pp. 122–125, 2016.

[10] C. D. Agardh, A. Aberg, and N. E. Norden, "Glucose levels and insulin secretion during a 75 g glucose challenge test in normal pregnancy," *Journal of Internal Medicine*, vol. 240, no. 5, pp. 303–309, 1996.

[11] B. E. Metzger, V. Ravnikar, R. A. Vileisis, and N. Freinkel, ""Accelerated starvation" and the skipped breakfast in late normal pregnancy," *The Lancet*, vol. 319, no. 8272, pp. 588–592, 1982.

[12] A. M. Guedj, "When should screening be performed for gestational diabetes?," *Diabetes & Metabolism*, vol. 36, no. 6, Part 2, pp. 652–657, 2010.

[13] H. D. McIntyre, D. A. Sacks, L. A. Barbour et al., "Issues with the diagnosis and classification of hyperglycemia in early pregnancy," *Diabetes Care*, vol. 39, no. 1, pp. 53-54, 2016.

[14] S. Riskin-Mashiah, G. Younes, A. Damti, and R. Auslender, "First-trimester fasting hyperglycemia and adverse pregnancy outcomes," *Diabetes Care*, vol. 32, no. 9, pp. 1639–1643, 2009.

[15] W. W. Zhu, H. X. Yang, Y. M. Wei et al., "Evaluation of the value of fasting plasma glucose in the first prenatal visit to diagnose gestational diabetes mellitus in China," *Diabetes Care*, vol. 36, no. 3, pp. 586–590, 2013.

[16] F. Corrado, R. D'Anna, M. L. Cannata, M. L. Interdonato, B. Pintaudi, and A. Di Benedetto, "Correspondence between first-trimester fasting glycaemia, and oral glucose tolerance test in gestational diabetes diagnosis," *Diabetes & Metabolism*, vol. 38, no. 5, pp. 458–461, 2012.

[17] N. Regnault, E. Moutengou, and S. Fosse-Edorh, "Differential materno-fetal outcomes according to the onset date of gestational diabetes mellitus: data from 788,494 deliveries in France in 2013," *EASD European Diabetes Epidemiology Group congress*, 2016.

[18] M. L. Alunni, H. A. Roeder, T. R. Moore, and G. A. Ramos, "First trimester gestational diabetes screening - change in incidence and pharmacotherapy need," *Diabetes Research and Clinical Practice*, vol. 109, no. 1, pp. 135–140, 2015.

[19] J. Harreiter, D. Simmons, G. Desoye et al., "IADPSG and WHO 2013 gestational diabetes mellitus criteria identify obese women with marked insulin resistance in early pregnancy," *Diabetes Care*, vol. 39, no. 7, pp. e90–e92, 2016.

[20] C. Capula, E. Chiefari, M. Borelli et al., "A new predictive tool for the early risk assessment of gestational diabetes mellitus," *Primary Care Diabetes*, vol. 10, no. 5, pp. 315–323, 2016.

[21] A. N. Sweeting, G. P. Ross, J. Hyett et al., "Gestational diabetes mellitus in early pregnancy: evidence for poor pregnancy outcomes despite treatment," *Diabetes Care*, vol. 39, no. 1, pp. 75–81, 2016.

[22] L. Bozkurt, C. S. Gobl, L. Pfligl et al., "Pathophysiological characteristics and effects of obesity in women with early and late manifestation of gestational diabetes diagnosed by the International Association of Diabetes and Pregnancy Study Groups criteria," *The Journal of Clinical Endocrinology & Metabolism*, vol. 100, no. 3, pp. 1113–1120, 2015.

[23] J. S. Hawkins, J. Y. Lo, B. M. Casey, D. D. McIntire, and K. J. Leveno, "Diet-treated gestational diabetes mellitus: comparison of early vs routine diagnosis," *American Journal of Obstetrics and Gynecology*, vol. 198, no. 3, pp. 287.e1–287.e6, 2008.

[24] J. L. Bartha, P. Martinez-Del-Fresno, and R. Comino-Delgado, "Gestational diabetes mellitus diagnosed during early pregnancy," *American Journal of Obstetrics and Gynecology*, vol. 182, no. 2, pp. 346–350, 2000.

[25] D. Boriboonhirunsarn and V. Kasempipatchai, "Incidence of large for gestational age infants when gestational diabetes mellitus is diagnosed early and late in pregnancy," *The Journal of Obstetrics and Gynaecology Research*, vol. 42, no. 3, pp. 273–278, 2016.

[26] S. Easmin, T. A. Chowdhury, M. R. Islam et al., "Obstetric outcome in early and late onset gestational diabetes mellitus," *Mymensingh Medical Journal*, vol. 24, no. 3, pp. 450–456, 2015.

[27] J. L. Mills, L. Jovanovic, R. Knopp et al., "Physiological reduction in fasting plasma glucose concentration in the first trimester of normal pregnancy: the diabetes in early pregnancy study," *Metabolism*, vol. 47, no. 9, pp. 1140–1144, 1998.

[28] P. M. Catalano, E. D. Tyzbir, N. M. Roman, S. B. Amini, and E. A. Sims, "Longitudinal changes in insulin release and insulin resistance in nonobese pregnant women," *American Journal of Obstetrics and Gynecology*, vol. 165, no. 6, Part 1, pp. 1667–1672, 1991.

[29] E. Cosson, P. Valensi, and L. Carbillon, "Screening for dysglycaemia during pregnancy: proposals conciliating International Association of Diabetes and Pregnancy Study Group (IADPSG) and US National Institutes of Health (NIH) panels," *Diabetes & Metabolism*, vol. 41, no. 3, pp. 239–243, 2015.

[30] E. Maury, J. Savel, V. Grouthier et al., "Is skin autofluorescence a marker of metabolic memory in pregnant women with diabetes?," *Diabetic Medicine*, vol. 32, no. 12, pp. 1575–1579, 2015.

[31] G. Rayanagoudar, A. A. Hashi, J. Zamora, K. S. Khan, G. A. Hitman, and S. Thangaratinam, "Quantification of the type 2 diabetes risk in women with gestational diabetes: a systematic review and meta-analysis of 95,750 women," *Diabetologia*, vol. 59, no. 7, pp. 1403–1411, 2016.

[32] E. Noctor, C. Crowe, L. A. Carmody et al., "Abnormal glucose tolerance post-gestational diabetes mellitus as defined by the International Association of Diabetes and Pregnancy Study Groups criteria," *European Journal of Endocrinology*, vol. 175, no. 4, pp. 287–297, 2016.

[33] K. V. Smirnakis, A. Martinez, K. H. Blatman, M. Wolf, J. L. Ecker, and R. Thadhani, "Early pregnancy insulin resistance and subsequent gestational diabetes mellitus," *Diabetes Care*, vol. 28, no. 5, pp. 1207-1208, 2005.

[34] C. L. Harrison, C. B. Lombard, C. East, J. Boyle, and H. J. Teede, "Risk stratification in early pregnancy for women at increased risk of gestational diabetes," *Diabetes Research and Clinical Practice*, vol. 107, no. 1, pp. 61–68, 2015.

[35] B. Pintaudi, G. Di Vieste, F. Corrado et al., "Improvement of selective screening strategy for gestational diabetes through a more accurate definition of high-risk groups," *European Journal of Endocrinology*, vol. 170, no. 1, pp. 87–93, 2014.

[36] B. Liu, H. Chen, Y. Xu et al., "Fetal growth is associated with maternal fasting plasma glucose at first prenatal visit," *PLoS One*, vol. 9, no. 12, article e116352, 2014.

[37] C. Wang, W. Zhu, Y. Wei et al., "The predictive effects of early pregnancy lipid profiles and fasting glucose on the risk of gestational diabetes mellitus stratified by body mass index," *Journal of Diabetes Research*, vol. 2016, Article ID 3013567, 8 pages, 2016.

[38] E. A. Huhn, T. Fischer, C. S. Gobl et al., "Screening of gestational diabetes mellitus in early pregnancy by oral glucose tolerance test and glycosylated fibronectin: study protocol for an international, prospective, multicentre cohort trial," *BMJ Open*, vol. 6, no. 10, article e012115, 2016.

[39] B. Liu, Y. Xu, Y. Zhang et al., "Early Diagnosis of Gestational Diabetes Mellitus (EDoGDM) study: a protocol for a prospective, longitudinal cohort study," *BMJ Open*, vol. 6, no. 11, article e012315, 2016.

[40] R. C. Hughes, M. P. Moore, J. E. Gullam, K. Mohamed, and J. Rowan, "An early pregnancy HbA_{1c} ≥5.9% (41 mmol/mol) is optimal for detecting diabetes and identifies women at increased risk of adverse pregnancy outcomes," *Diabetes Care*, vol. 37, no. 11, pp. 2953–2959, 2014.

[41] L. Mane, J. A. Flores-Le Roux, D. Benaiges et al., "Role of first trimester HbA1c as a predictor of adverse obstetric outcomes in a multi-ethnic cohort," *The Journal of Clinical Endocrinology & Metabolism*, vol. 102, no. 2, article jc20162581, 2016.

[42] L. R. Nielsen, P. Ekbom, P. Damm et al., "HbA_{1c} levels are significantly lower in early and late pregnancy," *Diabetes Care*, vol. 27, no. 5, pp. 1200-1201, 2004.

[43] E. Cosson, A. Benbara, I. Pharisien et al., "Diagnostic and prognostic performances over 9 years of a selective screening strategy for gestational diabetes mellitus in a cohort of 18,775 Subjects," *Diabetes Care*, vol. 36, pp. 598–603, 2013.

[44] V. Seshiah, A. Cynthia, V. Balaji et al., "Detection and care of women with gestational diabetes mellitus from early weeks of pregnancy results in birth weight of newborn babies appropriate for gestational age," *Diabetes Research and Clinical Practice*, vol. 80, no. 2, pp. 199–202, 2008.

[45] W. Y. Hong, J. R. Biggio, A. Tita, and L. M. Harper, "Impact of early screening for gestational diabetes on perinatal outcomes in high-risk women," *American Journal of Perinatology*, vol. 33, no. 8, pp. 758–764, 2016.

[46] A. Sweeting, F. Park, and J. Hyett, "The first trimester: prediction and prevention of the great obstetrical syndromes," *Best Practice & Research Clinical Obstetrics & Gynaecology*, vol. 29, no. 2, pp. 183–193, 2015.

[47] S. F. Ehrlich, Y. M. Crites, M. M. Hedderson, J. A. Darbinian, and A. Ferrara, "The risk of large for gestational age across increasing categories of pregnancy glycemia," *American Journal of Obstetrics and Gynecology*, vol. 204, no. 3, pp. 240.e1–240.e6, 2011.

[48] S. Riskin-Mashiah, A. Damti, G. Younes, and R. Auslander, "Normal fasting plasma glucose levels during pregnancy: a hospital-based study," *Journal of Perinatal Medicine*, vol. 39, no. 2, pp. 209–211, 2011.

[49] C. Song, J. Li, J. Leng, R. C. Ma, and X. Yang, "Lifestyle intervention can reduce the risk of gestational diabetes: a meta-analysis of randomized controlled trials," *Obesity Reviews*, vol. 17, no. 10, pp. 960–969, 2016.

25

Incidence and Contributing Factors of Persistent Hyperglycemia at 6–12 Weeks Postpartum in Iranian Women with Gestational Diabetes: Results from LAGA Cohort Study

Sedigheh Nouhjah,[1] Hajieh Shahbazian,[1] Nahid Shahbazian,[2] Alireza Jahanshahi,[1,3] Shayesteh Jahanfar,[4] and Bahman Cheraghian[5]

[1]*Diabetes Research Center, Health Research Institute, Ahvaz Jundishapur University of Medical Sciences, Ahvaz, Iran*
[2]*Department of Obstetrics and Gynecology, Fertility, Infertility and Perinatology Research Center, Imam Khomeini Hospital, Ahvaz Jundishapur University of Medical Sciences, Ahvaz, Iran*
[3]*Internal Medicine Ward, Golestan Teaching Hospital, Ahvaz Jundishapur University of Medical Sciences, Ahvaz, Iran*
[4]*School of Health Sciences, Central Michigan University, Building 2212, Room 2239, Mount Pleasant, MI 48859, USA*
[5]*Department of Epidemiology and Biostatistics, Faculty of Health, Ahvaz Jundishapur University of Medical Sciences, Ahvaz, Iran*

Correspondence should be addressed to Hajieh Shahbazian; hjb.shahbazian@gmail.com

Academic Editor: Daniela Foti

Background. A history of gestational diabetes is an important predictor of many metabolic disturbances later in life. *Method.* Life after gestational diabetes Ahvaz Study (LAGAs) is an ongoing population-based cohort study. Up to February 2016, 176 women with gestational diabetes underwent a 75 g oral glucose tolerance test (OGTT) at 6–12 weeks postpartum in Ahvaz (southwestern of Iran). Gestational diabetes was diagnosed according to the International Association of Diabetes and Pregnancy Study Groups (IADPSG) criteria and the American Diabetes Association (ADA) criteria applied for diagnosis of postpartum prediabetes and diabetes. Univariate and multivariate regression analysis were done. *Results.* Overall incidence of early postpartum glucose intolerance was 22.2% (95% CI, 16.3–29.0), 17.6% prediabetes (95% CI, 12.3–24.1) and 4.5% diabetes (95% CI, 2.0–8.8%). Independent risk factors for glucose intolerance were FPG ≥ 100 at the time of OGTT (OR 3.86; 95% CI; 1.60–9.32), earlier diagnosis of GDM (OR 0.92; 95% CI; 0.88–0.97), systolic blood pressure (OR 1.02; 95% CI; 1.002–1.04), and insulin or metformin therapy (OR 3.14; 95% CI; 1.20–8.21). *Conclusion.* Results determined a relatively high rate of glucose intolerance at 6–12 weeks after GDM pregnancy. Early postpartum screening of type 2 diabetes is needed particularly in women at high risk of type 2 diabetes.

1. Introduction

Gestational diabetes mellitus (GDM) is defined as any degree of glucose intolerance, onset or first recognition during pregnancy [1]. GDM is associated with adverse maternal and neonatal outcomes [2, 3]. The literature reports that GDM, through increased medical cost for prenatal care and excess cost of the newborn in the first year after birth, burdens a healthcare system. Based on a national report in the United States, GDM increased medical costs by $636 million ($596 million for maternal costs and $40 million for neonatal cost), although the long-term medical cost of GDM and related outcomes was not clarified [4].

Gestational diabetes mellitus, as a common metabolic disorder during pregnancy, affects between 1% and 28% of pregnancies [5] and global statistics indicate an even higher rate [6]. Incidence of GDM is increasing and this rise is attributed to obesity, type 2 diabetes and metabolic syndrome epidemic, advancing maternal age of pregnancy, and implementation of newly diagnosed criteria [1, 7, 8].

Prevalence of gestational diabetes in Iran varies from 1.3% to 18.6% based on Carpenter-Coustan criteria [9]. A Recent report shows high incidence of GDM in this area using new criteria (29.9%) [10].

A history of gestational diabetes is a strong predictor of many metabolic disturbances, particularly glucose intolerance later in life [11]. In the literature, the risk of diversion to type 2 diabetes increased during the 20-year period after the index pregnancy [12]. Reports have shown that the pattern can be changed and the interval shortened through changes in lifestyle [13, 14].

International guidelines recommend early screening of glucose status for development of prediabetes or diabetes in women with gestational diabetes at 6–12 weeks postpartum using the 75 g 2 h oral glucose tolerance test (OGTT) and thereafter [15–17]. But in most population, rates of women who return postpartum and screen are low [18, 19].

Potential predicators of future progression of prediabetes and/or diabetes in women with gestational diabetes are prepregnancy body mass index (BMI), higher blood glucose level in pregnancy, particular ethnic groups, earlier diagnosis of GDM, requirement of insulin therapy during pregnancy, and advanced maternal age, with high heterogeneity in reported risk factors [7, 20, 21].

Common universal features of GDM reported in recent decades include a rising trend in incidence of the condition [1] increasing prevalence of its risk factors [8, 11]; a high rate of metabolic and cardiovascular outcomes [11]; earlier progression to prediabetes and type 2 diabetes [13, 14], and suboptimal return of exposed women for postpartum screening and lifestyle interventions based on previous reports and our recent report in this area [18, 22] show this population is a high risk group for many metabolic outcomes. Therefore early identification of women with greater risk of progression to diabetes may provide opportunity for prevention and intervention program. Our motivation to conduct this study was lack of information on risk factors associated with early postpartum glucose intolerance following adoption of the International Association of Diabetes and Pregnancy Study Groups (IADPSG) criteria. we sought to estimate incidence of early postpartum glucose intolerance and to identify risk factors for future diabetes incidence among women with recent gestational diabetes.

2. Methods

2.1. Study Design and Settings. Life after gestational diabetes Ahvaz Study (LAGAs) is a population-based prospective cohort study to investigate potential short and long-term metabolic outcomes of gestational diabetes in mothers and their offspring. For this reason, the first gestational diabetes clinic in Khuzestan province was established as center of the cohort study on October 2013 in Golestan Hospital, the teaching hospital of Ahvaz Jundishapur University of Medical Sciences. Ahvaz is the capital of Khuzestan province, located in southwestern of Iran with high birth rate, high prevalence of obesity, metabolic syndrome, and type 2 diabetes [23–26].

2.2. Study Population. Pregnant women attending 25 urban public and private centers seeking prenatal care were recruited from March 2015. Single approach for screening, treatment, and management of GDM was applied. Initial screening was done in first trimester of pregnancy by fasting plasma glucose (FPG) test. Women with FPG ≥ 126 mg/dL and those who had pregestational diabetes type 1 or type 2 as defined by American Diabetes Association (ADA) criteria [27] were excluded. Women with FPG 100–125 mg/dL in first trimester of pregnancy received diet and physical activity program for 2 weeks and blood glucose check with 3 weeks interval. Based on results of blood test, women were referred for pharmacotherapy or continuing diet and physical activity. Women who refuse to continue and those planning to move from Ahvaz city within the subsequent 2 years were excluded.

75 g OGTT was performed between 24 and 32 weeks of gestation and based on IADPSG criteria, only one abnormal value equal to or greater than the known threshold value was detected as GDM values (≥92 for fasting, ≥180 and ≥153 mg/dL for 1-hour and 2-hour plasma glucose level, resp.) [28]. Women with impaired glucose metabolism, BMI ≥ 30 kg/m^2, history of diabetes mellitus in first relatives, and history of GDM in previous pregnancies underwent earlier OGTT before 14th week of gestation [16] and screening was repeated between 24 and 32 weeks of gestation if the result was normal.

All women with gestational diabetes received dietary and exercise counseling, individualized diet or pharmacotherapy (insulin or metformin), and clinical and biochemical reassessment with 2-3 weeks' interval. ADA recommendations were used for goals of treatment [29].

A list of women who were diagnosed as GDM with details of their address and contact information were sent for research team and women referred to Golestan Hospital if they verbally accepted participation in the study. Various methods of communication were used to encourage women to participate and for retention including direct contact by phone, SMS texts via phone line, and other social networks (Whats app and telegram). Messages and reminders were sent to the women themselves and/or to husbands or other relatives who had made their contact number available. Communications were made by Sedigheh Nouhjah who was able to respond to any questions presented by the participants. Clinical evaluation and blood tests were free of charge and a copy of their laboratory reports was submitted to the patients for future reference.

2.3. Data Collection. Questionnaires related to sociodemographic characteristics of women and their husbands, potential risk factors of GDM, pregnancy outcome for the fetus and mothers, obstetrics and medical history, physical activity, and food habits of participants during 6–12 weeks postpartum were filled by a trained questionnaire. A comprehensive second questionnaire will be used as a follow-up within 2 years of the date of entering the study, based on predicted plane, to identify postpartum problems among mothers or their infants. The questionnaires were completed by an independent and trained researcher at the prenatal care center and postpartum data were collected by a member of the research team in our cohort center. Short forms of delivery were completed during 3–5 days after delivery in 2 main centers for screening of neonatal hypothyroidism.

2.4. Postpartum Biochemical and Clinical Assessment. FPG and 75 g 2-hour oral glucose tolerance test were performed at 6–12 weeks after delivery and these tests will be repeated annually for up to two years postpartum. Fasting plasma glucose ≥ 126 mg/dL or 2 hour plasma glucose after a 75 g oral glucose load ≥ 200 mg/dL was defined as diabetes, and prediabetes was diagnosed with fasting plasma glucose between 100 and 125 mg/dL or 2 h post-glucose loading level between 140 and 199 mg/dL according to ADA criteria [30]. Diagnosis of diabetes was confirmed if a second test was positive using the same criteria.

Blood samples were transported to the laboratory at the Diabetes Research Center, where the research coordinator and two laboratory technicians evaluated blood samples using the standard methods. Prepregnancy weight was recorded using medical and health profile. Weight, height, waist circumference, blood pressure, and hip circumference were measured at each visit during pregnancy and postpartum follow-up.

2.5. Statistical Analysis. Statistical analysis was performed with Statistical Package for the *Social* Sciences (SPSS version 22). Clinical, biochemical, and sociodemographic characteristics of women who progressed to postpartum glucose intolerance compared with women with normal glucose tolerance using univariate logistic regression analysis. Risk factors with P value less than 0.05 were tested in multivariate backward regression model.

2.6. Ethics Statement. The study protocol was approved by the Ethics Committee of Ahvaz Jundishapur University of Medical Sciences and all participants signed written informed consent form in addition to the first verbal agreement to taking part in the baseline visit.

3. Results

Until now, of 800 women who were diagnosed as GDM, 176 women (22%) aged between 17–45 years underwent a postpartum OGTT at 6–12 weeks after delivery. About half of these participants had high school education. Most of them were housewives (92.4%). The mean prepregnancy BMI was 27.82 kg/m^2 (±4.41 SD). Records showing overweight or obesity were observed in 126/176 (71.6%) of participants based on prepregnancy BMI (Table 1). This rate was 79% (48.9% overweight and 30.1% obesity) using postpartum BMI. Birth weight ≥ 4000 gr was seen in 22 (12.5%) of newborns who had been exposed to GDM during the fetal period. A history of previous GDM was reported by 20.5% of multigravida participants.

Demographic and clinical characteristics associated with postpartum glucose test results are presented in Table 1. Mean gestational age at diagnosis of GDM was 19.83 weeks (range 4–37 weeks, ±8.46 SD). During oral glucose tolerance test, FPG ≥ 92 mg/dL, 1-hour plasma glucose level ≥ 180 mg/dL, and 2-hour plasma glucose concentration ≥153 mg/dL were detected in 65.9%, 34.7%, and 38.6% of women with gestational diabetes, respectively. Mean ± SD of clinical and laboratory characteristics of women with GDM based on results of postpartum 75 g OGTT are presented in Table 2.

The overall incidence of early postpartum glucose intolerance was 22.2% (95% CI, 16.3–29.0) inclusive of 17.6% prediabetes (95% CI, 12.3–24.1) and 4.5% diabetes (95% CI, 2.0–8.8%). Risk factors of persistent hyperglycemia at 6–12 weeks after GDM pregnancy were inclusive of FPG ≥ 100 at the time of OGTT in pregnancy, earlier diagnosis of GDM in pregnancy, systolic blood pressure, and the need for insulin inject or metformin therapy. Results of univariate and multivariate analysis using backward logistic regression are presented in Table 3.

4. Discussion

4.1. Postpartum Glucose Intolerance Rate. Incidence of glucose intolerance at 6–12 weeks after GDM pregnancy determined in this study was 22.5% (17.5% prediabetes and 4.5% type 2 diabetes).

These high estimated rates are consistent with results reported by Tovar et al. [31]. They reviewed 11 studies conducted between 2008 and 2010. Proportion of diabetes and prediabetes at 6–12 weeks postpartum were 1.2–4.5% and 12.2–36%, respectively. Rate of diabetes in our study was also consistent with that of Capula et al. [32] study on Caucasian women in Southern Italy at 6–12 weeks postpartum (4%) and Inturrisi et al. (4% to 9%) [33], but lower than previous reports in Asian women by Jang et al. (5–15%) [34, 35] and Korean women in Kwak et al. study (12.5%) [36].

In present study rate of prediabetes was in range with many previous reports [31] but lower than recent reports from Korea by Cho et al. (44.1%) [37] and that reported by Capula and colleagues (32.1%) [32].

Different ethnic groups with different backgrounds including prevalence of diabetes mellitus, obesity, metabolic syndrome, and variation in rate of severe hyperglycemia in pregnancy using different criteria for GDM diagnosis in pregnancy and classification of postpartum glucose intolerance may have caused this wide variation in rates.

4.2. Determinants of Postpartum Glucose Intolerance. Multivariate regression test showed that risk factors associated with persistent glucose intolerance 6–12 weeks postpartum were inclusive of earlier diagnosis of GDM, use of insulin or metformin for management of GDM, FPG ≥ 100 at the time of OGTT, and systolic blood pressure.

Various potential risk factors have been determined in other research for prediabetes or diabetes in early postpartum period previously [35, 38, 39]. Kwak et al. compared early and late clinical risk factors for progression of postpartum glucose intolerance. Except early detection of GDM and use of insulin, in early converters, no differences have been reported between the 2 groups (early and late *converters*) [36].

4.3. Gestational Age at Diagnosis. Consistent with results of this study, earlier diagnosis of GDM in pregnancy before increasing resistance to insulin between 16 and 26 weeks of gestation [7, 40] is reported as a common risk factor associated with progression to later glucose intolerance in

TABLE 1: Demographic and clinical characteristics associated with postpartum glucose test results among women with recent gestational diabetes at 6–12 weeks postpartum.

Characteristics	Total (*N* = 176) *N* (%)	NGT (*N* = 137) (%)	AGT (*N* = 39) *N* (%)	*P* value*
Education				
<high school	54 (30.7)	47 (34.3)	7 (17.9)	0.03
High school	81 (46.0)	56 (40.9)	25 (64.1)	
Collage	41 (23.3)	34 (24.8)	7 (17.9)	
Gravidity				
1	49 (27.8)	38 (27.7)	11 (28.2)	0.58
2	57 (32.4)	42 (30.7)	15 (38.5)	
3	40 (22.7)	31 (22.6)	9 (23.1)	
≥4	30 (17.0)	26 (19.0)	4 (10.3)	
Ethnicity				
Fars	63 (35.8)	47 (34.3)	16 (41.0)	0.29
Lor	33 (18.8)	29 (21.2)	4 (10.3)	
Arab	80 (45.5)	61 (44.5)	19 (48.7)	
*Prepregnancy BMI***				
Normal	50 (28.4)	43 (31.4)	7 (17.9)	0.20
Overweight	73 (41.5)	56 (40.9)	17 (43.6)	
Obesity	53 (30.1)	38 (27.7)	15 (38.5)	
Preterm delivery (<37 weeks' gestation)				
Yes	14 (8.0)	7 (5.1)	7 (17.9)	**0.009**
No	162 (92.0)	130 (94.9)	32 (82.1)	
Mode of delivery				
Vaginal	76 (43.2)	64 (46.7)	12 (30.8)	0.07
Cesarean section	100 (56.8)	73 (53.3)	27 (69.2)	
History of GDM in family				
Yes	64*** (46.7)	47 (42.7)	17 (63.0)	0.05
No	73 (53.3)	63 (57.3)	10 (37.0)	
History of diabetes in family				
Yes	98 (55.7)	76 (55.5)	22 (56.4)	0.57
No	78 (44.3)	61 (44.5)	17 (43.6)	
Hypertension in pregnancy				
Yes	26 (14.8)	17 (12.4)	9 (23.1)	0.09
No	150 (85.2)	120 (87.6)	30 (76.9)	
Nutrition of infant 6–12 weeks after birth				
Breast feeding	131 (74.4)	102 (74.5)	29 (74.4)	0.99
Formula or combined	45 (25.6)	35 (25.5)	10 (25.6)	
Treatment of GDM				
Nutrition	142 (80.7)	120 (87.6)	22 (56.4)	**<0.001**
Metformin	12 (6.8)	7 (5.1)	5 (12.8)	
Insulin	22 (12.5)	10 (7.3)	12 (30.8)	
Number of abnormal tests in pregnancy				
1	87 (49.4)	71 (51.8)	16 (41)	0.40
2	41 (23.3)	31 (22.6)	10 (25.6)	
3	27 (15.3)	18 (13.1)	9 (23.1)	
≥4	21 (11.9)	17 (12.4)	4 (10.3)	

NGT, normal glucose tolerance; AGT, abnormal glucose tolerance (prediabetes or diabetes); GDM, gestational diabetes mellitus.
*Using chi square test.
**Normal ≤ 29.9 kg/m^2, overweight ≥ 25kg/m^2, obesity ≥ 30 kg/m^2.
***Missing data are unknown history of GDM in family.

TABLE 2: Clinical and laboratory characteristics of women with GDM based on results of 6–12 weeks postpartum glucose tolerance using 75-g OGTT.

Characteristics	Women with GDM (N = 176) Mean (±SD)	Normal glucose tolerance (N = 137) Mean (±SD)	Abnormal glucose tolerance (N = 39) Mean (±SD)	P value*
Age (years)	29.68 (5.25)	29.71 (5.50)	29.56 (4.29)	0.87
Gestational age of diagnosis	19.83 (8.46)	21.29 (8.12)	14.71 (7.86)	**<0.001**
Total weight gain in pregnancy (kg)	10.88 (6.29)	10.85 (6.67)	10.98 (4.78)	0.90
Weight before pregnancy (kg)	71.51 (12.10)	71.08 (11.67)	73.05 (13.57)	0.37
Weight in last month of pregnancy (kg)	82.33 (12.92)	81.83 (12.51)	84.06 (14.32)	0.34
Gestational age at birth (weeks)	38.97 (1.36)	39.05 (1.29)	38.66 (1.54)	0.11
Birth weight of the child (g)	3378.70 (557.33)	3450.28 (549.61)	3250.21 (572.36)	0.10
Systolic BP pregnancy (mmHg)	114.11 (20.26)	111.89 (16.32)	121.92 (124.05)	**0.003**
Diastolic BP (mmHg)	69.28 (12.38)	68.10 (11.14)	73.46 (15.43)	**0.01**
FPG first visit pregnancy (g/dL)	92.41 (11.63)	91.15 (10.17)	96.84 (15.06)	**0.007**
FPG at time of OGTT (g/dL)	97.80 (19.44)	95.06 (17.23)	107.41 (23.57)	<0.001
1-hour pregnancy (g/dL)	160.75 (35.80)	158.69 (36.92)	167.97 (30.94)	0.15
2-hour pregnancy (g/dL)	139.74 (35.72)	136.21 (35.73)	152.12 (33.26)	**0.01**
FPG postpartum (g/dL)	91.81 (18.25)	85.78 (7.52)	112.97 (27.24)	**<0.001**
2-hour 75 gr OGTT postpartum (g/dL)	106.19 (41.70)	93.99 (19.09)	149.05 (65.70)	**<0.001**
Postpartum BMI (kg/m^2)	28.30 (4.43)	27.86 (4.21)	29.86 (4.86)	**0.01**

*Using t-test.
GDM, gestational diabetes mellitus; BP, blood pressure; FPG, fasting plasma glucose; OGTT, oral glucose tolerance test; BMI, body mass index, defined as weight (kg)/height (m)^2.

TABLE 3: Independent risk factors for glucose intolerance (prediabetes or diabetes) early postpartum using univariate and multivariate logistic regression analysis.

Variables	Unadjusted ORs	CI	P value	Adjusted ORs*	95% CI	P value
Gestational age at diagnosis	0.90	0.86–0.95	<0.001	0.92	0.88–0.97	0.006
FPG of first visit pregnancy	1.04	1.01–1.07	0.008	1.04	0.93–1.02	0.27
FPG on OGTT pregnancy ≥ 100	6.10	2.83–13.4	<0.001	3.86	1.60–9.32	0.003
2-hour plasma glucose pregnancy	1.01	1.002–1.022	0.016	1.005	0.99–1.01	0.45
BP systolic pregnancy	1.02	1.007–1.04	0.006	1.02	1.002–1.04	0.032
Insulin or metformin treatment	5.45	2.42–12.28	<0.001	3.14	1.20–8.21	0.020
Postpartum BMI	1.10	1.01–1.19	0.015	1.04	0.94–1.15	0. 39
Preterm delivery (<37 weeks gestation)	4.06	1.33–12.41	0.014	3.17	0.83–12.4	0.091

*The model is adjusted for covariates which had statistical P value less than 0.05 in the univariate analysis.

women with GDM. Results of a systematic review on 39 studies including 95,750 women demonstrated higher risk of progress to abnormal glucose tolerance in women diagnosed with GDM in early weeks of gestation (RR 2.13, 95% CI 1.52–3.56) [20]. Although there is strong evidence in support of these results, some controversy remains over screening high risk pregnant women in earlier weeks of gestation [40].

4.4. Use of Insulin or Metformin. In the present study, pharmacotherapy (use of insulin or metformin) for management of hyperglycemia in pregnancy was strong predictor of progression to abnormal glucose tolerance at 6–12 weeks postpartum (OR 3.14; 95% CI; 1.20–8.21). Rate of postpartum glucose intolerance in women who were treated with insulin was 54.4% versus 41.7% in women who had taken metformin while the same rate was 15.4% in diet-only group.

Need for treatment with insulin or metformin as an indicator of severity of hyperglycemia may reflect impairment in β-cell function in women exposed to gestational diabetes. Pellonperä et al. studied women with GDM with two or more abnormal glucose values at 2 h 75 g OGTT, for a period of one year postpartum. This study showed higher incidence of prediabetes in metformin and insulin users (19.1% and 15.6%, resp.) than women treated with diet only (7.1%, P = 0.039). Also, the rate of diabetes was lower in the diet treatment group (P = 0.027) [41]. In addition, findings reported by Ziegler et al. [42] showed 92.3% of German women who used insulin in pregnancy progressed to diabetes during the

15-year period after GDM pregnancy versus 39.7% in the diet treatment group. Median years of diabetes-free duration in women who had taken insulin was 2.1 years. This duration in the diet-only treatment group was 16.3 years.

4.5. FPG during OGTT. Another risk factor for progression of abnormal glucose tolerance in present study was a higher level of FPG (≥100) at the time of OGTT, during a 24–32 weeks' gestation period (OR 3.86; 95% CI; 1.60–9.32).

Fasting glucose on OGTT is a common risk factor associated with prediabetes and diabetes after GDM pregnancy [14, 43, 44]. Moreover, elevated fasting glucose level at the time of OGTT had been a strong factor associated with insulin therapy in pregnancy. Different cut-off values based on applied criteria for diagnosis of GDM were reported for this association [45–47]. Another report by Langer showed that fasting glucose > 105 mg/dL was associated with fetal macrosomia, hypoglycemia in newborn infants, cesarean delivery, and a need for insulin therapy [48]. Previous studies have failed to determine an association between fasting glucose and future progression to type 2 diabetes for several reasons as follows: it was not measured [49]; the variable was not entered in the statistical model [50]; or modeling excluded GDM women with high fasting glucose level [39, 51] in the studies [7, 52].

4.6. Blood Pressure. This study determined systolic blood pressure as another related risk factor. Hypertensive disorder in pregnancy (RR 1.38; 95% CI; 1.32–1.45) was associated with future diabetes based on the systematic review and meta-analysis reported in Rayanagoudar et al. [20]. Feig et al. showed that women with hypertensive disorder in pregnancy had a 2-fold increased risk of developing diabetes by 16.5 years after pregnancy, even in women without GDM [53]. In addition, women with preeclampsia and gestational hypertension had insulin resistance independent of obesity and abnormal glucose tolerance during pregnancy [54, 55].

4.7. Other Factors. In the present study there was no association of maternal age at pregnancy, maternal education and occupation, parity, and family history of diabetes with development of glucose intolerance in the early postpartum period. Some previous studies have shown an association of maternal age, parity, and a family history of diabetes with glucose intolerance, but reports are inconsistent [7, 39, 52].

No significant association was determined between total weight gain during pregnancy, BMI, and obesity before pregnancy and postpartum glucose intolerance at 6–12 weeks postpartum. Women with higher blood glucose levels, who had a high chance of early postpartum progression to abnormal glucose intolerance, usually received a strict diet program that controlled their weight gain during pregnancy [56]. Body mass index was also reported as a significant risk factor for progression to glucose intolerance after GDM pregnancy in previous studies, but there was no consistency after adjusting for other covariates. The studies that show this association resulted from long-term evaluation of a GDM group [57, 58]. Similar to results of this study, other research has reported no association between BMI and glucose intolerance in early postpartum follow-up [7].

In present study 56.8% of women with gestational diabetes underwent cesarean delivery. High rate of cesarean delivery (48%) in Iranian population is reported by Azami-Aghdash et al. [59]. Mean birth weight was 3378 gr (±557 gr SD) in GDM-exposed newborns. Results of a systematic review conducted by Mirmiran et al. showed mean weight of Iranian newborns at birth has been 3152 gr (95% CI = 3114–3189) [60].

Moreover, based on our results, rate of preterm delivery was 8%. This rate in general population reported 9.2% (95% CI: 7.6–10.7) by Vakilian et al. [61], based on the random effect model in a systematic meta-analysis.

Preterm delivery was associated with higher risk of progression to postpartum glucose intolerance using univariate analysis but was not determined as a risk factor when adjusted in the multivariate model. Rayanagoudar et al. showed preterm delivery increases risk of diabetes in women with GDM (RR 1.81; 95% CI; 1.35–2.43) [20]. Our results related to preterm delivery could probably reach a significant level with increased number of subjects during future months of the study. Also, the role of some variables may change in a long-term follow-up.

4.8. Limitation and Strength. There were two main limitations in this study. Despite using different methods of communication, the rate of postpartum return for glucose testing and follow-up was low. This may be a source of bias. Participants in this study were compared in terms of sociodemographic and clinical characteristics and those who did not return for follow-up. There were no significant differences between the two groups. A similar problem has been reported in several previous studies [18, 19]. Another limitation was the relative small sample size. Ongoing sampling in future months may change the chances of some variables as significant risk factors and improve a wide range of confidence interval (CI) in multivariate analysis.

The strength of this study was that it involved husbands of patients at follow-up in order to decrease the chance of attrition bias. In addition, using a combination of different methods for recall and by sending reminders, this study benefited from its use of social media. To the best our knowledge, this study is the first population-based prospective cohort study in this area to follow postpartum metabolic outcome of gestational diabetes in mothers and their offspring that included several variables.

5. Conclusion

Gestational diabetes is a risk factor for postpartum progression to glucose intolerance. Short-term postpartum follow-up of women with GDM showed a relatively high rate of glucose intolerance among women in this population. This finding highlighted the need for early postpartum screening and implementation of an intervention program to prevent type 2 diabetes, particularly in women whose GDM was diagnosed during the earlier weeks of gestation, mothers with higher fasting glucose level at the time of OGTT, higher blood pressure in pregnancy, and patients who required pharmacotherapy for management of hyperglycemia.

Competing Interests

The authors declare that there are no competing interests regarding the publication of this paper.

Acknowledgments

The authors gratefully acknowledge all of the participants in the studies. Our sincere appreciation goes to public health students and public and private prenatal care personnel and staff at the Diabetes Research Center at Ahvaz Jundishapur University of Medical Sciences for their assistance in collecting data. This manuscript is a part of a Ph.D. thesis written by Nouhjah which was approved and granted by Ahvaz Jundishapur University of Medical Sciences (Registration no. D-9405, Ethic code: IR.AJUMS.REC.1394.252).

References

[1] A. Ferrara, "Increasing prevalence of gestational diabetes mellitus: a public health perspective," *Diabetes Care*, vol. 30, no. 2, pp. S141–S146, 2007.

[2] T. A. Hillier, K. L. Pedula, M. M. Schmidt, J. A. Mullen, M.-A. Charles, and D. J. Pettitt, "Childhood obesity and metabolic imprinting: the ongoing effects of maternal hyperglycemia," *Diabetes Care*, vol. 30, no. 9, pp. 2287–2292, 2007.

[3] B. E. Metzger, "Long-term outcomes in mothers diagnosed with gestational diabetes mellitus and their offspring," *Clinical Obstetrics and Gynecology*, vol. 50, no. 4, pp. 972–979, 2007.

[4] Y. Chen, W. W. Quick, W. Yang et al., "Cost of gestational diabetes mellitus in the united states in 2007," *Population Health Management*, vol. 12, no. 3, pp. 165–171, 2009.

[5] A. Jiwani, E. Marseille, N. Lohse, P. Damm, M. Hod, and J. G. Kahn, "Gestational diabetes mellitus: results from a survey of country prevalence and practices," *Journal of Maternal-Fetal and Neonatal Medicine*, vol. 25, no. 6, pp. 600–610, 2012.

[6] A. Duran, S. Sáenz, M. J. Torrejón et al., "Introduction of IADPSG criteria for the screening and diagnosis of gestational diabetes mellitus results in improved pregnancy outcomes at a lower cost in a large cohort of pregnant women: the St. Carlos Gestational Diabetes Study," *Diabetes Care*, vol. 37, no. 9, pp. 2442–2450, 2014.

[7] E. Noctor and F. P. Dunne, "Type 2 diabetes after gestational diabetes: the influence of changing diagnostic criteria," *World Journal of Diabetes*, vol. 6, no. 2, pp. 234–244, 2015.

[8] Y. Xu, S. Shen, L. Sun, H. Yang, B. Jin, and X. Cao, "Metabolic syndrome risk after gestational diabetes: a systematic review and meta-analysis," *PLOS ONE*, vol. 9, no. 1, Article ID e87863, 2014.

[9] M. Jafari-Shobeiri, M. Ghojazadeh, S. Azami-Aghdash et al., "Prevalence and risk factors of gestational diabetes in Iran: a systematic review and meta-analysis," *Iranian Journal of Public Health*, vol. 44, no. 8, pp. 1036–1044, 2015.

[10] H. Shahbazian, S. Nouhjah, N. Shahbazian et al., "Gestational diabetes mellitus in an Iranian pregnant population using IADPSG criteria: incidence, contributing factors and outcomes," *Diabetes and Metabolic Syndrome: Clinical Research and Reviews*, vol. 10, no. 4, pp. 242–246, 2016.

[11] J. H. Moon, S. H. Kwak, and H. C. Jang, "Prevention of type 2 diabetes mellitus in women with previous gestational diabetes mellitus," *The Korean Journal of Internal Medicine*, vol. 32, no. 1, pp. 26–41, 2017.

[12] J. B. O'Sullivan, "Gestational diabetes: factors influencing the rates of subsequent diabetes," in *Carbohydrate Metabolism in Pregnancy and the Newborn 1978*, pp. 425–435, Springer, Berlin, Germany, 1979.

[13] L. Bellamy, J.-P. Casas, A. D. Hingorani, and D. Williams, "Type 2 diabetes mellitus after gestational diabetes: a systematic review and meta-analysis," *The Lancet*, vol. 373, no. 9677, pp. 1773–1779, 2009.

[14] C. Kim, K. M. Newton, and R. H. Knopp, "Gestational diabetes and the incidence of type 2 diabetes: a systematic review," *Diabetes Care*, vol. 25, no. 10, pp. 1862–1868, 2002.

[15] "Gestational diabetes mellitus," *Diabetes Care*, vol. 27, S1, pp. S88–S90, 2004.

[16] B. E. Metzger, T. A. Buchanan, D. R. Coustan et al., "Summary and recommendations of the fifth international workshop-conference on gestational diabetes mellitus," *Diabetes Care*, vol. 30, no. 2, pp. S251–S260, 2007.

[17] American Diabetes Association, "Standards of medical care in diabetes—2013," *Diabetes Care*, vol. 36, supplement 1, pp. S11–S66, 2013.

[18] A. Ferrara, T. Peng, and C. Kim, "Trends in postpartum diabetes screening and subsequent diabetes and impaired fasting glucose among women with histories of gestational diabetes mellitus: a report from the translating research into action for diabetes (TRIAD) study," *Diabetes Care*, vol. 32, no. 2, pp. 269–274, 2009.

[19] C. Kim, B. P. Tabaei, R. Burke et al., "Missed opportunities for type 2 diabetes mellitus screening among women with a history of gestational diabetes mellitus," *American Journal of Public Health*, vol. 96, no. 9, pp. 1643–1648, 2006.

[20] G. Rayanagoudar, A. A. Hashi, J. Zamora, K. S. Khan, G. A. Hitman, and S. Thangaratinam, "Quantification of the type 2 diabetes risk in women with gestational diabetes: a systematic review and meta-analysis of 95,750 women," *Diabetologia*, vol. 59, no. 7, pp. 1403–1411, 2016.

[21] A. H. Xiang, B. H. Li, M. H. Black et al., "Racial and ethnic disparities in diabetes risk after gestational diabetes mellitus," *Diabetologia*, vol. 54, no. 12, pp. 3016–3021, 2011.

[22] H. Shahbazian, S. Nouhjah, S. Jahanfar, and M. Nasiri, "Recall for postpartum follow-up of women with gestational diabetes mellitus: climbing a mountain," *Journal of Diabetes and Metabolic Disorders*, vol. 15, no. 1, article 20, 2016.

[23] S. Nouhjah, E. Amiri, A. Khodai, A. Yazdanpanah, and M. N. Baghu, "Popular contraceptive methods in women aged 35 years and older attending health centers of 4 cities in Khuzestan province, Iran," *Iranian Red Crescent Medical Journal*, vol. 15, no. 10, 2013.

[24] S. Nouhjah, M. Nadi-Baghu, M. Salehi, and H. Ghajari, "Prevalence of overweight, obesity and the related factors in women aged 35—57 years in Khuzestan Province of Iran," *Advanced Studies in Biology*, vol. 4, no. 2, pp. 57–65, 2012.

[25] S. M. Latifi, M. Karandish, H. Shahbazian, and L. Hardani Pasand, "Incidence of prediabetes and type 2 diabetes among people aged over 20 years in ahvaz: a 5-year perspective study (2009–2014)," *Journal of Diabetes Research*, vol. 2016, Article ID 4908647, 6 pages, 2016.

[26] H. Shahbazian, S. M. Latifi, and S. Nouhjah, "Cut-off point of waist circumference used for the diagnosis of metabolic

syndrome among adult population in ahvaz, Southwestern Iran," *Jentashapir Journal of Health Research*, vol. 6, no. 4, Article ID e30588, 2015.

[27] American Diabetes Association, "Diagnosis and classification of diabetes mellitus," *Diabetes Care*, vol. 32, S1, pp. S62–S67, 2008.

[28] B. E. Metzger, "International association of diabetes and pregnancy study groups recommendations on the diagnosis and classification of hyperglycemia in pregnancy," *Diabetes Care*, vol. 33, no. 3, pp. 676–682, 2010.

[29] American Diabetes Association, "Gestational diabetes mellitus," *Diabetes Care*, vol. 26, no. Supplement 1, pp. S103–S105, 2003.

[30] "Report of the Expert Committee on the Diagnosis and Classification of Diabetes Mellitus," *Diabetes Care*, vol. 20, no. 7, pp. 1183–1197, 1997.

[31] A. Tovar, L. Chasan-Taber, E. Eggleston, and E. Oken, "Postpartum screening for diabetes among women with a history of gestational diabetes mellitus," *Preventing Chronic Disease*, vol. 8, no. 6, article A124, 2011.

[32] C. Capula, E. Chiefari, A. Vero, D. P. Foti, A. Brunetti, and R. Vero, "Prevalence and predictors of postpartum glucose intolerance in Italian women with gestational diabetes mellitus," *Diabetes Research and Clinical Practice*, vol. 105, no. 2, pp. 223–230, 2014.

[33] M. Inturrisi, N. C. Lintner, and K. A. Sorem, "Diagnosis and treatment of hyperglycemia in pregnancy," *Endocrinology and Metabolism Clinics of North America*, vol. 40, no. 4, pp. 703–726, 2011.

[34] K. S. L. Lam, D. F. Li, I. J. Lauder, C. P. Lee, A. W. C. Kung, and J. T. C. Ma, "Prediction of persistent carbohydrate intolerance in patients with gestational diabetes," *Diabetes Research and Clinical Practice*, vol. 12, no. 3, pp. 181–186, 1991.

[35] H. C. Jang, C.-H. Yim, K. O. Han et al., "Gestational diabetes mellitus in Korea: prevalence and prediction of glucose intolerance at early postpartum," *Diabetes Research and Clinical Practice*, vol. 61, no. 2, pp. 117–124, 2003.

[36] S. H. Kwak, S. H. Choi, H. S. Jung et al., "Clinical and genetic risk factors for type 2 diabetes at early or late post partum after gestational diabetes mellitus," *The Journal of Clinical Endocrinology & Metabolism*, vol. 98, no. 4, pp. E744–E752, 2013.

[37] G. J. Cho, J.-J. An, S.-J. Choi et al., "Postpartum glucose testing rates following gestational diabetes mellitus and factors affecting testing non-compliance from four tertiary centers in Korea," *Journal of Korean Medical Science*, vol. 30, no. 12, pp. 1841–1846, 2015.

[38] H. C. Jang, "Gestational diabetes in Korea: incidence and risk factors of diabetes in women with previous gestational diabetes," *Diabetes & Metabolism Journal*, vol. 35, no. 1, pp. 1–7, 2011.

[39] B. E. Metzger, N. H. Cho, S. M. Roston, and R. Radvany, "Prepregnancy weight and antepartum insulin secretion predict glucose tolerance five years after gestational diabetes mellitus," *Diabetes Care*, vol. 16, no. 12, pp. 1598–1605, 1993.

[40] K. Stanley, R. Fraser, and C. Bruce, "Physiological changes in insulin resistance in human pregnancy: longitudinal study with the hyperinsulinaemic euglycaemic clamp technique," *British Journal of Obstetrics and Gynaecology*, vol. 105, no. 7, pp. 756–759, 1998.

[41] O. Pellonperä, T. Rönnemaa, U. Ekblad, T. Vahlberg, and K. Tertti, "The effects of metformin treatment of gestational diabetes on maternal weight and glucose tolerance postpartum—a prospective follow-up study," *Acta Obstetricia et Gynecologica Scandinavica*, vol. 95, no. 1, pp. 79–87, 2016.

[42] A.-G. Ziegler, M. Wallner, I. Kaiser et al., "Long-term protective effect of lactation on the development of type 2 diabetes in women with recent gestational diabetes mellitus," *Diabetes*, vol. 61, no. 12, pp. 3167–3171, 2012.

[43] B. E. Metzger, D. E. Bybee, N. Freinkel, R. L. Phelps, R. M. Radvany, and N. Vaisrub, "Gestational diabetes mellitus. Correlations between the phenotypic and genotypic characteristics of the mother and abnormal glucose tolerance during the first year postpartum," *Diabetes*, vol. 34, supplement 2, pp. 111–115, 1985.

[44] S. L. Kjos, R. K. Peters, A. Xiang, O. A. Henry, M. Montoro, and T. A. Buchanan, "Predicting future diabetes in Latino women with gestational diabetes: utility of early postpartum glucose tolerance testing," *Diabetes*, vol. 44, no. 5, pp. 586–591, 1995.

[45] Y. Zhang, J. Shao, F. Li, and X. Xu, "Factors in gestational diabetes mellitus predicting the needs for insulin therapy," *International Journal of Endocrinology*, vol. 2016, Article ID 4858976, 5 pages, 2016.

[46] J. Juutinen, A.-L. Hartikainen, R. Bloigu, and J. S. Tapanainen, "A retrospective study on 435 women with gestational diabetes: fasting plasma glucose is not sensitive enough for screening but predicts a need for insulin treatment," *Diabetes Care*, vol. 23, no. 12, pp. 1858–1859, 2000.

[47] O. Bakiner, E. Bozkirli, K. Ozsahin, C. Sariturk, and E. Ertorer, "Risk factors that can predict antenatal insulin need in gestational diabetes," *Journal of Clinical Medicine Research*, vol. 5, no. 5, pp. 381–388, 2013.

[48] O. Langer, "Maternal glycemic criteria for insulin therapy in gestational diabetes mellitus," *Diabetes Care*, vol. 21, supplement 2, pp. B91–B98, 1998.

[49] A. E. B. Åberg, E. K. Jönsson, I. Eskilsson, M. Landin-Olsson, and A. H. Frid, "Predictive factors of developing diabetes mellitus in women with gestational diabetes," *Acta Obstetricia et Gynecologica Scandinavica*, vol. 81, no. 1, pp. 11–16, 2002.

[50] M. W. O'Reilly, G. Avalos, M. C. Dennedy, E. P. O'Sullivan, and F. Dunne, "Atlantic DIP: high prevalence of abnormal glucose tolerance post partum is reduced by breast-feeding in women with prior gestational diabetes mellitus," *European Journal of Endocrinology*, vol. 165, no. 6, pp. 953–959, 2011.

[51] T. A. Buchanan, A. H. Xiang, S. L. Kjos, E. Trigo, W. P. Lee, and R. K. Peters, "Antepartum predictors of the development of type 2 diabetes in Latino women 11-26 months after pregnancies complicated by gestational diabetes," *Diabetes*, vol. 48, no. 12, pp. 2430–2436, 1999.

[52] Ö. S. Kerimoglu, S. Yalvaç, D. Karçaaltinçaba, and Ö. Kandemir, "Incidence of diabetes mellitus at postpartum six to twelve months following the diagnosis of gestational diabetes mellitus," *Journal of the Turkish German Gynecology Association*, vol. 11, no. 2, pp. 89–94, 2010.

[53] D. S. Feig, B. R. Shah, L. L. Lipscombe et al., "Preeclampsia as a risk factor for diabetes: A Population-Based Cohort Study," *PLOS Medicine*, vol. 10, no. 4, Article ID e1001425, 2013.

[54] E. Parretti, A. Lapolla, M. Dalfrà et al., "Preeclampsia in lean normotensive normotolerant pregnant women can be predicted by simple insulin sensitivity indexes," *Hypertension*, vol. 47, no. 3, pp. 449–453, 2006.

[55] J. Sierra-Laguado, R. G. García, J. Celedón et al., "Determination of insulin resistance using the homeostatic model assessment

(HOMA) and its relation with the risk of developing pregnancy-induced hypertension," *American Journal of Hypertension*, vol. 20, no. 4, pp. 437–442, 2007.

[56] M. G. Dalfrà, A. Lapolla, M. Masin et al., "Antepartum and early postpartum predictors of type 2 diabetes development in women with gestational diabetes mellitus," *Diabetes and Metabolism*, vol. 27, no. 6, pp. 675–680, 2001.

[57] K. Löbner, A. Knopff, A. Baumgarten et al., "Predictors of postpartum diabetes in women with gestational diabetes mellitus," *Diabetes*, vol. 55, no. 3, pp. 792–797, 2006.

[58] N. W. Cheung and D. Helmink, "Gestational diabetes: the significance of persistent fasting hyperglycemia for the subsequent development of diabetes mellitus," *Journal of Diabetes and its Complications*, vol. 20, no. 1, pp. 21–25, 2006.

[59] S. Azami-Aghdash, M. Ghojazadeh, N. Dehdilani, M. Mohammadi, and R. Asl Amin Abad, "Prevalence and causes of cesarean section in Iran: systematic review and meta-analysis," *Iranian Journal of Public Health*, vol. 43, no. 5, pp. 545–555, 2014.

[60] P. Mirmiran, N. Moslehi, G. Asghari, S. Jambarsang, Y. Mehrabi, and F. Azizi, "Secular trends in size at birth of Iranian neonates: meta-analyses of published and unpublished studies," *Annals of Human Biology*, vol. 40, no. 1, pp. 75–82, 2013.

[61] K. Vakilian, M. Ranjbaran, M. Khorsandi, N. Sharafkhani, and M. Khodadost, "Prevalence of preterm labor in Iran: a systematic review and meta-analysis," *Iranian Journal of Reproductive Medicine*, vol. 13, no. 12, pp. 743–748, 2015.

26

Th1/Th2 Dichotomy in Obese Women with Gestational Diabetes and their Macrosomic Babies

A. Seck,[1] A. Hichami,[2] S. Doucouré,[3] F. Diallo Agne,[4] H. Bassène,[3] A. Ba,[1,5] C. Sokhna,[3] N. A. Khan,[2] and A. Samb[1,5]

[1]*Laboratory of Physiology and Functional Explorations, Faculty of Medicine, Pharmacy and Odontology, Cheikh Anta Diop University, 5005 Dakar-Fann, Senegal*
[2]*U1231 INSERM/Université de Bourgogne-Franche Comté (UBFC)/Agro-Sup, Physiologie de la Nutrition & Toxicologie, Dijon 21000, France*
[3]*Institute of Research for Development, VITROME Aix Marseille Univ, IRD, AP-HM, SSA, VITROME, IHU-Mediterranean Infection, CP18524 Dakar, Senegal*
[4]*Laboratory of Biochemistry and Molecular Biology, Faculty of Medicine, Pharmacy and Odontology, Cheikh Anta Diop University, 5005 Dakar-Fann, Senegal*
[5]*UMI 3189, "Environnement, Santé, Sociétés", CNRS, CNRST, Université Bamako-UCAD, Dakar, Senegal*

Correspondence should be addressed to A. Seck; aichaseck75@yahoo.fr

Academic Editor: Jonathan M. Peterson

The aim of the study was to assess T cell differentiation and the modulation of inflammatory cytokines in obese and gestational diabetes mellitus (GDM) women and their macrosomic newborns. Hence, immediately after delivery, blood samples were collected through the mother's arm vein and the umbilical cordon vein. Biochemical parameters measured were HbA1C, glucose, insulin, triglyceride (TG), total cholesterol (Tchol), HDL cholesterol (HDLchol), and LDL cholesterol (LDLchol). T lymphocytes were purified from the total blood with Ficoll-Paque. The mRNA expression of inflammatory markers in T cells was determined by RT-qPCR. We observed that diabetic mothers exhibited higher HbA1C, glycemia, insulinemia, TG, Tchol, HDLchol, and LDLchol levels than control mothers. Glycemia was not significantly different between macrosomic and control newborns. However, insulinemia was high in macrosomic babies. TG, Tchol, HDLchol, and LDLchol were not significantly different between macrosomic and control babies. In diabetic mothers, mRNA expression of the Th1 cell subtype was significantly increased. Th1 markers were upregulated in babies born to diabetic women than in control newborns. However, expression of two Th2 markers (GATA3 and IL-4) was not significantly different between control and GDM women and between their respective newborns. Interestingly, IL-10 mRNA expression was decreased in diabetic mothers and their offsprings. The Th1/Th2 cytokine ratio was increased in GDM obese mothers and their macrosomic newborns, suggesting a proinflammatory status in these subjects.

1. Introduction

Gestational diabetes mellitus (GDM) is defined as a state of glucose intolerance during pregnancy [1]. A sedentary and the modern lifestyle in developing countries contributes to the increased prevalence of the GDM. In studies, the global prevalence of GDM was estimated to be 1%–14% according to the population studied [2–5]. Gestational diabetes mellitus is also associated with increased risk for a mother and her offspring in the short and long term. About 50% of GDM women develop type II diabetes in 5–10 years after their pregnancy [4]. Gestational diabetes is responsible for perinatal complexities such as fetal malformations, growth anomalies, and miscarriages induced by high blood pressure and preeclampsia [6]. Several studies support the hypothesis that maternal hyperglycemia in the second half of pregnancy may lead to an increased fetal weight. Indeed, some authors have reported the relationship between gestational diabetes and fetal macrosomia [7, 8]. Macrosomia is observed in 50% of pregnancies with gestational diabetes, being one of the main reasons of increased perinatal morbidity and mortality [8, 9]. In the long term, children born to gestational diabetic women present a high risk to develop obesity and type II diabetes in adolescence [2]. It has been clearly established that both obese and type II diabetic subjects suffer from having a proinflammatory status [10, 11]. Adipose tissue of obese people has been shown to release several cytokines such as IL-6 and TNF-α favouring inflammation and insulin resistance [12, 13].

The immune system is composed of two major subdivisions, the innate immune system and the adaptive immune system. The innate immune cells control the adaptive immune response through the activation and induction of differentiation of naive T helper (Th0) cells to Th1, Th2, Treg, or Th17 effector cells. Th1 cells, by the production of IL-2 and IFN-γ, trigger a cell-mediated immunity response through the activation of macrophages and cytotoxic T cells, whereas Th2 cells trigger a humoral immune response by the production IL-4, IL-5, and IL-13 which activate IgE antibody-producing B cells [13]. Thus, it has also been shown that the immune system, particularly T helper lymphocytes (Th cells), by their capacity to differentiate into either pro- or anti-inflammatory Th cells, plays a pivotal role during the development of insulin resistance [13].

Differentiation of Th cells into Th1 and Th2 cells involves the activation of Th1 and Th2 transcription factors, T-bet and GATA3, respectively [14, 15]. It has been reported that abnormalities of humoral and cell-mediated immunity in type I diabetic women during pregnancy may complicate immune-fetal interaction leading to fetal overgrowth and alteration in the immune system of a newborn which persist till adulthood [16, 17].

With regard to gestational diabetes, several reports have analysed the expression of cytokines by ELISA in serum or by RT-PCR in the pancreas and spleen of gestational diabetes rats [18] and mice [19]. A few studies have reported in nonobese human GDM the production of proinflammatory cytokines measured either by ELISA in serum or by RT-PCR in the placenta [19–21]. The originality of our study is that we selected only obese GDM mothers and their macrosomic offsprings and we determined Th1/Th2 lymphocyte differentiation by measuring their respective mRNA in purified T cell lymphocytes from these subjects.

2. Subjects and Methods

2.1. Subjects and Protocol

2.1.1. Subjects. This study was conducted at the gynecology department of Roi Baudouin Guediawaye Hospital, Dakar Principal Hospital, and Health Center Dakar Plateau between July 2016 and April 2017. The study protocol was approved by the National Ethical Committee of Senegal. All subjects were informed about the procedure and purpose of the study. The written informed consent was obtained from all the participants.

We recruited 20 pregnant women and their newborns ($n = 20$). Women aged from 24 to 39 years were between their 20th and 30th week of gestational period. These subjects were divided into two groups; (i) the first group (G1), considered the control group, included normoglycemic pregnant subjects without any history of illness or risk factors for gestational diabetes and (ii) the second group (G2) included women with gestational diabetic mellitus (GDM) diagnosed during pregnancy by the oral glucose tolerance test (OGTT) and they had not received insulin treatment. All pregnant women included in this study had no history of smoking and were not taking decoction or medicine, which could disturb the pregnancy evolution.

Immediately after delivery, blood samples were collected through the mother's arm vein and the umbilical cord vein.

2.1.2. Experimental Protocol

(1) Blood Samples. After delivery, fasting venous samples were collected in either EDTA or dry tubes (without anticoagulant). The blood collected in the EDTA tube was used for determination of the HbA1C (glycated hemoglobin) level. Blood samples in the dry tube or in EDTA were centrifuged to obtain, respectively, serum and plasma. Samples were aliquoted and frozen at −80°C for determination of other biochemical parameters.

(2) Determination of Biochemical Parameters. Biochemical parameters were analysed by using an automatic spectrometer (chemistry module LEc4000 of architect system ci4100). We determined plasma glucose concentrations and serum levels of insulinemia, triglyceride (TG), total cholesterol (Tchol), and high-density lipoprotein cholesterol (HDLchol). Low-density lipoprotein cholesterol (LDLchol) concentrations were calculated by the Friedewald formula: LDLchol = Tchol − HDLchol − TG/5.

(3) T Cell Isolation. PBMC were isolated from the blood with EDTA using Ficoll-Paque™. T lymphocytes were isolated from PBMC by panning as described elsewhere [22]. Briefly, PBMC were washed once with PBS-containing bovine serum albumin (2 g/L) and seeded in a Petri dish. After 2 h, nonadherent cells were gently decanted and transferred to antihuman IgG-coated Petri dishes. This allowed adhesion of B lymphocytes to the substratum of the Petri dishes. After one hour of incubation, T lymphocyte-rich supernatant was decanted and washed twice with PBS-BSA and resuspended in RPMI 1640 medium. This technique provided us with an enriched T cell population (99%), verified by flow cytofluorometry (data not shown).

(4) Detection of mRNA Expression of Inflammatory Markers in T Cells by RT-qPCR. Total RNA of T lymphocytes was extracted using TRIzol® Reagent, the quality of RNA was evaluated with the optical density (OD) at 260 nm–280 nm, and the RNA/DNA ratio was measured by spectrophotometry (Jenway Genova).

Real-time qPCR (RT-qPCR) was performed with StepOne software V2.3 using Power SYBR Green PCR Master Mix (Thermo Fisher Scientific) and oligonucleotide human primers (Table 1). We used β-actin as the reference gene since it has shown the most relative stability. The relative

TABLE 1: Sequences of PCR primers.

Genes amplified	Human primer sequences
Actin	Forward 5′ATG ATA TCG CCG CGC TCG TCG TC 3′ Reverse 5′AGG TCC CGG CCA GCC AGG TCC AG 3′
T-bet	Forward 5′TGT CCT ACT ACC GAG GCC AG 3′ Reverse 5′ATC TCA GTC CAC ACC AAG GG 3′
IFN-γ	Forward 5′AGC ACT GGC TCA GAT TGC AGG C3′ Reverse 5′ATC TCA GGG GCC AAC TAG GCA G3′
IL-2	Forward 5′CAC TAA TTC TTG CAC TTG TCA C 3′ Reverse 5′CCT TCT TGG GCA TGT AAA ACT 3′
GATA3	Forward 5′CTC ATT AAG CCC AAG CGA AG 3′ Reverse 5′TCT GAC AGT TCG CAC AGG AC 3′
IL-4	Forward 5′ TGC-CGG-CAA-CTT-TGT-CCA-CG 3′ Reverse 5′ TGG-TGG-CTG-TAG-AAC-TGC-CGG-A 3′
IL-10	Forward 5′ AGG-AGG-TGA-TGC-CCC-AAG-CTG-A 3′ Reverse 5′ TTC-TTC-ACC-TGC-TCC-ACG-GCC-T 3′

gene expression was determined using the ΔΔCt method. The normalized delta cycle threshold (ΔCt) was calculated by subtracting the cycle threshold (Ct) value of the genes of interest from the β-actin cycle threshold value ($\Delta Ct = Ct\beta - \text{actin} - \text{Ctgene}$). Comparative gene expression between two independent samples (ΔΔCt) was obtained by subtracting the delta cycle threshold of the control group from the delta cycle threshold of the group of interest (obese or macrosomic).

(5) Statistical Analysis. Samples were analysed using GraphPad Prism version 5.2. Data expressed as mean ± standard deviation (SD) were evaluated by one-way ANOVA. The Fisher test and the Student t-test were used to compare the values between two groups. Differences were considered significant when the p value was <0.05.

3. Results

3.1. Medical and Obstetrical Background. Regarding the medical and obstetrical background, GDM women presented more obstetrical complications than their preceding pregnancy. Recurrent spontaneous abortions were frequent in GDM mothers (70%). Miscarriage and stillbirth were ranged from 20% to 30% on gestational diabetes. Other previous complications such as preeclampsia and high blood pressure were less frequent (10%) (Table 2).

3.2. Anthropometrical Parameters. We observed that the control group (mothers and their newborns) had normal BMI. All of gestational diabetic women included in the study were obese, and their newborns were macrosomic with a birth weight over 4 kg. The cranial perimeter of macrosomic newborns was significantly higher than that of the control newborns (Table 3).

TABLE 2: Medical and obstetrical background of women.

Background	Control mothers	GDM mothers
Previous gestational diabetes	—	1 (10%)
High blood pressure	—	1 (10%)
Preeclampsia	—	1 (10%)
Miscarriage	2 (20%)	3 (30%)
Recurrent spontaneous abortions	—	7 (70%)
Stillbirth	1 (10%)	2 (20%)

%: the percentage of the occurrence of previous obstetric complications; $n = 10$ control mothers; $n = 10$ gestational diabetes mellitus (GDM) mothers.

3.3. Biochemical Parameters. Diabetic mothers exhibited a higher level of fasting glycemia and insulinemia than control mothers. Compared to nondiabetic mothers, blood HbA1C percentage was increased in gestational diabetic women. Plasma glycemia was not significantly different between macrosomic and control newborns. However, the serum insulinemia level was high in the macrosomic babies.

As regards the lipid parameters, gestational diabetic women had significantly higher levels of triglycerides, total cholesterol, HDL cholesterol, and LDL cholesterol compared to nondiabetic women. Serum triglycerides, total cholesterol, HDL cholesterol, and LDL cholesterol were not significantly different between macrosomic newborns and babies born to control mothers (Table 3).

3.4. Expression of Pro- and Anti-Inflammatory mRNA Markers (Th1/Th2) in T Cells. In T cells of diabetic gestational mothers, the mRNA expression of Th1 transcriptional factor (T-bet) and Th1 cytokines (IL-2 and IFN-γ) was significantly higher compared to that in T cells of nondiabetic mothers (Figure 1(a)). Th1 markers were more expressed in babies born to gestational diabetic women than in newborns of control mothers (Figure 1(b)). Analysis of mRNA expression of Th2 transcriptional factor (GATA3) and IL-4 (Th2 cytokine) showed that there was no significant difference between control and diabetic women and between their respective newborns (Figures 2(a) and 2(b)). However, IL-10 expression (Th2 cytokine) was decreased in T lymphocytes from diabetic gestational mothers and in their offsprings (Figures 2(a) and 2(b)).

In gestational diabetic mothers and control mothers and their corresponding babies, the Th1/Th2 ratios were calculated: T-bet/GATA3, IL-2/IL-4, IL-2/IL-10, IFN-γ/IL-4, and IFN-γ/IL-10. The obtained ratio showed that the profile of Th1 transcriptional factor and Th1 cytokines was upregulated, while Th2 markers were downregulated, in T lymphocytes from both obese gestational diabetic mothers and their macrosomic newborns, compared to their respective controls (Table 4).

Table 3: Anthropometrical and biochemical parameters.

Parameters	Mothers		Babies	
	Control	GDM	Control	Macrosomic
Age	30.6 ± 3.47	32.3 ± 4.3	H1	H1
Weight (kg)[a,b]	63.4 ± 3.9	$84.4 \pm 2.4^*$	3.29 ± 0.33	$4.585 \pm 0.46^*$
Height (m)	1.65 0.04	1.67 ± 0.04	0.493 ± 0.011	0.51 ± 0.009
BMI (kg/m^2)[c]	23.21 ± 1.27	$30.25 \pm 1.9^*$	—	—
Cranial perimeter (cm)	—	—	32.9 ± 1.45	$35.5 \pm 1.78^*$
Glycemia (g/L)	0.70 ± 0.23	$1.26 \pm 0.24^*$	0.908 ± 0.26	0.78 ± 0.065
Insulinemia (μU/mL)	3.59 ± 2.26	$17.02 \pm 5.63^*$	2.73 ± 1.77	$5.81 \pm 4.4^*$
HbA1C (%)	4.46 ± 0.18	5.27 ± 0.18	—	—
Triglycerides (g/L)	0.51 ± 0.19	$1.47 \pm 0.31^*$	0.31 ± 0.13	0.55 ± 0.25
Total cholesterol (g/L)	0.64 ± 0.29	$2.33 \pm 0.68^*$	0.51 ± 0.15	0.42 ± 0.13
HDL cholesterol (g/L)	0.39 ± 0.15	$0.84 \pm 0.19^*$	0.30 ± 0.08	0.36 ± 0.10
LDL cholesterol (g/L)	0.15 ± 0.16	$1.2 \pm 0.52^*$	0.061 ± 0.04	0.14 ± 0.08

*Significant difference between diabetic mothers and macrosomic newborns and their corresponding controls; $^*P < 0.05$. [a]Mother's weight measured in the first trimester of pregnancy. [b]Babies weight measured in the first hour after birth. [c]Body mass index (BMI) of mothers, calculated with the following formula: BMI (kg/m^2) = weight/(height)^2. H1 = first hour after birth.

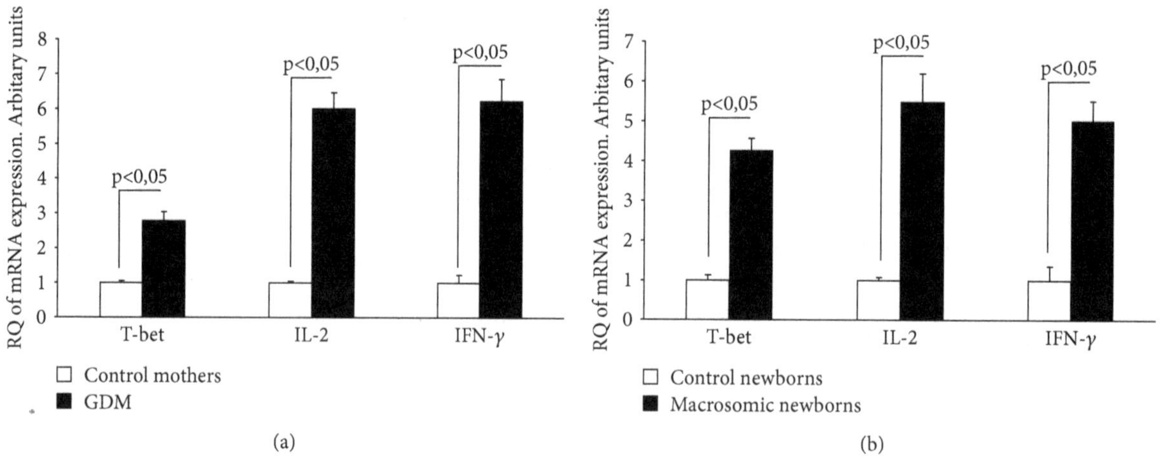

Figure 1: Th1 markers in T cells: mRNA expression of Th1 transcriptional factor (T-bet) and Th1 cytokines (IL-2, IFN-γ) in GDM and control mothers (a) and their newborns (b). Relative quantity (RQ) of mRNA in different groups was determined as described in Subjects and Methods.

4. Discussion

Both obesity and gestational diabetes mellitus (GDM) complications during pregnancy can substantially influence the development of offspring during fetal life and postnatally. Several complications have been associated with gestational diabetes as well as with macrosomia, including metabolic abnormalities, alteration in antioxidant status, and dysregulation of the immune system [23].

This study was conducted to investigate Th1/Th2 T cell polarisation in obese mothers with GDM and their macrosomic offspring. GDM confers a risk of obstetrical complications during pregnancy [2]. The high frequency of obstetrical background observed in our gestational diabetic women corroborates the observations of several studies that have reported links between gestational diabetes and high risk of obstetrical complications during pregnancy [2, 24].

By the anthropometric view, GDM mothers of the study population were obese and their newborns were macrosomic. Biochemical data obtained in the present study showed that gestational diabetic women were hyperglycemic, hyperinsulinemic with HbA1C, and lipidic with levels higher than those of control mothers. The HbA1C elevation shows that glycemic balance was better in the control group than in the gestational diabetic one. Hyperglycemia associated with hyperinsulinemia observed in GDM mothers represents an insulin-resistant state as shown in several reports [20, 25]. Obesity constitutes a favourable situation for diabetes development. Moreover, gestational diabetes mellitus and obesity during pregnancy significantly influence the development of offspring during fetal life and postnatally. Indeed, animal and human studies indicated that fetuses from mothers with gestational diabetes are at high risk of developing fetal macrosomia and they are prone to adverse side effects

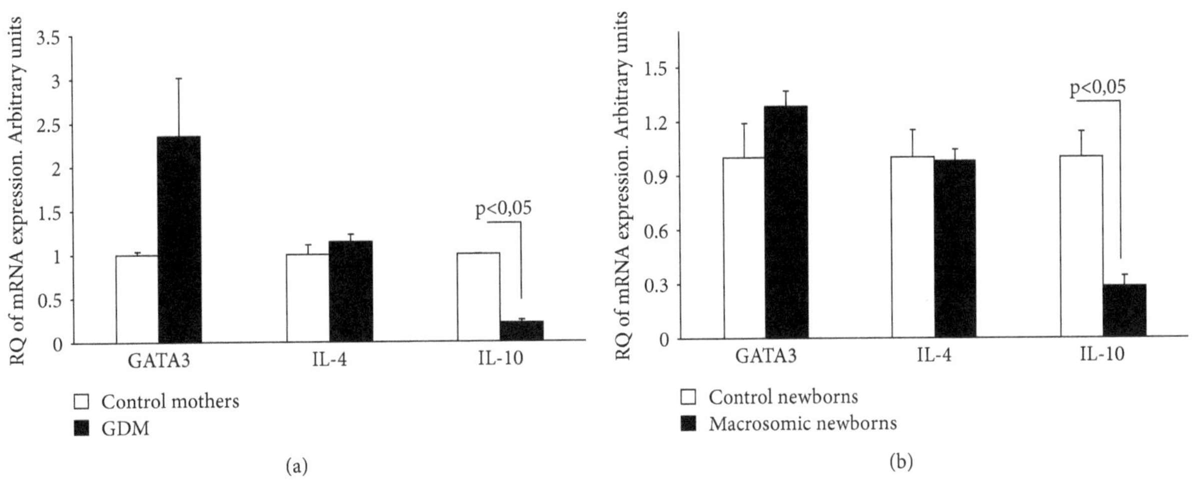

Figure 2: Th2 markers in T cells: mRNA expression of Th2 transcriptional factor (GATA3) and Th2 cytokines (IL-4, IL-10) in GDM and control mothers (a) and their newborns (b). Relative quantity (RQ) of mRNA in different groups was determined as described in Subjects and Methods.

Table 4: Ratio of Th1/Th2 mRNA of transcription factors and cytokines.

Th1/Th2 ratio	Mothers Control	Mothers Diabetic	Newborns Control	Newborns Macrosomic
T-bet/GATA3	4.73	6.44*	1.031	5.48*
IL-2/IL-4	1.093	5.74*	0.36	2.03*
IL-2/IL-10	0.034	0.95*	0.03	0.57*
IFN-γ/IL-4	4.16	22.7*	0.22	1.14*
IFN-γ/IL-10	0.13	3.76*	0.018	0.32*

Relative quantity of mRNA in different groups was determined, and RQ values were used to calculate the Th1/Th2 mRNA ratio in mothers (control and gestational diabetic) and newborns (control and macrosomic). *Significant difference between diabetic mothers and macrosomic newborns as compared to their corresponding controls.

strongly associated with prematurity, birth trauma, respiratory distress syndrome, and fetal death [24].

Macrosomic newborns were normoglycemic but hyperinsulinemic and had increased lipid levels compared to the control newborns. According to several studies, high glucose level of a gestational diabetic mother may induce the release of insulin from the fetal pancreas, leading to fetal hyperinsulinemia [25–27]. Besides, Grissa et al. demonstrated correlations with obesity in maternal levels of amino acids, triglycerides, fatty acids, and birth weight [28]. These substances might modulate insulin secretion and insulin sensitivity and increase fetal growth [28–30]. The hyperinsulinemia, associated with other growth factors like IGF-1 and IGF-2, could be responsible for hypoglycemic accidents of newborns [28].

Commonly, macrosomic newborns of diabetic mothers used to be hypoglycemic after birth as a consequence of their hyperinsulinemia. In our study, the hyperglycemic babies from obese diabetic pregnancies showed normoglycemia. Studies have shown that, compared to pregnancies in nonobese diabetic subjects, gestational diabetes in obese subjects is characterized by lower weight gain and higher baseline glucose [31]. This fact could explain the normoglycemic status of the newborns from obese diabetic mothers.

T cells (responsible for cell-mediated immunity) have been shown to play a critical role in GDM and macrosomia [13, 17, 18]. T cells can be divided into two subsets: T helper cells (CD4+) and T cytotoxic cells (CD8+). Prolonged stimulation of Th0 cells with a specific antigen allows their differentiation into two phenotypes: Th1 or Th2, characterized by different profiles of cytokines. Th1 cells (IFN-γ) inhibit the proliferation of Th2 cells, whileTh2 cells (IL-10) block the Th1 cytokine processing. T cell differentiation into Th1 and Th2 phenotypes is dependent, respectively, on T-bet and GATA3. Two transcriptional factors allow the transcriptional activation of cytokine genes [14].

In the present study, T-bet and Th1 cytokines were increased in both gestational diabetic mothers and macrosomic newborns, while, except for the downregulation of IL-10, there was no significant modulation of GATA3 and IL-4, the Th2 markers, in both diabetic women and their macrosomic offsprings. IL-10 is mainly produced by activated macrophages and Treg and Th2 cells. IL-10 inhibits the production of IFN-γ by Th1 cells, which shifts immune responses toward a Th2 type [15, 31].

Also, Mayer and Hudrisier [32] reported that pregnancies in obese women have a dysregulated maternal cytokine profile with a significant rise in proinflammatory cytokines [32–34]. These observations suggest the inflammatory state in obese GDM women.

In normal pregnancy, Th1 cytokines are downregulated whereas cytokines belonging to Th2 cells are upregulated at the end of the first trimester and at delivery [35]. Besides, a shift of a Th1 phenotype to Th2 during pregnancy has been shown to encourage vigorous production of antibodies that not only combat infections during pregnancy but also offer passive immunity to the fetus [36]. In this present study, the fetal passive immunity might be compromised by the decrease in the Th2 phenotype in gestational diabetic mothers.

Atègbo et al. [20] have demonstrated the downregulation of the Th1 phenotype. Contrary to that, in our obese gestational diabetes women and their macrosomic newborns, the Th1/Th2 ratio reveals the upregulation of the Th1 phenotype. Obesity of mothers might involve a Th1 increase. Our idea can be supported by observations of Khan et al. who developed an animal model of macrosomic offspring of rats which become obese and diabetic in adulthood. They observed a very high level of proinflammatory cytokines, IFNg and IL2, in obese and diabetic animals [18]. In gestational diabetic women, some authors have shown that low Th1 concentrations and high IL-10 levels may be implicated in maintaining the pregnancy [13, 17, 20]. Besides, recent data have suggested the protective role of IL-10 against inflammation in adipose tissue and insulin resistance [37–39].

Furthermore, some authors [17, 40] have reported spontaneous abortion cases and patients with recurrent miscarriage are associated with lower systemic IL-10 compared to normal pregnancies. Jasper et al. [41] have shown that adoptive transfer of T lymphocytes depleted of Treg cells in pregnant T cell-deficient mice led to a failure of gestation due to immunological rejection of the fetus [17, 41].

In our study, the increase in Th1 and decrease in IL-10 can be also explained by the status of GDM mothers with multiple background of recurrent miscarriage and spontaneous abortion.

We have not observed any significant variation in GATA3 and IL-4, which is in line with previous reports [18–20]. The lack of decrease in mRNA expression of GATA3 and IL-4 would lead to a successful pregnancy in these obese women with GDM.

5. Conclusion

In the context of gestational diabetes with obesity and multiple background of recurrent abortion, Th1 transcriptional factor and cytokines are upregulated while GATA3 and IL-4 (belonging to the Th2 phenotype) are not altered in diabetic mothers and their newborns. IL-10, belonging to both Treg and Th2, is decreased. The modulation of Th1/Th2 balance during pregnancy could explain the proinflammatory status observed in diabetic mothers and their offsprings.

Abbreviations

HbA1C: Glycated hemoglobin
TG: Triglyceride
Tchol: Total cholesterol
HDLchol: High-density lipoprotein cholesterol
LDLchol: Low-density lipoprotein cholesterol
RT-qPCR: Quantitative reverse transcription-polymerase chain reaction
T-bet: Trans-acting T cell-specific transcription factor T-bet
IL-2: Interleukin-2
IFN-γ: Interferon-γ
GATA3: Trans-acting T cell-specific transcription factor GATA3
IL-4: Interleukin-4
IL-10: Interleukin-10.

Conflicts of Interest

All of the authors have nothing to declare as far as the conflict of interests is concerned.

Acknowledgments

We express our sincere thanks to the gynecological department of Roi Baudouin Hospital Center, Dakar Principal Hospital, Dakar Plateau, and Wakhinane Health Center. We gratefully acknowledge the Office of Cooperation and Cultural Action (SCAC) of the French Embassy at Senegal that granted a doctoral scholarship to one of the authors (A. Seck).

References

[1] T. A. Buchanan, A. Xiang, S. L. Kjos, and R. Watanabe, "What is gestational diabetes?," *Diabetes Care*, vol. 30, Supplement 2, pp. S105–S111, 2007.

[2] American Diabetes Association, "Gestational diabetes mellitus," *Diabetes Care*, vol. 27, Supplement 1, pp. S88–S90, 2004.

[3] J. C. Hill, G. V. Krishnaveni, I. Annamma, S. D. Leary, and C. H. D. Fall, "Glucose tolerance in pregnancy in South India: relationships to neonatal anthropometry," *Acta Obstetricia et Gynecologica Scandinavica*, vol. 84, no. 2, pp. 159–165, 2005.

[4] L. J. England, P. M. Dietz, T. Njoroge et al., "Preventing type 2 diabetes: public health implications for women with a history of gestational diabetes mellitus," *American Journal of Obstetrics and Gynecology*, vol. 200, no. 4, pp. 365.e1–365.e8, 2009.

[5] H. Yang, Y. Wei, X. Gao et al., "Risk factors for gestational diabetes mellitus in Chinese women: a prospective study of 16,286 pregnant women in China," *Diabetic Medicine*, vol. 26, no. 11, pp. 1099–1104, 2009.

[6] F. P. Dunne, "Pregestational diabetes mellitus and pregnancy," *Trends in Endocrinology & Metabolism*, vol. 10, no. 5, pp. 179–182, 1999.

[7] D. Kyne-Grzebalski, L. Wood, S. M. Marshall, and R. Taylor, "Episodic hyperglycaemia in pregnant women with well-controlled type 1 diabetes mellitus: a major potential factor underlying macrosomia," *Diabetic Medicine*, vol. 16, no. 8, pp. 702–706, 1999.

[8] J. Lepercq, P. Taupin, D. Dubois-Laforgue et al., "Heterogeneity of fetal growth in type 1 diabetic pregnancy," *Diabetes & Metabolism*, vol. 27, no. 3, pp. 339–344, 2001.

[9] J. Star and M. W. Carpenter, "The effect of pregnancy on the natural history of diabetic retinopathy and nephropathy," *Clinics in Perinatology*, vol. 25, no. 4, pp. 887–916, 1998.

[10] P. Dandona, A. Aljada, and A. Bandyopadhyay, "Inflammation: the link between insulin resistance, obesity and diabetes," *Trends in Immunology*, vol. 25, no. 1, pp. 4–7, 2004.

[11] P. Dandona, A. Aljada, A. Chaudhuri, P. Mohanty, and R. Garg, "Metabolic syndrome: a comprehensive perspective based on interactions between obesity, diabetes, and inflammation," *Circulation*, vol. 111, no. 11, pp. 1448–1454, 2005.

[12] I. Mothe-Satney, C. Filloux, H. Amghar et al., "Adipocytes secrete leukotrienes: contribution to obesity-associated inflammation and insulin resistance in mice," *Diabetes*, vol. 61, no. 9, pp. 2311–2319, 2012.

[13] N. A. Khan, "Inflammation et immunité: implications dans l'obésité et le diabète de type 2," *Oléagineux, Corps gras, Lipides*, vol. 13, no. 5, pp. 343–351, 2006.

[14] F. Nasta, V. Ubaldi, L. Pace, G. Doria, and C. Pioli, "Cytotoxic T-lymphocyte antigen-4 inhibits GATA-3 but not T-bet mRNA expression during T helper cell differentiation," *Immunology*, vol. 117, no. 3, pp. 358–367, 2006.

[15] A. K. Abbas, A. H. Lichtman, and S. Pillai, *Les bases de l'immunologie fondamentale et clinique. Traduit de la 3éme édition anglaise*, P. L. Masson, Ed., p. 328, Elsevier Masson, 2016.

[16] C. Giordano, "Immunobiology of normal and diabetic pregnancy," *Immunology Today*, vol. 11, no. 9, pp. 301–303, 1990.

[17] A. Hichami, O. Grissa, I. Mrizak, C. Benammar, and N. A. Khan, "Role of T-cell polarization and inflammation and their modulation by n-3 fatty acids in gestational diabetes and macrosomia," *Journal of Nutrition and Metabolism*, vol. 2016, Article ID 3124960, 10 pages, 2016.

[18] N. Khan, A. Yessoufou, M. Kim, and A. Hichami, "N-3 fatty acids modulate Th1 and Th2 dichotomy in diabetic pregnancy and macrosomia," *Journal of Autoimmunity*, vol. 26, no. 4, pp. 268–277, 2006.

[19] A. Yessoufou, A. Hichami, P. Besnard, K. Moutairou, and N. A. Khan, "Peroxisome proliferator-activated receptor α deficiency increases the risk of maternal abortion and neonatal mortality in murine pregnancy with or without diabetes mellitus: modulation of T cell differentiation," *Endocrinology*, vol. 147, no. 9, pp. 4410–4418, 2006.

[20] J.-M. Atègbo, O. Grissa, A. Yessoufou et al., "Modulation of adipokines and cytokines in gestational diabetes and macrosomia," *The Journal of Clinical Endocrinology & Metabolism*, vol. 91, no. 10, pp. 4137–4143, 2006.

[21] I. Mrizak, O. Grissa, B. Henault et al., "Placental infiltration of inflammatory markers in gestational diabetic women," *General Physiology and Biophysics*, vol. 33, no. 2, pp. 169–176, 2014.

[22] C. Triboulot, A. Hichami, A. Denys, and N. A. Khan, "Dietary (n-3) polyunsaturated fatty acids exert antihypertensive effects by modulating calcium signaling in T cells of rats," *The Journal of Nutrition*, vol. 131, no. 9, pp. 2364–2369, 2001.

[23] A. Yessoufou and K. Moutairou, "Maternal diabetes in pregnancy: early and long-term outcomes on the offspring and the concept of "metabolic memory"," *Experimental Diabetes Research*, vol. 2011, Article ID 218598, 12 pages, 2011.

[24] A. Yessoufou, M. P. Nekoua, A. Gbankoto, Y. Mashalla, and K. Moutairou, "Beneficial effects of omega-3 polyunsaturated fatty acids in gestational diabetes: consequences in macrosomia and adulthood obesity," *Journal of Diabetes Research*, vol. 2015, Article ID 731434, 11 pages, 2015.

[25] P. M. Catalano, J. P. Kirwan, S. Haugel-de Mouzon, and J. King, "Gestational diabetes and insulin resistance: role in short- and long-term implications for mother and fetus," *The Journal of Nutrition*, vol. 133, no. 5, pp. 1674S–1683S, 2003.

[26] P. M. Catalano, L. Huston, S. B. Amini, and S. C. Kalhan, "Longitudinal changes in glucose metabolism during pregnancy in obese women with normal glucose tolerance and gestational diabetes mellitus," *American Journal of Obstetrics and Gynecology*, vol. 180, no. 4, pp. 903–916, 1999.

[27] P. M. Catalano, "Trying to understand gestational diabetes," *Diabetic Medicine*, vol. 31, no. 3, pp. 273–281, 2014.

[28] O. Grissa, A. Yessoufou, I. Mrisak et al., "Growth factor concentrations and their placental mRNA expression are modulated in gestational diabetes mellitus: possible interactions with macrosomia," *BMC Pregnancy and Childbirth*, vol. 10, no. 1, p. 7, 2010.

[29] H. Pribylova and L. Dvorakova, "Long-term prognosis of infants of diabetic mothers: relationship between metabolic disorders in newborns and adult offspring," *Acta Diabetologica*, vol. 33, no. 1, pp. 30–34, 1996.

[30] H. Merzouk, S. Madani, D. Chabane Sari, J. Prost, M. Bouchenak, and J. Belleville, "Time course of changes in serum glucose, insulin, lipids and tissue lipase activities in macrosomic offspring of rats with streptozotocin-induced diabetes," *Clinical Science*, vol. 98, no. 1, pp. 21–30, 2000.

[31] R. Comtois, M. C. Séguin, N. Aris-Jilwan, M. Couturier, and H. Beauregard, "Comparison of obese and non-obese patients with gestational diabetes," *International Journal of Obesity and Related Metabolic Disorders*, vol. 17, no. 10, pp. 605–608, 1993.

[32] G. Mayer and D. Hudrisier, "Cytokines and Immunoregulation," in *Immunology - chapter thirteen – Page maintained by Richard Hunt-last changed on Wednesday, November 08, 2017*, In Microbiology and Immunology On-line. University of south Carolina School of Medicine, http://www.microbiologybook.org/bowers/imm-reg-ver2.htm, Consulted on Wednesday, May 02, 2018.

[33] N. Jayabalan, S. Nair, Z. Nuzhat et al., "Cross talk between adipose tissue and placenta in obese and gestational diabetes mellitus pregnancies via exosomes," *Frontiers in Endocrinology*, vol. 8, no. 239, 2017.

[34] C. Ingvorsen, S. Brix, S. E. Ozanne, and L. I. Hellgren, "The effect of maternal inflammation on foetal programming of metabolic disease," *Acta Physiologica*, vol. 214, no. 4, pp. 440–449, 2015.

[35] A. M. Martin, H. Berger, R. Nisenbaum et al., "Abdominal visceral adiposity in the first trimester predicts glucose intolerance in later pregnancy," *Diabetes Care*, vol. 32, no. 7, pp. 1308–1310, 2009.

[36] R. Raghupathy, "Pregnancy: success and failure within the Th1/Th2/Th3 paradigm," *Seminars in Immunology*, vol. 13, no. 4, pp. 219–227, 2001.

[37] G. Reinhard, A. Noll, H. Schlebusch, P. Mallmann, and A. V. Ruecker, "Shifts in the TH1/TH2 balance during human pregnancy correlate with apoptotic changes," *Biochemical and Biophysical Research Communications*, vol. 245, no. 3, pp. 933–938, 1998.

[38] M. Feuerer, L. Herrero, D. Cipolletta et al., "Lean, but not obese, fat is enriched for a unique population of regulatory T cells that affect metabolic parameters," *Nature Medicine*, vol. 15, no. 8, pp. 930–939, 2009.

[39] J. Deiuliis, Z. Shah, N. Shah et al., "Visceral adipose inflammation in obesity is associated with critical alterations in T regulatory cell numbers," *PLoS One*, vol. 6, no. 1, article e16376, 2011.

[40] M. P. Nekoua, R. Fachinan, A. K. Atchamou et al., "Modulation of immune cells and Th1/Th2 cytokines in insulin-treated type 2 diabetes mellitus," *African Health Sciences*, vol. 16, no. 3, pp. 712–724, 2016.

[41] M. J. Jasper, K. P. Tremellen, and S. A. Robertson, "Primary unexplained infertility is associated with reduced expression of the T-regulatory cell transcription factor Foxp3 in endometrial tissue," *Molecular Human Reproduction*, vol. 12, no. 5, pp. 301–308, 2006.

Permissions

All chapters in this book were first published in JDR, by Hindawi Publishing Corporation; hereby published with permission under the Creative Commons Attribution License or equivalent. Every chapter published in this book has been scrutinized by our experts. Their significance has been extensively debated. The topics covered herein carry significant findings which will fuel the growth of the discipline. They may even be implemented as practical applications or may be referred to as a beginning point for another development.

The contributors of this book come from diverse backgrounds, making this book a truly international effort. This book will bring forth new frontiers with its revolutionizing research information and detailed analysis of the nascent developments around the world.

We would like to thank all the contributing authors for lending their expertise to make the book truly unique. They have played a crucial role in the development of this book. Without their invaluable contributions this book wouldn't have been possible. They have made vital efforts to compile up to date information on the varied aspects of this subject to make this book a valuable addition to the collection of many professionals and students.

This book was conceptualized with the vision of imparting up-to-date information and advanced data in this field. To ensure the same, a matchless editorial board was set up. Every individual on the board went through rigorous rounds of assessment to prove their worth. After which they invested a large part of their time researching and compiling the most relevant data for our readers.

The editorial board has been involved in producing this book since its inception. They have spent rigorous hours researching and exploring the diverse topics which have resulted in the successful publishing of this book. They have passed on their knowledge of decades through this book. To expedite this challenging task, the publisher supported the team at every step. A small team of assistant editors was also appointed to further simplify the editing procedure and attain best results for the readers.

Apart from the editorial board, the designing team has also invested a significant amount of their time in understanding the subject and creating the most relevant covers. They scrutinized every image to scout for the most suitable representation of the subject and create an appropriate cover for the book.

The publishing team has been an ardent support to the editorial, designing and production team. Their endless efforts to recruit the best for this project, has resulted in the accomplishment of this book. They are a veteran in the field of academics and their pool of knowledge is as vast as their experience in printing. Their expertise and guidance has proved useful at every step. Their uncompromising quality standards have made this book an exceptional effort. Their encouragement from time to time has been an inspiration for everyone.

The publisher and the editorial board hope that this book will prove to be a valuable piece of knowledge for researchers, students, practitioners and scholars across the globe.

List of Contributors

Elżbieta Poniedziałek-Czajkowska, Radzisław Mierzyński, Dariusz Szymula, Bożena Leszczyńska-Gorzelak and Jan Oleszczuk
Chair and Department of Obstetrics and Perinatology, Medical University of Lublin, Jaczewskiego 8, 20-954 Lublin, Poland

Fatemeh Sedaghat and Nila Ghanei
Department of Basic Medical Sciences, Faculty of Nutrition Sciences and Food Technology, National Nutrition and Food Technology Research Institute, Shahid Beheshti University of Medical Sciences, Tehran, Iran

Mahdieh Akhoondan, Mehdi Ehteshami and Bahram Rashidkhani
Department of Community Nutrition, Faculty of Nutrition Sciences and Food Technology, National Nutrition and Food Technology Research Institute, Shahid Beheshti University of Medical Sciences, Tehran, Iran

Vahideh Aghamohammadi
Department of Paramedical Sciences, Ahvaz Jundishapur University of Medical Sciences, Ahvaz, Iran

Parvin Mirmiran
Nutrition and Endocrine Research Center, Research Institute for Endocrine Sciences, Shahid Beheshti University of Medical Sciences, Tehran, Iran

Gülen Yerlikaya, Veronica Falcone, Tina Stopp, Peter Husslein, Wolfgang Eppel and Christian S. Göbl
Department of Obstetrics and Gynecology, Division of Obstetrics and Feto-Naternal Medicine, Medical University of Vienna, Vienna, Austria

Martina Mittlböck
Center of Medical Statistics, Informatics and Intelligent Systems, Section for Clinical Biometrics, Medical University of Vienna, Vienna, Austria

Andrea Tura
Metabolic Unit, Institute of Neuroscience, National Research Council, Padova, Italy

Marica Franzago and Liborio Stuppia
Laboratory of Molecular Genetics, Department of Psychological, Health and Territorial Sciences, School of Medicine and Health Sciences, "G. d'Annunzio" University, Chieti-Pescara, Via dei Vestini 31, 66013 Chieti, Italy
Ce.S.I-Met, "G. d'Annunzio" University, Chieti-Pescara, Via Colle dell'Ara No. 1, 66100 Chieti, Italy

Federica Fraticelli and Ester Vitacolonna
Ce.S.I-Met, "G. d'Annunzio" University, Chieti-Pescara, Via Colle dell'Ara No. 1, 66100 Chieti, Italy
Department of Medicine and Aging, School of Medicine and Health Sciences, "G. d'Annunzio" University, Chieti-Pescara, Chieti, Italy

Claudio Celentano and Marco Liberati
Department of Medicine and Aging, School of Medicine and Health Sciences, "G. d'Annunzio" University, Chieti-Pescara, Chieti, Italy

Antonio Nicolucci
Center for Outcomes Research and Clinical Epidemiology (CORE), Pescara, Italy

Diana L. Lip-Sosa, Eva Meler and Jordi Clotet
Fetal i+D Fetal Medicine Research Center, BC Natal-Barcelona Center for Maternal-Fetal and Neonatal Medicine (Hospital Clínic and Hospital Sant Joan de Déu), IDIBAPS, University of Barcelona, Spain

Raigam J. Martinez-Portilla
Fetal i+D Fetal Medicine Research Center, BC Natal-Barcelona Center for Maternal-Fetal and Neonatal Medicine (Hospital Clínic and Hospital Sant Joan de Déu), IDIBAPS, University of Barcelona, Spain
Maternal-Fetal Medicine and Therapy Research Center Mexico in behalf of the Iberoamerican Research Network in Translational, Molecular and Maternal-Fetal Medicine, Mexico

Jose R. Villafan-Bernal
Mexican Consortium of Biomedicine, Biotechnology and Health Dissemination-Consortium BIO2-DIS, Mexico
CONACYT Researcher at the Department of Surgery, Health Science Center, Autonomous University of Aguascalientes, Mexico
Center for Health Sciences, Autonomous University of Aguascalientes, Mexico

Francisco J. Serna-Vela
Center for Health Sciences, Autonomous University of Aguascalientes, Mexico

Sergio Velazquez-Garcia
CIMeTA Research Unit-ISSEA, Mexico

Leopoldo C. Serrano-Diaz
Women's Hospital of the State of Aguascalientes-ISSEA, Mexico

Francesc Figueras
Fetal i+D Fetal Medicine Research Center, BC Natal-Barcelona Center for Maternal-Fetal and Neonatal Medicine (Hospital Clínic and Hospital Sant Joan de Déu), IDIBAPS, University of Barcelona, Spain
Center for Biomedical Research on Rare Diseases (CIBER-ER), Madrid, Spain

Ruth Martis, Julie Brown and Caroline A. Crowther
Liggins Institute, The University of Auckland, Auckland 1142, New Zealand

Joan C. Lo, Jingrong Yang, Erica P. Gunderson, Mohammad K. Hararah, Joel R. Gonzalez and Assiamira Ferrara
Division of Research, Kaiser Permanente Northern California, Oakland, CA, USA

Hui Li, Lulu Song, Lijun Shen, Bingqing Liu, Xiaoxuan Zheng, Lina Zhang and Youjie Wang
Department of Maternal and Child Health, School of Public Health, Tongji Medical College, Huazhong University of Science and Technology, Wuhan, Hubei 430030, China

Zhongqiang Cao
Wuhan Children's Hospital (Wuhan Maternal and Child Healthcare Hospital), Tongji Medical College, Huazhong University of Science and Technology, Wuhan, Hubei 430030, China

Shunqing Xu
Key Laboratory of Environment and Health, Ministry of Education & Ministry of Environmental Protection and State Key Laboratory of Environmental Health, School of Public Health, Tongji Medical College, Huazhong University of Science and Technology, Wuhan, Hubei 430030, China

Per Glud Ovesen, Jens Fuglsang, Mette Bisgaard Andersen, Charlotte Wolff and Olav Bjørn Petersen
Department of Obstetrics and Gynecology, Aarhus University Hospital, Aarhus, Denmark

H. David McIntyre
Faculty of Medicine, University of Queensland, Brisbane, QLD, Australia
Danish Diabetes Academy, Odense University Hospital, Odense, Denmark

Ulrika Andersson-Hall, Carolina Gustavsson, Louise Joelsson and Agneta Holmäng
Institute of Neuroscience and Physiology, Sahlgrenska Academy, University of Gothenburg, Gothenburg, Sweden

Anders Pedersen and Daniel Malmodin
Swedish NMR Centre, University of Gothenburg, Gothenburg, Sweden

Zhongwei Zhou, Hongmei Chen, Mingzhong Sun and Huixiang Ju
Department of Clinical Laboratory, Affiliated Yancheng Hospital, School of Medicine, Southeast University, Yancheng, Jiangsu 224001, China

Thamudi D. Sundarapperuma
Department of Nursing, University of Ruhuna, Galle 80000, Sri Lanka

Champa J. Wijesinghe
Department of Community Medicine, University of Ruhuna, Galle 80000, Sri Lanka

Priyadarshika Hettiarachchi
Department of Physiology, University of Sri Jayewardenepura, Nugegoda 11222, Sri Lanka

Sudharshani Wasalathanthri
Department of Physiology, University of Colombo, Colombo 00800, Sri Lanka

Hayfaa Wahabi
Chair of Evidence-Based Healthcare and Knowledge Translation, College of Medicine, King Saud University, Saudi Arabia

Lucia Borsari, Carlotta Malagoli and Marcella Malavolti
Department of Biomedical, Metabolic and Neural Sciences, Environmental, Genetic and Nutritional Epidemiology Research Center (CREAGEN), University of Modena and Reggio Emilia, Modena 41125, Italy

Marco Vinceti
Department of Biomedical, Metabolic and Neural Sciences, Environmental, Genetic and Nutritional Epidemiology Research Center (CREAGEN), University of Modena and Reggio Emilia, Modena 41125, Italy
Clinical and Experimental Medicine PhD Program, University of Modena and Reggio Emilia, Modena, Italy
Department of Epidemiology, Boston University School of Public Health, Boston, MA 02118, USA

Martha M. Werler
Clinical and Experimental Medicine PhD Program, University of Modena and Reggio Emilia, Modena, Italy
Department of Epidemiology, Boston University School of Public Health, Boston, MA 02118, USA

Kenneth J. Rothman
Clinical and Experimental Medicine PhD Program, University of Modena and Reggio Emilia, Modena, Italy
Department of Epidemiology, Boston University School of Public Health, Boston, MA 02118, USA
Research Triangle Institute, Research Triangle Park, NC 27709, USA

Rossella Rodolfi and Fausto Nicolini
Local Health Authority of Reggio Emilia, Reggio Emilia 42122, Italy

Gianfranco De Girolamo
Department of Public Health, Unit of Epidemiology and Risk Communication, Local Health Authority of Modena, Modena 41126, Italy

Alice S. Ryan
VA Maryland Health Care System, Research Service, Department of Medicine, Division of Gerontology and Geriatric Medicine, University of Maryland School of Medicine and Baltimore Geriatric Research Education and Clinical Center (GRECC), Baltimore, MD 21201, USA

Sumaiya Adam
Department of Obstetrics and Gynecology, University of Pretoria, Pretoria, South Africa

Paul Rheeder
Department of Internal Medicine, University of Pretoria, Pretoria, South Africa

Colin W. Binns and Andy H. Lee
School of Public Health, Curtin University, Perth, WA, Australia

Cong Luat Nguyen
School of Public Health, Curtin University, Perth, WA, Australia
National Institute of Hygiene and Epidemiology, Hanoi, Vietnam

Ngoc Minh Pham
School of Public Health, Curtin University, Perth, WA, Australia
Thai Nguyen University of Medicine and Pharmacy, Thai Nguyen, Vietnam

Dat Van Duong
United Nations Population Fund, Hanoi, Vietnam

Marica Franzago, Federica Fraticelli, Claudio Celentano, Marco Liberati and Ester Vitacolonna
Department of Medicine and Aging, School of Medicine and Health Sciences, "G. d'Annunzio" University, Chieti-Pescara, Chieti, Italy

Marta Di Nicola
Laboratory of Biostatistics, Department of Medical, Oral and Biotechnological Sciences, "G. d'Annunzio" University, Chieti-Pescara, Chieti, Italy

Francesco Bianco and Raffaele De Caterina
Institute of Cardiology, School of Medicine and Health Sciences, "G. d'Annunzio" University, Chieti-Pescara, Chieti, Italy

Daniela Marchetti and Liborio Stuppia
Department of Psychological, Health and Territorial Sciences, School of Medicine and Health Sciences, "G. d'Annunzio" University, Chieti-Pescara, Chieti, Italy

Patrícia Damé, Kadhija Cherubini, Pâmella Goveia, Geórgia Pena and Maria Angélica Nunes
Postgraduate Program in Epidemiology, School of Medicine, Federal University of Rio Grande do Sul, Porto Alegre, RS, Brazil

Leony Galliano
Postgraduate Program in Physical Education, Superior School of Physical Education, Federal University of Pelotas, Pelotas, RS, Brazil

Cristina Façanha
Integrated Center for Diabetes and Hypertension, Ceará State Health Department, Fortaleza, CE, Brazil
School of Medicine, Unichristus University Center, Fortaleza, CE, Brazil

Anastasia Katsarou, Nael Shaat and Kerstin Berntorp
Department of Clinical Sciences, Lund University, Malmö, Sweden
Department of Endocrinology, Skåne University Hospital, Malmö, Sweden

Rickard Claesson
Department of Clinical Sciences, Lund University, Malmö, Sweden
Department of Obstetrics and Gynaecology, Office for Healthcare "Kryh", Ystad, Sweden

Claes Ignell
Department of Clinical Sciences, Lund University, Malmö, Sweden
Department of Obstetrics and Gynaecology, Office for Healthcare "Sund", Helsingborg, Sweden

Åse Ruth Eggemoen and Christin Wiegels Waage
Department of General Practice, Institute of Health and Society, University of Oslo, Oslo, Norway

Line Sletner
Department of Child and Adolescence Medicine, Akershus University Hospital, Lørenskog, Norway

Hanne L. Gulseth
Department of Endocrinology, Morbid Obesity and Preventive Medicine, Oslo University Hospital, Oslo, Norway
Department of Non communicable Diseases, Norwegian Institute of Public Health, Oslo, Norway

Kåre I. Birkeland
Department of Transplantation Medicine, Oslo University Hospital, Oslo, Norway
Institute of Clinical Medicine, Faculty of Medicine, University of Oslo, Oslo, Norway

Anne Karen Jenum
General Practice Research Unit (AFE), Department of General Practice, Institute of Health and Society, University of Oslo, Oslo, Norway

Daniela Marchetti and Mario Fulcheri
Department of Psychological Health and Territorial Sciences, "G. d'Annunzio" University of Chieti-Pescara, Chieti, Italy

Danilo Carrozzino
Department of Psychological Health and Territorial Sciences, "G. d'Annunzio" University of Chieti-Pescara, Chieti, Italy
Psychiatric Research Unit, Psychiatric Centre North Zealand, Copenhagen University Hospital, Hillerød, Denmark

Federica Fraticelli and Ester Vitacolonna
Department of Medicine and Aging, "G. d'Annunzio" University of Chieti-Pescara, Chieti, Italy

Akihiro Katayama and Jun Wada
Department of Nephrology, Rheumatology, Endocrinology and Metabolism, Okayama University Graduate School of Medicine, Dentistry and Pharmaceutical Sciences, Okayama 700 8558, Japan

Mayu Watanabe and Daisuke Ogawa
Department of Nephrology, Rheumatology, Endocrinology and Metabolism, Okayama University Graduate School of Medicine, Dentistry and Pharmaceutical Sciences, Okayama 700 8558, Japan
Department of Internal Medicine, Japanese Red Cross Society Himeji Hospital, Himeji, Hyogo 670-8540, Japan

Hidetoshi Kagawa
Department of Internal Medicine, Japanese Red Cross Society Himeji Hospital, Himeji, Hyogo 670-8540, Japan

P. Valensi
Department of Endocrinology-Diabetology-Nutrition, AP-HP, Jean Verdier Hospital, Paris 13 University, Sorbonne Paris Cité, CRNH-IdF, CINFO, Bondy, France

E. Cosson
Department of Endocrinology-Diabetology-Nutrition, AP-HP, Jean Verdier Hospital, Paris 13 University, Sorbonne Paris Cité, CRNH-IdF, CINFO, Bondy, France
Sorbonne Paris Cité, UMR U1153 Inserm/U1125 Inra/Cnam/Université Paris 13, Bobigny, France

L. Carbillon
Department of Gynecology-Obstetrics, AP-HP, Jean Verdier Hospital, Paris 13 University, Sorbonne Paris Cité, Bondy, France

Sedigheh Nouhjah and Hajieh Shahbazian
Diabetes Research Center, Health Research Institute, Ahvaz Jundishapur University of Medical Sciences, Ahvaz, Iran

Nahid Shahbazian
Department of Obstetrics and Gynecology, Fertility, Infertility and Perinatology Research Center, Imam Khomeini Hospital, Ahvaz Jundishapur University of Medical Sciences, Ahvaz, Iran

Alireza Jahanshahi
Diabetes Research Center, Health Research Institute, Ahvaz Jundishapur University of Medical Sciences, Ahvaz, Iran
Internal Medicine Ward, Golestan Teaching Hospital, Ahvaz Jundishapur University of Medical Sciences, Ahvaz, Iran

Shayesteh Jahanfar
School of Health Sciences, Central Michigan University, Building 2212, Room 2239, Mount Pleasant, MI 48859, USA

Bahman Cheraghian
Department of Epidemiology and Biostatistics, Faculty of Health, Ahvaz Jundishapur University of Medical Sciences, Ahvaz, Iran

A. Seck
Laboratory of Physiology and Functional Explorations, Faculty of Medicine, Pharmacy and Odontology, Cheikh Anta Diop University, 5005 Dakar-Fann, Senegal

A. Hichami and N. A. Khan
U1231 INSERM/Université de Bourgogne-Franche Comté (UBFC)/Agro-Sup, Physiologie de la Nutrition & Toxicologie, Dijon 21000, France

S. Doucouré, H. Bassène and C. Sokhna
Institute of Research for Development, VITROME Aix Marseille Univ, IRD, AP-HM, SSA, VITROME, IHUMediterranean Infection, CP18524 Dakar, Senegal

F. Diallo Agne
Laboratory of Biochemistry and Molecular Biology, Faculty of Medicine, Pharmacy and Odontology, Cheikh Anta Diop University, 5005 Dakar-Fann, Senegal

A. Ba and A. Samb
Laboratory of Physiology and Functional Explorations, Faculty of Medicine, Pharmacy and Odontology, Cheikh Anta Diop University, 5005 Dakar-Fann, Senegal
UMI 3189, "Environnement, Santé, Sociétés", CNRS, CNRST, Université Bamako-UCAD, Dakar, Senegal

Index

www.ingramcontent.com/pod-product-compliance
Lightning Source LLC
LaVergne TN
LVHW060602210926
848485LV00005B/1355
9781639271177